A Comprehensive Manual of
Pediatric Nursing Procedures

2nd Edition

A Comprehensive Manual of
Pediatric Nursing Procedures

Kavitha K MSc(N), PhD, SCEM
Professor and Head
Department of Child Health Nursing
BLDEA's Shri BM Patil Institute of Nursing Sciences
Vijayapura, Karnataka, India

Foreword
Asha P Shetty

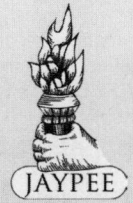

JAYPEE

JAYPEE BROTHERS MEDICAL PUBLISHERS
The Health Sciences Publisher
New Delhi | London

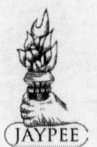 **Jaypee Brothers Medical Publishers (P) Ltd**

Headquarters
Jaypee Brothers Medical Publishers (P) Ltd
4838/24, Ansari Road, Daryaganj
New Delhi 110 002, India
Phone: +91-11-43574357
Fax: +91-11-43574314
Email: jaypee@jaypeebrothers.com

Overseas Office
J.P. Medical Ltd
83 Victoria Street, London
SW1H 0HW (UK)
Phone: +44 20 3170 8910
Fax: +44 (0)20 3008 6180
Email: info@jpmedpub.com

Website: www.jaypeebrothers.com
Website: www.jaypeedigital.com

© 2021, Jaypee Brothers Medical Publishers

The views and opinions expressed in this book are solely those of the original contributor(s)/author(s) and do not necessarily represent those of editor(s) of the book.

All rights reserved. No part of this publication may be reproduced, stored or transmitted in any form or by any means, electronic, mechanical, photocopying, recording or otherwise, without the prior permission in writing of the publishers.

All brand names and product names used in this book are trade names, service marks, trademarks or registered trademarks of their respective owners. The publisher is not associated with any product or vendor mentioned in this book.

Medical knowledge and practice change constantly. This book is designed to provide accurate, authoritative information about the subject matter in question. However, readers are advised to check the most current information available on procedures included and check information from the manufacturer of each product to be administered, to verify the recommended dose, formula, method and duration of administration, adverse effects and contraindications. It is the responsibility of the practitioner to take all appropriate safety precautions. Neither the publisher nor the author(s)/editor(s) assume any liability for any injury and/or damage to persons or property arising from or related to use of material in this book.

This book is sold on the understanding that the publisher is not engaged in providing professional medical services. If such advice or services are required, the services of a competent medical professional should be sought.

Every effort has been made where necessary to contact holders of copyright to obtain permission to reproduce copyright material. If any have been inadvertently overlooked, the publisher will be pleased to make the necessary arrangements at the first opportunity. The **CD/DVD-ROM** (if any) provided in the sealed envelope with this book is complimentary and free of cost. **Not meant for sale.**

Inquiries for bulk sales may be solicited at: jaypee@jaypeebrothers.com

A Comprehensive Manual of Pediatric Nursing Procedures

First Edition: 2015
Second Edition: **2021**

ISBN 978-93-5465-147-2

Printed at: Sterling Graphics Pvt. Ltd.

Dedicated to
My parents-in-laws
Shri JB Sikandar
&
Smt Beyama Sikandar

Foreword

> "Your life can only get better when you do. Do something every day to improve your key skill areas."
> —**Brian Tracy**—

There is nothing heart-rending than seeing a sick infant or child. As pediatric nurses, it takes a very special set of clinical and bedside skills to deal with challenges. It takes a pediatric nurse with a great bedside manner to be there to provide care.

As a teacher and principal of an institute of eminence, I would be remiss if I do not appreciate the efforts Professor Kavitha K has taken up in writing this book entitled *A Comprehensive Manual of Pediatric Nursing Procedures*. Having read this book in entirely, I am of the opine that she has made a full-scale effort to keep the book crisp and brief, while covering all procedures related to pediatric nursing practice.

The breadth and depth of information presented is ample, organized and well expressed. The author has extensively covered the pediatric nursing procedure to its widest extent possible. The illustration adds up the beauty.

I am pretty confident; this manual will appeal to a wide audience within nursing profession, pediatric practitioners in specific and is to be recommended in any nurse's library portfolio. So, read this book, do it and stick to it.

Best wishes!

Dr Asha P Shetty
Professor cum Principal
College of Nursing
All India Institute of Medical Sciences (AIIMS)
Bhubaneswar, Odisha

Preface to the Second Edition

The overwhelming response of nursing students, faculty, and staff nurses regarding the first edition of this book motivated the author to bring out the second edition.

The technologies in care of newborn and pediatric clients are advancing day by day. Hence, the second edition is mainly focused on including the recent advances in care of this precious age group. One chapter has been completely devoted for this.

Topics, such as administration of vaccines, newborn history taking, and guidelines for breast milk storage are newly added to this edition. Apart from this, the contents of various procedures are updated relevant to present scenario and research evidences.

Further, the incorporation of figures, tables and flowcharts in various chapters will serve as a valuable tool in understanding the procedures in a holistic way. At the beginning of every chapter, the learning objectives and keywords are stated. The key points of the topics are summarized as highlights. To have self-assessment of learning outcomes, memory exercise is given.

I believe that this book will serve as a valuable guide for the nurses and students in enhancing their knowledge and skills of pediatric nursing procedures.

Kavitha K

Preface to the First Edition

The health care of pediatric age group is being delivered in a new service formats and a range of settings. These demand the nurses to equip with thorough knowledge, big attitude and high, level skills in caring this age group.

I believe that this manual will help the student nurses of both undergraduate as well as postgraduate and the staff nurses working in pediatric setting to equip with the thorough knowledge and techniques of common pediatric nursing procedures.

A sincere effort is made to incorporate the modern trends in pediatric nursing, such as atraumatic care, family centered care, etc., in carrying out the procedures.

I hope this manual will serve as a valuable guide to all the nurses, who provide a comprehensive care to the most precious pediatric age group.

Kavitha K

Acknowledgments

- I pay my humble tribute to Lord Almighty, for His showers of blessing in all my endeavors.
- I extend my sincere gratitude to my godmother Dr (Lt Col) N Premakumari, Founder Principal, Meenakshi College of Nursing, Chennai, Tamil Nadu, India, for her prayers and blessings, constant moral support, guidance and motivation in all my ventures.
- I owe my sense of deep gratitude to Dr Asha P Shetty, Professor cum Principal, College of Nursing, All India Institute of Medical Sciences (AIIMS), Bhubaneshwar, Odisha, India, for her exemplary peer review and writing foreword for this manual.
- I am most grateful to all my teachers of Meenakshi College of Nursing, Chennai, who sown a seed of wisdom in me.
- My sincere thanks to the Management, Principal and Faculty of BLDEA's Shri BM Patil Institute of Nursing Sciences, Vijayapura, Karnataka, India, for their support and encouragement in accomplishing this task.
- My sincere thanks to M/s Jaypee Brothers Medical Publishers (P) Ltd, New Delhi, India, who helped and guided me, especially Shri Jitendar P Vij (Group Chairman), Mr Ankit Vij (Managing Director), Mr MS Mani (Group President), Dr Madhu Choudhary (Publishing Head–Education), Ms Pooja Bhandari (Production Head), Ms Sunita Katla (Executive Assistant to Group Chairman and Publishing Manager), Ms Samina Khan (Executive Assistant to Publishing Head–Education), Mr Rajesh Sharma (Production Coordinator), Ms Seema Dogra (Cover Visualizer), Mr Kapil Dev Sharma (Typesetter), Mr Vakil Khan (Proofreader), Mr Rajesh Gurkundi (Graphic Designer), and their team members, for giving me an opportunity to bring out the second edition of this manual.
- Above all, I am grateful to my beloved husband Mr Basheerahamed and my sweet sons Master Mohammed Eshan and Mohammed Arsh, for their unconditional love and support in balancing the glorious professional career and most beautiful personal life.
- I am indebted to my co-sisters Mrs Raziya and Mrs Fatima, for being my source of support and reducing my burden, so that I could concentrate on professional advancement.
- I also acknowledge the prayers of my beloved sisters Mrs Kannagi and Mrs Kalaiselvi.
- I extend my sincere thanks to my brother-in-laws Mr Abdul Rahman and Mr Mubarak, for their motivation and encouragement.
- I thank all the readers who have given wonderful feedback about the first edition, which motivated me to bring out this edition even better.

Contents

1. **Newborn Care** — 1
   - Neonatal Resuscitation 1
   - Neonatal Examination 7
   - Format for Newborn History Taking 19
   - Baby Bath 20
   - Kangaroo Mother Care 24
   - Radiant Warmer 26
   - Phototherapy 28
   - Incubator 31
   - Apnea Monitor 33

2. **Assessment Procedures** — 36
   - Admission Procedure 36
   - History Taking 38
   - Mission Indradhanush 42
   - Vital Signs 44
   - Anthropometric Measurements 51
   - Abdominal Girth 58
   - Physical Examination 59
   - Developmental Assessment 72
   - Neurological Examination 76
   - Documentation 80

3. **Assisting in Diagnostic Procedures** — 83
   - Collection of Blood Sample (Venipuncture) 83
   - Arterial Puncture 86
   - Blood Gas Analysis 88
   - Capillary Blood Sampling 90
   - Urine Specimen Collection 93
   - Stool Specimen Collection 95
   - Lumbar Puncture 96
   - Liver Biopsy 99
   - Kidney Biopsy 101
   - Bone Marrow Aspiration 102
   - Cardiac Catheterization 104
   - Electrocardiogram 108
   - Fine Needle Aspiration 112

4. **Meeting Nutritional Needs** — 115
   - Assisting in Breastfeeding 115
   - Cleaning and Sterilization of Feeding Articles 121
   - Formula Feeding 121
   - Gavage Feeding 123
   - Gastrostomy Feeding 126
   - Jejunostomy Feeding (Postpyloric or Transpyloric Feeding) 129
   - Total Parenteral Nutrition 131

5. **Respiratory Care** — 136
   - Steam Inhalation 136
   - Nebulization 137
   - Oxygen Therapy 140
   - Low-flow Delivery System 141
   - Chest Physiotherapy 146
   - Incentive Spirometry 149

6. **Administration of Medications and Vaccines** — 152
   - Introduction to Administration of Medications in Children 152
   - Oral Medications 154
   - Intramuscular Injection 158
   - Intradermal Injection 160
   - Subcutaneous Administration of Medications 161
   - Intravenous Therapy 162

Instillation 168
Topical Applications 171
Administration of Vaccines 173

7. Elimination Needs 176

Urinary Catheterization 176
Suprapubic Catheterization 181
Enema 185
Colostomy Care 187
Colonic Irrigation 189
Double Diapering 190
Ureterostomy Care 191
Insertion of Suppository 192
Enterostomy Care 193

8. Emergency Procedures 195

Manual Removal of Foreign Body from the Airway 195
Tracheostomy Care 202
Pulse Oximetry 212
Abdominal Paracentesis 214
Blood Transfusion 216
Exchange Blood Transfusion 221
Gastric Lavage 225
Umbilical Vein Catheterization 226
Thoracentesis 228

9. Safety and Recreation 230

Play Therapy 230
Restraints 234

10. Care of Child with Fracture 240

Traction Care 240
Cast Care 244

11. Care of Child Undergoing Surgery 248

Pre- and Postoperative Nursing Care 248
Surgical Dressing 253
Removal of Sutures 254

12. Meeting Children's Hygiene Needs 257

Benefits of Good Hygiene 257
Main Areas for Consideration 257
Oral Hygiene 258
Eye Care 258
Ear Care 259
Bathing 260

13. Recent Advances in Prenatal, Neonatal, and Pediatric Care 262

Laminar Flow Hoods 262
Transcutaneous Bilimeter 265
Giraffe Incubator 266
Bubble CPAP 267
Body Cooling 271

Appendix 275

Index 283

CHAPTER 1

Newborn Care

LEARNING OBJECTIVES

Upon the completion of this chapter, the learners will be able to:
- Define the key terms of newborn care.
- List the indications for various neonatal procedures.
- Prepare the articles appropriately.
- Communicate with the parents regarding importance of carrying out the procedures as appropriate to the newborn condition.
- Demonstrate the various aspects of newborn care.

Keywords: newborn, resuscitation, assessment, golden minute, bathing, thermoregulation, examination, skin-to-skin contact, closed system, open system, reflexes.

NEONATAL RESUSCITATION

Definition
Neonatal resuscitation is defined as a set of interventions done at the time of birth to support the establishment of breathing and circulation.

Purpose
- To ensure clear and open airway
- To ensure there is spontaneous or assisted breathing
- To ensure there is adequate circulation of oxygenated blood

Indications
The conditions that necessitate neonatal resuscitation can be prenatal, intranatal, and postnatal factors (**Table 1.1**).

Table 1.1: Indications for neonatal resuscitation.

Period	Conditions	Manifestations that necessitate neonatal resuscitation
Prenatal	Toxemia, pregnancy-induced hypertension, medications	Decreased fetal movements, deceleration of fetal heart rate, passage of meconium
Intranatal	Prolonged first and second stage of labor, pressure over umbilical vessels	Absent or reduced respiratory effort, cyanosis, decreased muscle tone, decreased heart rate

Contd...

Contd...

Period	Conditions	Manifestations that necessitate neonatal resuscitation
	■ Meconium aspiration syndrome ■ Instrumental delivery ■ Birth injuries, medications	
Postnatal	Metabolic abnormality, prematurity, hypoglycemia, cardiac anomalies, persistent pulmonary hypertension, neurological abnormalities	Reduced oxygenation, hypoxia, decreased perfusion of heart

Equipment Needed

- Radiant warmer
- In-built suction and intermittent positive pressure
- Pencil handle laryngoscope with infant (0 and 1) size blade with light source and battery
- Disposable endotracheal (ET) tubes with internal diameter of 2.5, 3.0, 3.5, 4.0 mm mounted with adapters (**Table 1.2**)
- Electrical outlets
- Different size suction catheters (6, 8, 10, and 12 Fr)
- Meconium aspiration device
- Plastic oral airway
- Syringes and needles
- 7.5% sodium bicarbonate
- Epinephrine 1:10,000
- Neonatal nalorphine (1 mg/1 mL)
- Naloxone hydrochloride (0.4 mg/mL)
- Ampules of distilled water
- Normal saline
- 10% dextrose
- Sterile neonatal delivery pack containing bowl, scissors, cotton swabs, and umbilical cord ties
- Umbilical vessel catheterization supplies
- Warm clean bassinet
- Stop clock
- Cardiac monitor and pulse oximeter

Table 1.2: Selection of ET tube and suction catheter.

Weight of newborn (g)	Gestational age (weeks)	ET tube size (inside diameter)	Catheter size (Fr)
<1,000	<28	2.5	5
1,000–2,000	28–34	3.0	6
2,000–3,000	34–38	3.5	8
>3,000	>38	3.5–4	8

Preparation

- The resuscitation kit should be ready before the baby is born.
  - Assemble the bag and connect to oxygen source.
  - If self-inflating bag is used, attach oxygen reservoir and adjust flow to 5–10 L/min.
  - Anticipate bag size and keep ready appropriate size of mask.
- Check the equipment for working condition.
  - Check the light source of laryngoscope: check the batteries and bulb is working. Bulb should be tightly screwed to avoid flickering.

Chapter 1: Newborn Care

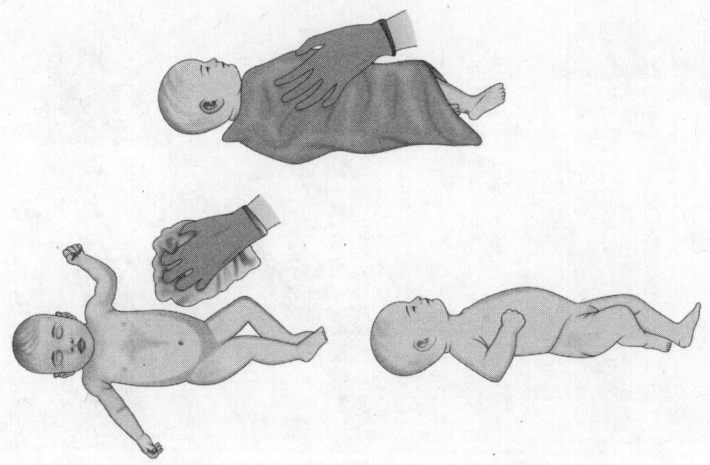

Fig. 1.1: Drying and positioning of newborn.

- The radiant warmer should be put on and plenty of sterile prewarmed linen should be available.

Initial Steps in Resuscitation

1. Perform hand hygiene and wear gloves.
2. The baby should be received in a warm sheet.
3. Place the baby under radiant warmer.
4. The baby should be placed supine or lying on side, with the head in a neutral or slightly extended position (**Fig. 1.1**).
5. The infant's mouth, oropharynx, hypopharynx and nose are sucked using thick 10 Fr suction catheter with gentle intermittent suction.
   Note: The nose should not be sucked first as it would leads to reflex breathing with risk of aspiration of secretions contained in the oral cavity (**Fig. 1.2**).
6. The baby should be dried effectively and wet linen should be removed.
7. If an infant is not breathing or breathing efforts are sluggish, he should be stimulated by flicking the soles or rubbing the back (**Fig. 1.3**).

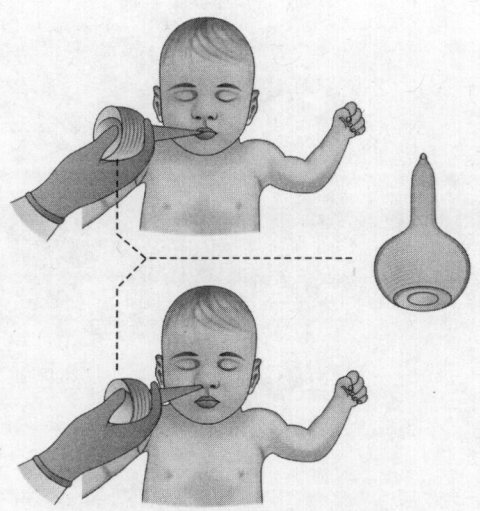

Fig. 1.2: Correct method for suctioning.

Note: The tactile stimulation should not be continued beyond 3-4 flicks and when it is ineffective.

8. The baby should be promptly ventilated with a bag and mask (**Fig. 1.4**).
   Note: Evaluate the infant every 30 seconds by simultaneously observing respirations, heartbeat, and color to decide the need for further steps.

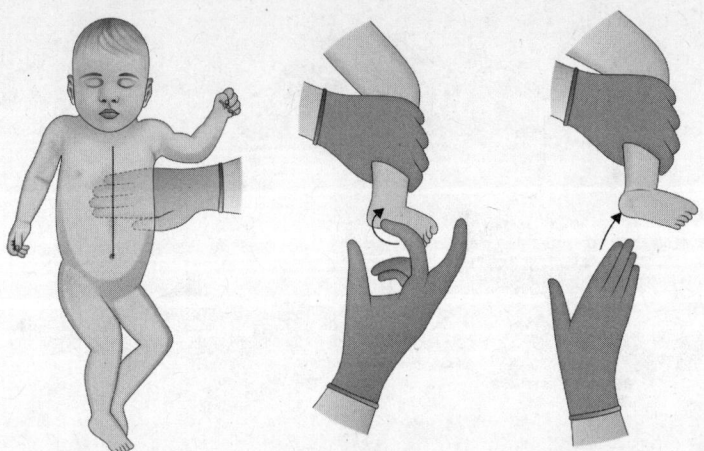

Fig. 1.3: Techniques for stimulating the newborn.

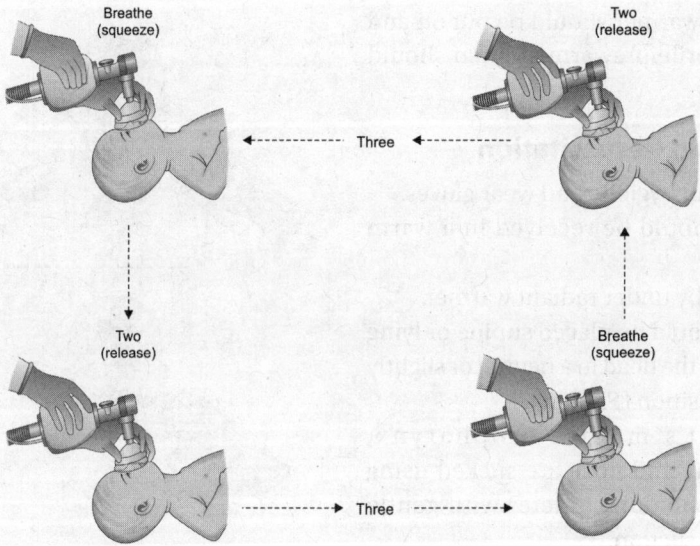

Fig. 1.4: Timing the rate of ventilation (4 event cycle/2 seconds).

Resuscitation Procedure

- Position the infant supine by placing a roll of towel under the shoulders in order to extend the neck and open the airways.
- Thorough suctioning should be done.
- Rightly fit the mask on the face enclosing nose and mouth of the baby.
- The oxygen reservoir should be attached to the bag.
- Ventilate the infant at a rate of 40–60 breaths/min; the pressure should be 15–20 cm of water. In the case of collapsed alveoli, few initial inflation pressure of 30–40 cm of water is recommended.

- There should be noticeable rise and fall of the chest during each ventilation.
- Monitor the heart rate (HR) q30 seconds. To save the time, the heart rate can be counted for 6 seconds and multiplied by 10 to get the heart rate per minute.
- In spite of effective bag and mask ventilation, heart rate is not coming up or it further slows down and drops below 80/min, the newborn should be intubated (**Fig. 1.5**).
- The ET tube should be suctioned before starting positive pressure ventilation.
- The ventilation can be stopped as soon as the baby establishes spontaneous breathing and heart rate is maintained above 100/min.

External Cardiac Massage

- External cardiac massage (ECM) is indicated for babies in whom heart rate drops below 60/min despite effective ventilation with 100% O_2 for 30 seconds.
- The ventilation should be continued by an assistant and simultaneously heart should be massaged either by using two fingers of one hand or encircling the chest of baby with both the hands and applying sternal compressions with two thumbs (**Fig. 1.6**).
- Press the lower part of the sternum just above the xiphoid cartilage to a depth of one-third of the anterior–posterior diameter of the chest at a rate of 90 compression and 30 ventilations (3:1 ratio)/min.
- The thumb and tip of the fingers should remain in contact with the sternum all the time and they should not be lifted off after each compression.
- Check the heart rate after q30 seconds and chest compression may be stopped when heart rate goes above 60/min.

Medications

- If HR is not picking up despite effective ventilation and ECM, administer 0.1–0.3 mL/kg of 1:10,000 solution (0.01–0.03 mg/kg) of epinephrine through the umbilical vein or ET tube.
- The dose of the epinephrine may be repeated after every 3–5 minutes as indicated.
- If the baby is in shock, consider the use of plasma expander [blood, normal saline (NS), or RL] in a dose of 10 mL/kg slow IV push over 5–10 minutes.
- Monitor the blood acid–base parameters.
- Sodium bicarbonate 5–10 mL of 7.5% solution (adequately diluted with equal volume of distilled water or double volume of 5% dextrose) should be administered intravenously slowly at the rate of 1 mL/min to babies in whom effective ventilation is not established even by 10 minutes or later (Apgar score <7).

Postresuscitation Care

- Infants with birth asphyxia (Apgar score of <4 at 5 minutes) should be admitted to the special care neonatal unit for observation and management during the next 12–48 hours.
- Those babies who require ET intubation, chest compressions, or medications should be shifted to newborn intensive care unit (NICU) for careful observation and clinical monitoring.
- The baby should be attached to a vital signs monitor and pulse oximeter or arterial blood gas (ABG) should be monitored to assess oxygenation and acid–base balance.
- A stomach wash should be done with NS and vitamin K 0.5–1 mg should be given intramuscularly (IM).
- The newborn should be nursed in a thermoneutral environment.
- IV infusion with 10% dextrose should be started immediately to prevent any hypoglycemia.
- Fluid volume should be restricted to two-third of maintenance fluid.
- Infants with prolonged birth asphyxia

Chapter 1: Newborn Care

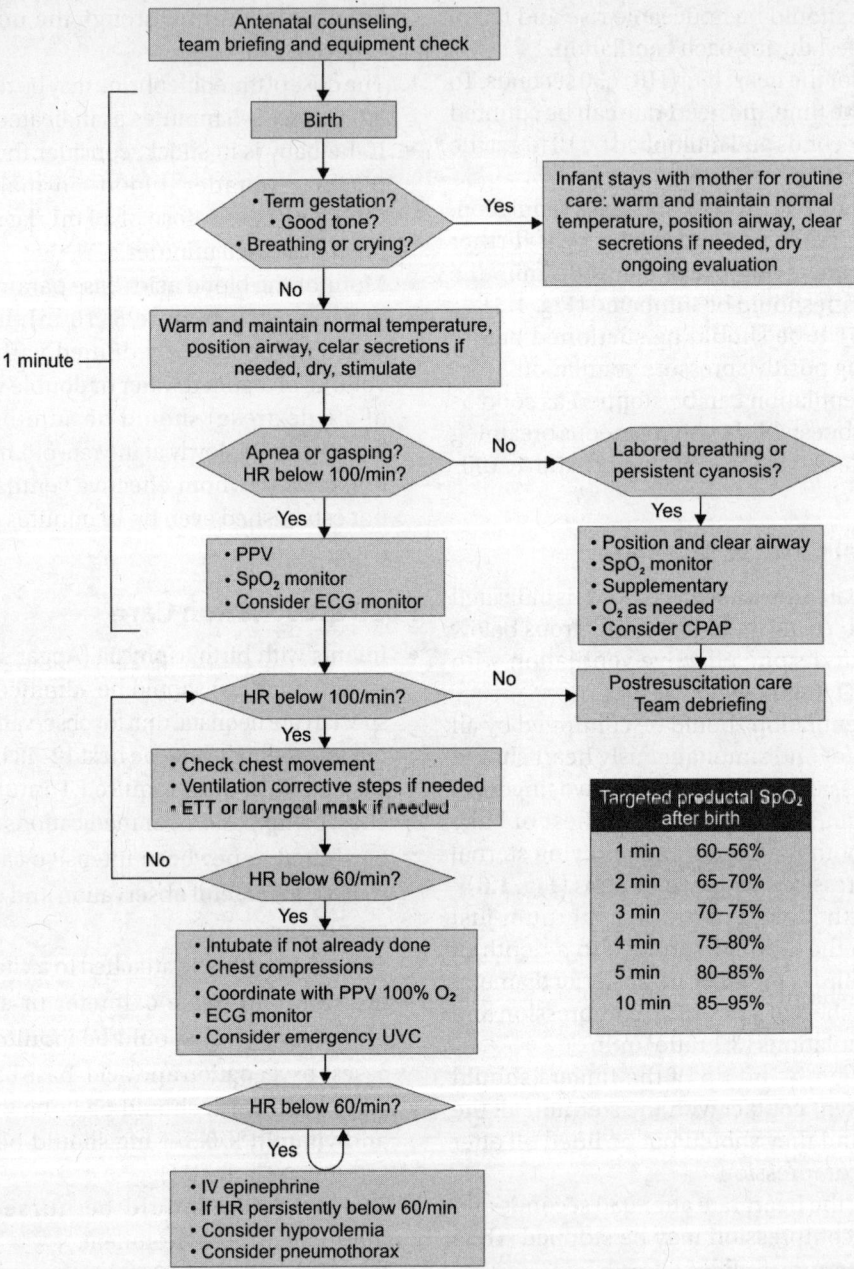

Fig. 1.5: Neonatal resuscitation algorithm.
Source: American Heart Association (2015).

(HR: heart rate; ETT: endotracheal tube; PPV: positive pressure ventilation; UVC: umbilical venous catheter; SpO_2: oxygen saturation; ECG: electrocardiogram; IV: intravenous; CPAP: continuous positive airway pressure)

Chapter 1: Newborn Care

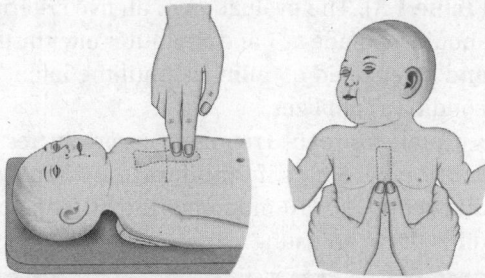

Fig. 1.6: Methods of external cardiac massage.

should be given 7.5% sodium bicarbonate 2–3 mL/kg diluted with equal volume of distilled water or double volume of 5% dextrose slowly to correct any acidosis.
- Hypovolemic shock should be corrected by the administration of 10 mL/kg of fresh "O" Rh –ve blood or NS or RL.
- Dopamine infusion (6 mg/kg/mL) should be started if tissue perfusion is unsatisfactory due to hypotension.
- Antibiotics are administered if perinatal high-risk factors for the development of congenital bacterial infection coexist.
- A skiagram (X-ray) of chest should be taken.
- The infant should be closely monitored to detect any manifestations of hypoxic damage to various organs.
- Urine should be checked for red blood cells (RBCs) and protein to rule out acute tubular necrosis.
- Urine output, body weight, serum electrolytes, and blood glucose should be monitored frequently.
- Seizures should be promptly managed by correction of any metabolic disturbances and by administration of phenobarbitone 20 mg/kg IV slowly over 10 minutes.
- The neurological behavior of the neonate should be watched.
- Enteral feeding should be delayed for 48 hours and started when ventilation and tissue perfusion are adequate.

Highlights ● ● ● ●

- Neonatal resuscitation is defined as a set of intervention at the time of birth to support the establishment of breathing and circulation.
- The main aim of this procedure is to ensure clear and open airway, spontaneous or assisted breathing, and adequate circulation of oxygenated blood.
- The conditions that necessitate neonatal resuscitation can be prenatal, intranatal, and postnatal factors.
- Initial steps of neonatal resuscitation include drying, suctioning of mouth and nose, warmth, and stimulation.
- If not spontaneous breathing, start back and mask ventilation.
- Provide external cardiac massage.
- Assess the heart rate and respiratory rate every 30 seconds.
- Follow AHA algorithm for neonatal resuscitation.

NEONATAL EXAMINATION

Neonatal examination refers to a complete assessment of the newborn after birth.

Aim of Neonatal Examination
- To detect congenital anomalies
- To provide information and education, recognizing and supporting parents
- As a part of routine screening

Equipment Needed
A tray containing:
- Pair of gloves
- Bright pen light with a pinpoint beam
- Tape measure
- Pneumatic otoscope with small head
- Ophthalmoscope
- Standardized sound source (wrist watch)
- Tongue blade
- A clear, flexible ruler
- Pediatric stethoscope
- BP cuff pediatric size (optional)
- A bowl with sterile cotton balls
- Weighing machine

- Infantometer
- Bright colorful objects
- Vital signs tray
- Examination chart

Principles of Examination

- Provision should be made to prevent neonatal heat loss during the physical assessment.
- A rapid overall assessment of the baby will be done at the time of birth, with a more detailed assessment completed on admissions.
- Where possible, the parents should be present during the assessment.
- Sequence of examination include:
  - *Inspection:* Body proportion, posture, and skin, amount of subcutaneous fat, facial appearance, respiration, sleep status, movement, and responsiveness
  - *Auscultation:* Heart, lung, and bowel sounds
  - *Palpation:* Cranium, peripheral pulses, abdomen, liver, spleen, and kidneys
  - *Neurologic reflexes:* Sucking/rooting, Moro, grasping, Babinski, etc.
  - *Others:* Vital signs and measurement.

The assessment of newborn can be divided into four phases.
1. Initial assessment
2. Transitional assessment
3. Assessment of gestational age
4. Comprehensive physical examination of the newborn, including newborn reflexes

Initial Assessment

The aim of examination of the baby at birth is to ensure and assess that lungs have expanded and that air passages are not obstructed and to make an early diagnosis of life-threatening congenital malformations and birth injuries.

The most frequently used method to assess the newborn at birth is Apgar score (**Table 1.3**). The evaluation of all five criteria should be made at 1 and 5 minutes after birth and is repeated q5 minutes until the infant's condition stabilizes.

Total score of 0–3 represent severe distress, score of 4–6 signify moderate difficulty, and score of 7–10 moderate the absence of difficulty in adjusting extrauterine life.

Table 1.3: Apgar score.

Criteria	0	1	2
Heart rate	Absent	Slow (<100)	>100
Respiratory effort	Absent	Slow, irregular	Good, crying
Muscle tone	Limp	Some flexion of extremities	Active motion
Reflex	No response	Grimace	Cough or sneeze
Color	Blue, pale	Body pink, extremities blue	Complete pink

Transitional Assessment

Periods of reactivity during the first 24 hours after birth, the changes in heart rate, respiration, motor activity, color, mucus production, and bowel activity occur in an orderly predictable sequence. For the first 6–8 hours after birth, the newborn is in the first period of reactivity. During the first 30 minutes, the infant is alert, cries vigorously, may suck his or her fingers or fist, and appears interested in the environment. At this time, the neonate's eyes are usually open, thus is an excellent opportunity for mother, father, and child to see each other. The newborn usually grasp the nipple quickly, satisfying both mother and child. Physiologically the respiratory rate may reach 80 breaths/min, crackles may be heard, heart rate may reach 80 beats/min, bowel sounds are active, mucus secretions are increased, and temperature may decrease slightly. After this, the infant enter the second stage of the first reactive period, which generally lasts 2-4 hours. Heart and respiratory rates decrease, temperature continues to fall, mucus production decreases, and urine or stool is usually not passed. The infant is in the state of sleep and relatively calm. Any attempt at stimulation usually elicits a minimal response.

The second period of reactivity begins when the infant wakes from this deep sleep, it lasts about 2-5 hours and provides another excellent opportunity for child and parent to interact. The infant is again alert and responsive, heart and respiratory rates increase, and the gag reflex is active. Gastric and respiratory secretions are increased and passage of meconium commonly occurs. This period is usually over when the amount of respiratory mucus decreased. After this stage is a period of stabilization of physiologic systems and vacillating pattern of sleep and activity.

Clinical Assessment of Gestational Age

To assess the gestational age "new Ballard scale" can be used. It assesses six external physical and six neuromuscular signs. Each sign has a number score and the cumulative score correlates with a maturity rating of 26-44 weeks of gestation (**Figs. 1.7A and B**).

Neuromuscular maturity

The neurological assessment is based on five fundamental observations.

1. *Muscle tone:* Progressively increases in utero as maturity proceeds. The tone in the newborn baby is assessed by three parameters: (1) posture or attitude, (2) passive tone is evaluated by assessing popliteal angle and scarf sign, and (3) active tone is assessed by traction response and recoil.
2. *Joint mobility:* The degree of flexion at ankle and wrist (square window) is limited in preterm babies because of relatively greater stiffness of joints in early gestation. As term approaches the joints become more flexible and relaxed to allow for easy molding during delivery.
3. Certain automatic reflexes appear at specific ages of gestational maturity, for example, Moro reflex appears as early as 28-30 weeks but lacks complete adduction phase till 38 weeks of gestation. Response of pupils to light is present after 30 weeks and baby may turn his head toward diffuse light during 32-36 weeks of gestation. Grasp response makes its appearance around 30 weeks, but a strong grasp can be elicited after 36 weeks. Neck flexors are able to contract in response to traction around 33 weeks of maturity. Rooting and coordinated sucking efforts are present by 34 weeks of gestation.
4. *Fundus examination:* The disappearance of the anterior vascular capsule of the lens has been used to assess the gestational age. After 34 weeks of maturity, anterior capsular vessels are almost completely atrophies with graded changes in babies between 28 and 34 weeks of gestation.
5. Elicitation of the signs.
   - *Square window:* Hand is flexed on the forearm between thumb and index finger of examiner is relatively stiff, which limits the flexion at the wrist (**Fig. 1.8**).
   - *Arm recoil:* The arm is extended and brought close to the trunk. When released, it briskly recoils or flexes in a term infant (**Fig. 1.9**).
   - *Popliteal angle:* Thigh is held in knee chest position and examiner tries to extend the knee with gentle pressure behind the ankle. The angle is 90° or less in a term infant, 120° among babies of 33-36 weeks of gestation, and almost 180° in a neonate <32 weeks (**Fig. 1.10**).
   - *Scarf sign:* The baby lies supine and head is maintained in the midline. Arm is held at the wrist and pulled across the chest toward the opposite shoulder. In a preterm baby, elbow readily goes beyond the midline of the chest (**Fig. 1.11**).

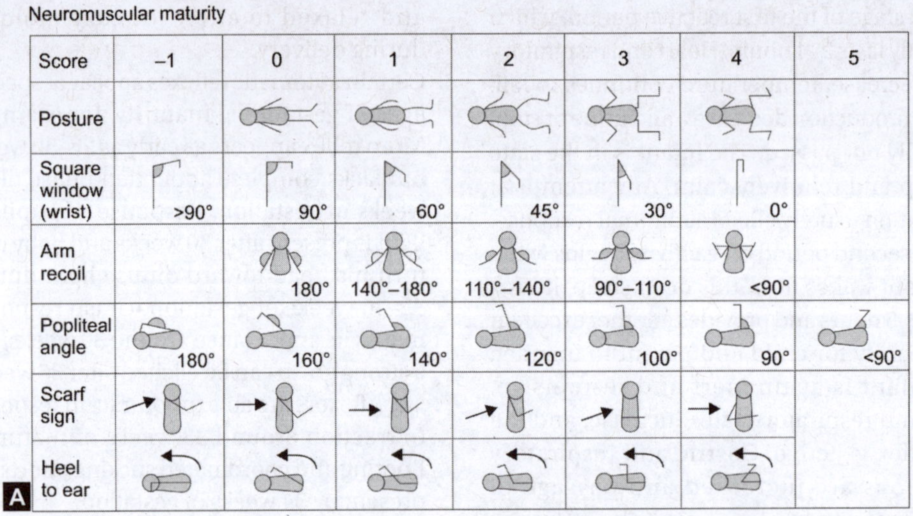

Neuromuscular maturity

Score	-1	0	1	2	3	4	5
Posture							
Square window (wrist)	>90°	90°	60°	45°	30°	0°	
Arm recoil		180°	140°–180°	110°–140°	90°–110°	<90°	
Popliteal angle	180°	160°	140°	120°	100°	90°	<90°
Scarf sign							
Heel to ear							

A

Physical maturity

								Maturity rating	
Skin	Sticky, friable, transparent	Gelatinous, red, translucent	Smooth, pink; visible veins	Superficial peeling and or rash few veins	Cracking, pale areas rare veins	Parchment deep cracking, no vessels	Leathery cracked, wrinkled	Score	Weeks
Lanugo	None	Sparse	Abundant	Thinning	Bald areas	Mostly bald		-10	20
Plantar surface	Heel–toe 40–50 mm; -1 <40 mm; -2	>50 mm, no crease	Faint red marks	Anterior transverse crease only	Creases anterior 2/3	Creases over entire sole		-5	22
								0	24
Breast	Imperceptible	Barely perceptible	Flat areola, no bud	Stipped areola, 1–2 mm bud	Raised areola, 3–4 mm bud	Full areola, 5–10 mm bud		5	26
								10	28
Eye/ear	Lids fused loosely—1 tightly—2	Lids open pinna flat stays folded	Slightly curved pinna, soft slow recoil	Well curved pinna soft but ready recoil	Formed and firm instant recoil	Thick cartilage, ear stift		15	30
								20	32
								25	34
Genitals (male)	Scretum flat, smooth	Scretum empty, faint rugae	Testes in upper canal, rare rugae	Tests descending few rugae	Tests down good rugae	Tests pendulous deep rugae		30	36
								35	38
								40	40
Genitals (female)	Clitoris prominent, labia flat	Clitoris prominent, small labia minora	Clitoris prominent, enlarging minora	Majora and minora equally prominent	Majora large, minora small	Majora cover clitoris and minora		45	42
								50	44

B

Figs. 1.7A and B: New Ballard chart for the assessment of gestational age of newborn.

Physical Examination

A thorough head-to-foot examination of newborn is done to assess the general condition of baby in detail. This should be done in a systematic manner. The scheme of assessment is presented in **Table 1.4**.

Elicitation of reflexes

Reflexes are involuntary movements of the body parts. Some reflexes occur spontaneously where as other movements occur as a response to specific stimuli. Examination of reflex should be done as part of newborn assessment

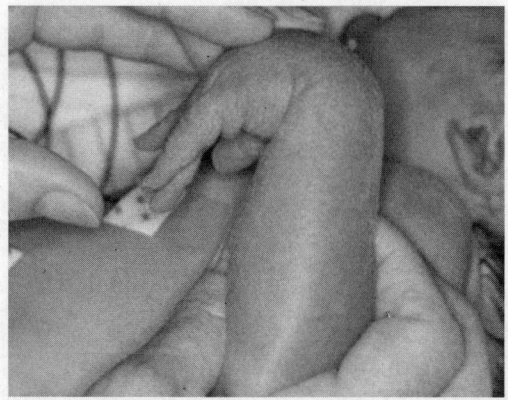

Fig. 1.8: Square window sign.

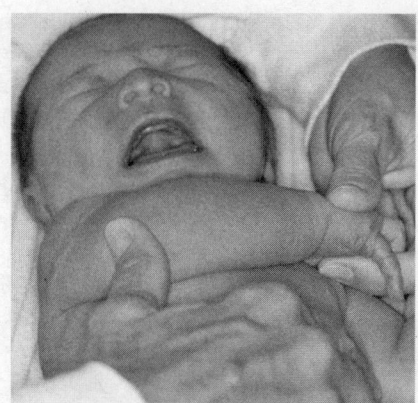

Fig. 1.11: Scarf sign.

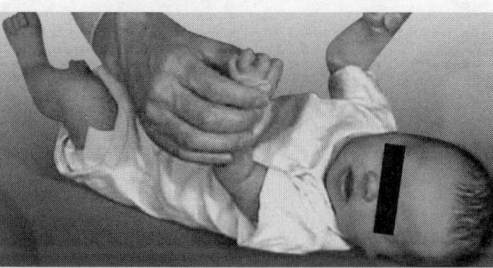

Fig. 1.9: Arm recoil sign.

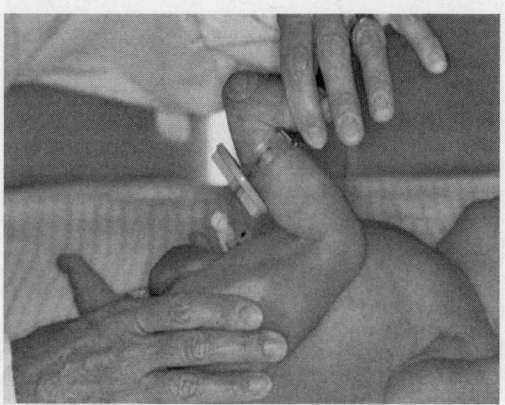

Fig. 1.10: Popliteal angle sign.

to determine the brain and nervous system function. Some of the newborn reflexes that are commonly elicited is given in **Table 1.5**.

Highlights ●●●●

+ Neonatal examination refers to a complete assessment of the newborn after birth.
+ The purposes of newborn examination are to detect congenital anomalies, to provide information and education, recognizing and supporting parents and as a part of routine screening.
+ The assessment of newborn can be divided into four phases: initial assessment, transitional assessment, assessment of gestational age, and comprehensive physical examination of the newborn, including newborn reflexes.
+ The most frequently used method to assess the newborn at birth is Apgar score.
+ Transitional assessment notes the periods of reactivity during the first 24 hours after birth, the changes in heart rate, respiration, motor activity, color, mucus production, and bowel activity.
+ To assess the gestational age "new Ballard scale" can be used. It assesses six external physical and six neuromuscular signs. Each sign has a number score and the cumulative score correlates with a maturity rating of 26–44 weeks of gestation.
+ A thorough and systematic head-to-foot examination of newborn is done to assess the general condition of baby in detail.
+ Examination of reflex should be done as part of newborn assessment to determine the brain and nervous system function.

Table 1.4: Scheme assessment of newborn.

Assessment items	Norms
Parent–infant interaction	Assess for signs of affection or mutual responsiveness between parent and newborn
Sleep	12–16 hours of sleep/24 hours; pattern variable
Feeding	On an average, normal newborn takes 8–12 breastfeedings in a 24-hour period. In the case of formula feeding, 14–31 oz/24-hour period. The baby takes feed with interest and without difficulty
Elimination	<ul><li>Newborn should pass urine within the first 12–24 hours after birth. One wet diaper every 8 hours on day 2, 4–6 wet diapers in 24 hours on days 3 and 4, by day 5 should have 6–8 wet diapers/24-hour period</li><li>Newborn should pass first stool within 48 hours after birth (meconium)</li><li>Stools progress from thick, tarry, black to thin, brown to green (transitional stool) to yellow, gold, soft or mush for breastfed babies or pale yellow foam and pasty for formula-fed babies</li><li>Breastfed newborn should have 3–4 stools/day or more and the formula-fed newborn may have 1–2 stools/day</li></ul>
Well-being	<ul><li>Alert and responsive to environment</li><li>Cry is lusty and vigorous</li><li>Feeding well</li><li>Respirations normal</li><li>Temperature stable</li><li>Apical pulse normal</li></ul>
Weight	<ul><li>2.5–3 kg</li><li>10% weight loss over first 5–7 days of life is normal. Most of the neonates regain weight within 10–14 days of life</li></ul>
Tactile stimulation	Consolable, quiet when held
Movement and muscle tone symmetry	Partially flexed extremities with knees up toward abdomen, active uncoordinated symmetrical bilateral movements of the extremities
Skin color	<ul><li>Pink, cyanosis of hands and feet (acrocyanosis) is seen in the first 24–48 hours of life and may last up to 10 days; mottling</li><li>Circumoral cyanosis with crying, possibly with feeding</li><li>No pallor</li><li>Physiologic jaundice occurs after 24 hours of birth (onset by the end of second or beginning of third day and ending around seventh day)</li><li>Progression: Jaundice first appears on the head and face progressing downward to the trunk and extremities and finally to the sclera of the eyes</li></ul>
Hydration	<ul><li>Falls quickly into place without residual marks after gently lifting up a fold of skin</li><li>Localized edema may be noted in a presenting part due to trauma</li></ul>

Contd...

Contd...

Assessment items	Norms
General appearance	- Swelling of breasts, genitals common (due to maternal hormones) - Normally skin is dry and peeling - Vernix caseosa—cheesy white layer of skin formed in uterus and lubricates the skin of the newborn - Milia—multiple yellow/pearly white papules, located on the face due to retained sebum, disappear in a few weeks - Miliaria (heat rash)—superficial grouped vesicles without erythema or red grouped papules, usually found in forehead skin, scalp, creases, or groin area caused by obstruction of sweat ducts from excessively warm and hurried environment - Erythema toxicum—blotchy, red papule with central yellow/white elevations, located generally on face, trunk, or extremities, appears suddenly on the first or second day and disappears in a few hours to few days; often called newborn rash or flea bite dermatitis - Forceps marks on face, cheeks and jaw, usually disappear in a day or two in the case of forceps delivery - Stork bites (telangiectatic nevi)—pale pink or red spots found on the eyelids, nose, lower occipital bone, and nape of the neck, usually fade by second birthday - Strawberry marks (nevus vasculosus)—raised, clearly delineated, dark red, rough-surfaced birthmark commonly found in head region. Grow often rapidly for several months and become fixed in size by 8 months. Then begin to shrink and resolve spontaneously. About 90% cases resolved by 9 years of age - Mongolian spots—dark blue or purple, bruise-like spots usually over sacrum found in darker complexioned infants. Gradually fade during first or second year of life - Port-wine stains (nevus flammeus): nonelevated, red to purple area (in infants of African descent it may appear on the face). It does not grow in size, does not fade with time, and does not blanch as a rule
Head symmetry	- Minor asymmetry is common and should equalize by approximately 4 months - Cephalohematomas emerge between the first and second day, may be unilateral or bilateral, and do not cross suture lines - Caput succedaneum (the fluid in a caput) is reabsorbed within 12 hours or a few days after birth
Fontanels (assess when newborn not crying)	- Anterior: 2- to 3-cm wide, 3- to 4-cm long, closes at 1.5 years - Posterior: 1–2 cm may be almost closed at birth and closes at 6–8 weeks - Sutures felt as depressed ridges in a newborn, molding can be overriding of the cranial bones. The suture lines become palpable within the few days after birth when this overriding diminishes
Condition of scalp cradle cap	Clean scalp, native lanugo, dense and silky hair growth
Face	Normal configuration
Ears—appearance and response to sound	Normally ears are placed with the top of the ear in line with inner and outer canthi respond to sound and voice

Contd...

Contd...

Assessment items	Norms
Eyes	
Appearance	- Bruised and/or puffy eyelids are normal - Sclera white to bluish white; slightly brownish in newborns of African descent - Small conjunctival, scleral, and retinal hemorrhages are common (*Note:* Erythromycin and tetracycline are now frequently used prophylactically instead of silver nitrate. If silver nitrate drops are used, it may cause edema and chemical conjunctivitis, which may appear a few hours after instillation and disappear in 1–2 days.)
Visual activity	- Blinks - Response to face or object - Should be alert with decrease in random activity, a focus on object in the line of vision; follows an arc, brightens (change in facial expression), widens eyes, jagged respiration
Discharge	Nil
Nose	
Shape	Symmetrical
Patency of nares	Breathes easily through either nostril with lips closed
Discharge	- May have temporary plugging - Sneezing is a natural reflex that clears nostrils
Facial skin	- Smooth pink/white milia present - Chin is poorly developed in relation to face
Mouth	
Hard and soft palate	Intact soft and hard palate
Lips and buccal mucosa	- Sucking callus on lips - Whitish appearance on roof of the mouth (cartilage) - Epstein's pearl
Tongue (frenulum)	Allows good mobility of tongue
Smile	Smiles at 3–4 weeks
Rooting and sucking reflexes	Present at birth and disappear at 6 weeks to 4 months (see the neonatal reflex)
Neck	
Traction response appearance	Contraction of the shoulder and arm muscles, followed by flexion of the neck and minimal head lag when pulling infant from a supine to sitting position
Hands	
Palmar grasp reflex	The newborn grasps the examiner's finger when palm is stimulated and holds momentarily
Chest	
Nipples, breast	May have some enlargement due to the presence of witch's milk (maternal hormone effect)

Contd...

Contd...

Assessment items	Norms
Cardiovascular	Apical pulse normal range for neonate: 100–160 beats/min, peripheral pulses equal to apical
Respiratory	30–60 breaths/min
Abdomen	<ul><li>Slight protrusion</li><li>Palpation: Liver 2 cm below costal margin</li><li>Auscultation: Bowel sounds normally can be heard</li></ul>
Umbilicus	Dried cord remnant up to 2–3 weeks of age; occasionally small amounts of bloody discharge
Back	
Spine	Spine straight
Gluteal folds	Symmetrical
Hips	Range of motion adequate
Genitalia (male)	
Scrotum	<ul><li>Two testes can be felt in scrotum, hydrocele is common in newborns</li><li>Genitalia may have edema due to maternal hormones, which should decrease in a few days</li></ul>
Penis	Foreskin normally adherent; cannot be completely retracted until 2 years of age
Genitalia (female)	
Hymen	Hymenal tag is a common neonatal variation that usually disappears after few weeks
Discharge	During the first week of life, the baby may have vaginal discharge composed of thick whitish mucus, which can be tinged with blood (pseudomenstruation) due to maternal hormone
Anus	Patent
Extremities	Normal activity, normal tone, normal deep tendon reflexes

Table 1.5: Newborn reflexes.

Reflex	Stimulation	Expected response	Age of disappearance	Figures
Rooting	Touching or stroking the cheek near the corner of the mouth	Head turns in direction of stimulation, when the breast touches the cheek, the neonate turns toward the nipple	<ul><li>When awake: 3–4 months</li><li>When sleep: 7–8 months</li></ul>	

Contd...

Chapter 1: Newborn Care

Contd...

Reflex	Stimulation	Expected response	Age of disappearance	Figures
Sucking	Touching the lips with the nipple of the breast or bottle	Sucking movements that enable the newborn to take food	After 6 months	
Swallowing	Accompanies the sucking reflex	Food reaching the posterior of the mouth is swallowed	Does not disappear	
Gagging	When more is taken into the mouth than can be successfully swallowed	Immediate return of undigested food	Does not disappear	
Sneezing and coughing	Foreign substances entering the upper or lower airways	Clearing of the upper air passages by sneezing, the lower air passages by coughing	Does not disappear	
Extrusion	Substance placed on anterior portion of tongue	Extrusion of the substance to prevent swallowing	4 months	

Contd...

Contd...

Reflex	Stimulation	Expected response	Age of disappearance	Figures
Blinking	Exposure of eye to bright light or sudden movement of object toward eye	Eyelid closure	Does not disappear	
Glabellar reflex	Repeatedly tapping between the eyebrows of newborn	Eyes blink	Does not disappear	
Doll's eye	Turn the newborn's head slowly to the right or left side	Normally eyes do not move	When fixation develops	
Palmar grasp	Objects placed in newborn's palm	Grasping of object by closing finger around it, reflex may be too strong that a neonate grasping the examiner's fingers can be lifted from the supine to standing position	6 weeks to 3 months	
Plantar grasp	Touching the sole of the foot at the base of the toes	Toes grasp around very small object	8–9 months	

Contd...

Contd...

Reflex	Stimulation	Expected response	Age of disappearance	Figures
Dancing (stepping place)	Hold neonate in a vertical position with the feet touching a flat, firm surface	Rapid alternating flexion and extension of the legs as if stepping	3–4 weeks	
Babinski	Stroking the lateral aspect of the sole of the foot with a relatively sharp objects from the heel up toward the little toe and across the foot to the big toe	Fans the toes	3 months of age, variable	
Tonic neck (fencing position)	Turning the head quickly to one side while the infant is supine	Arm and leg on the side, the head is turned toward extend. Arm and leg on the opposite side flex. Both hands may make a fist	18–20 weeks	
Moro (startle)	Startle the infant with a loud voice or apparent loss of support due to a change in equilibrium; the neonate is held supine position above the table or bed, the nurse supports the upper back and head with one hand and lower back with the other,	Generalized muscular activity symmetric abduction and extremities of the arms and legs with fanning of the fingers. The thumb and index finger on each hand form a C shape, the extremities then flex and adduct, the baby may cry	3–4 months	

Contd...

Contd...

Reflex	Stimulation	Expected response	Age of disappearance	Figures
	the newborn's head is suddenly allowed to drop backward an inch or so			
Swimming	Placed face down as if in water	Makes coordinate swimming movements	6–7 months	
Prone crawl	Place the baby prone on a flat surface	The neonate will attempt to crawl forward using arms and legs	3–4 months	

FORMAT FOR NEWBORN HISTORY TAKING

I. *Newborn's profile*
 – Name: B/O ___ (mother's name)
 – Date of birth: (if the baby is <72-hour old, then time of birth should be asked)
 – Gender: Male/female
 – Gestational age: To calculate the gestational age, last menstrual period (LMP) and (expected date of delivery (EDD) of mother can be asked
 – Weight of newborn
 – Type: Identify whether the baby's weight is small for gestational age (SGA), appropriate for gestational age (AGA), or large for gestational age (LGA)
 – Place and type of delivery: Institutional/ home; normal vaginal/instrumental/ cesarean
 – Address of the client
 – Maternal age, gravida, para, and number of live births and abortions if any
 – Informant: Mother/father/significant others
 – Reliability: Determine whether the information provided by the person is reliable or not

II. *Antenatal history*
Ask about the age of mother at marriage as well as conception. Details of medications taken and immunization, total number of antenatal visits, and history of any infection, such as fever, rash, and urinary tract infection should be noted. In the case of high-risk newborn, detailed history of antenatal events can be collected.
 – *First trimester:* History of vomiting (hyperemesis gravidarum), fever with rash (e.g., rubella), intake of teratogenic drugs, and exposure to X-rays or radiation.
 – *Second trimester:* Inquire about gestational week at which mother felt first fetal movement (quickening), TT

injection, and intake of iron and folic acid supplements.
- *Third trimester:* History of decreased fetal movements, premature rupture of membranes and color of liquor, fever, and foul smelling vaginal discharge.

Details regarding onset and duration of labor, maternal medications and induction and history of maternal complications, such as hemorrhage, obstructed labor, rupture of uterus, and sepsis are noted.

III. *Natal history*
- Date and time and mode of delivery of baby: Ask the informant whether the baby is delivered in hospital or at home. Inquire about mode of delivery, i.e., normal vaginal delivery or cesarean section. In the case of cesarean, reason should be known.
- Birth weight on newborn.
- Time of cry, Apgar score (if known), and any history of birth asphyxia.
- Any complications associated with umbilical cord like cord around the neck.

IV. *Neonatal history:* Collect information regarding the following:
- Time of voiding urine and meconium: Normally newborns will pass urine within 48 hours and meconium within 24 hours.
- History of seizures: Ask regarding signs and symptoms of neonatal seizure, such as abnormal cyclic movement of limbs and uprolling of eyes.
- Umbilical cord fall: Usually umbilical cord will fall off after 7-10 days. Ask the informant about any discharge, color changes, and pustules around the umbilical cord of newborn.
- History of shock, infection, temperature instability (hypothermia/hyperthermia), and congenital anomalies.
- Details of admission to NICU.
- Feeding: Time of first feed, any prelacteal feed (such as sugar water and honey) given to the baby, frequency of feeding, and any difficulties in feeding should be gathered from the mother.
- Immunization: History of vaccinations at birth (BCG, polio).

V. *Maternal health:* Neonatal health and welfare is associated with the health condition of mothers. Hence, it is mandatory to collect information about mother's health status. The information elicited should include the following:
- Systematic disorders (renal, cardiac, diabetes mellitus, etc.)
- Maternal drug abuse (alcohol, tobacco, cocaine, heroin, marijuana, etc.)
- Obstetrical complications in previous pregnancies
- Nutritional status (anemia, malnutrition)

Highlights ● ● ●

✦ Elicitation of newborn history includes newborn profile, antenatal history, intranatal history, and postnatal history.
✦ Maternal health status during pregnancy should be included in newborn history taking.

BABY BATH

Definition

Baby bath is a procedure to maintain hygiene of the baby to prevent colonization of harmful organisms.

Purposes

- To keep the baby's skin clean
- To refresh the baby
- To stimulate circulation
- To increase bonding between the mother and the child
- To prevent the baby from infection

- To provide an opportunity for mother to explore the baby for any abnormalities.

Types of Bathing

- *Sponging:* Sponge baths are given to infants who are acutely ill. Bath is given on the bed using soft sponge cloth.
- *Tub bath:* This is the common method of giving bath to a baby. The baby is submerged into the water in a tub or basin.
- *Lap bath:* When tub baths are not possible, mother keeps the baby on her lap and gives the bath.
- *Oil bath:* Premature babies and sick babies are given oil bath. Oil is applied all over the body and it is wiped off with cotton balls or rag pieces. When the baby's body is covered with vernix caseosa, an oil bath is given to remove it.

Ideal Time for Bath

Baby should not be bathed within an hour after feed because moving may cause vomit. Most babies go to sleep soon after feeding. The babies are bathed before the second feeding. Take care that the baby is not tired or hungry.

General Considerations during Baby Bath

An infant can be bathed in much the same as an adult, by a sponge bath or in a small tub. However, the nurse should take special precaution because an infant's temperature control mechanisms are still immature. Prolonged exposure of body parts may cause rapid heat loss. Some considerations are:

- Fitting baths into families schedule: Give bath at any time convenient to the family members but not immediately after feeding because increase handling may cause regurgitation of the feed.
- Preventing heat loss before starting the procedure: Put off the fans and close the doors and windows. The temperature of the room should be free from draughts. Bath the infant quickly. Expose only a portion of the baby at a time and thoroughly dry the body parts. Ideally, the initial bath is given, when the infant's skin temperature is 36.5°C (97°F) or the core temperature is 37°C (98°F).
- Preservation of the skin acid mantle: At birth, the skin pH is acidic around 5 (pH <5). This is bacteriostatic, so soap is used. Select mild soap, the soap containing less alkali.
- Preventing the skin trauma: Too vigorous handling can injure the fragile skin of the baby. If stool or other skin debris has dried and caked on the skin, soak the area to remove it and do not attempt to rub it off.
- Care of the cord: The cord is allowed to remain open and to get dried and shed of naturally.

Points to be Remembered

- Ensure that before giving the bath the infant's temperature should be normal. Bathing should be avoided for at least 2–6 hours after birth until cardiorespiratory status are stabilized.
- Babies <2,500 g are not to be given bath.
- Demonstrate baby bath at least once to the mother before discharge from the hospital.
- Vigorous cleaning of vernix is not recommended as it will fall off in few days. It acts as an insulator for the preterm babies and helps to prevent risk of infection.

Nurse's Responsibility in Giving a Tub Bath

Preliminary Assessment

- Check the neonatologist's order for the specific precautions to be taken if any.
- Assess the infant need for bathing.
- Check the temperature, respiration, and color of the skin.

- Check whether the child has taken the feed in previous 1 hour.
- Check the articles available in the unit.
- Check the weight of the baby.

Equipment Needed

A clean-lined tray/trolley containing:
- Bath basin or tub: To bath the baby
- Jugs 2: To keep hot and cold water
- Buckets 2: One for collecting the dirty water and another for soiled linen
- Mackintosh and towel: To protect the bed/table
- Bath blanket: To wrap the baby
- Towels 2: One big and one small: to wrap and dry the baby, respectively
- Soap in a soap dish: To remove dirt from the skin
- Sterile cotton balls in a bowl: To clean the ears, eyes, and nose
- Oil in a container: For oil massage
- Baby powder: To prevent bad odor
- Baby's dress: To prevent baby from chill after bath
- Kidney tray and paper bag: To collect waste
- Apron for the nurse: To prevent wetting of clothing

Massaging

- Take a few drops of oil, such as coconut oil, olive oil, or sweet almond oil into your warm hands and begin massaging the soles of the baby's feet. Use firm, gentle, slow strokes from the heel toward the toes.
- Continue with long smooth strokes up baby's legs, massage from the ankle up to the thigh and over the hip.
- Massaging upper body: Start the upper body massage with your hands on the baby's shoulders and make gentle strokes toward the chest.
- Massage the arms by stroking from the shoulders toward the wrist. Try not to get oil on baby's hands but if that happens, wipe his fingers clean before he sucks them.
- If baby's tummy feels soft (not hard or full) massage his belly using circular, clockwise strokes. Baby's tummy is sensitive, so if he becomes unsettled move on to next step.
- Use your fingertips to massage baby's face. Stroke from the middle of his face and toward cheeks.
- If baby is still relaxed, once you have finished front of his body, you can turn him onto his tummy and use long strokes from head to toe.
- Use respectful touch and stop massaging if baby is not enjoying himself or showing any signs of being uncomfortable. It is also best to avoid a massage if you are very tense, or if baby is agitated or upset.

Preparation of the Infant and the Unit

- Check the infant's conditions, i.e., feeding time, general conditions, such as temperature, drowsiness, and lethargy.
- Check the room temperature and warm it if necessary.
- Close the windows and switch off the fan to prevent draughts.
- Explain the mother what you are going to do.
- Wash hands prior to touching the baby.
- Set the articles.
- Adjust the position of the bath table to prevent the baby from falling.
  - Keep the table against the wall.
  - Place the tub or basin on one end of the table and place the tray and clothing on another end, so that the baby will be protected on three sides and there is less chance for the baby to roll and fall from the table.
  - Prepare an L-shaped setting of the trolley; on the main trolley, procedure is done and the trolley on the other side placed in L position contains weighing machine and TPR tray.

- Place the mackintosh on the table.
- Keep all the articles ready before beginning the procedure, so as to avoid leaving the child unnecessarily until the procedure has been completed.
- Wash hands and wear apron. Bring the baby to the bath table wrapped in bath blankets.
- Check whether the baby is wet with urine or stool. If wet, clean the baby.
- Undress the baby and wrap in big towel.

Procedure

- Clean the perineum if dirty.
- Wash hands after cleaning the perineum.
- Check the temperature of the baby.
- Check the weight of the baby.
- Take the baby into the bath trolley.
- First oil massage should be done. Massage the head in circulatory manner with oil and then massage the face, arms, chest, abdomen, legs, and back. Expose the needed areas only.
- Wrap the baby in clean dry towel.
- Attend to the infant's face, ears, and scalp.
- Wipe eyes from the inner canthus to outer canthus using separate wisp of cotton for each eye. Use one wisp for one stroke. If the secretions are crusted in the nostrils, take a rolled wisp of cotton and gently introduce into the nostrils and rotate. The baby will sneeze and bring out the secretions.
- Clean the mouth by using wet rag piece. Clean the thrush if present.
- The inside of the ears are cleaned with rolled wisp of cotton.
- With the wet hand clean the face and behind the ears. Do not apply soap on the face. Dry the face by patting not by rubbing.
- Pick up the baby securely by sliding your hand until the baby's head is well supported in your palm. Hold the baby's head over

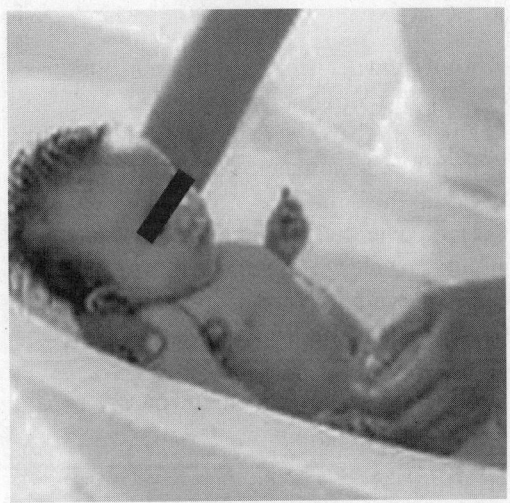

Fig. 1.12: Bathing newborn in tub.

the basin, apply ear plug, wet the head preventing water entering into the ears, apply soap, rinse it with water, and dry it thoroughly (**Fig. 1.12**).
- Discard the water and take fresh water. Keep one mug of water aside.
- Unwrap the baby, hold the baby securely, supporting head, neck, and shoulder. Apply soap all over the body, giving special attention to the neck, arms, axillae, groins, fingers, and toes. Rinse well.
- Turn the baby carefully; hold the baby securely supporting the head, neck, and shoulders. Apply soap over the back and buttocks. Rinse well.
- Take the baby up from the tub and pour the mug full of water over baby's body preventing the entry of water into the mouth.
- Take the baby from the water and dry him/her by patting gently. Special attention is given to clean the body creases.
- Change the towel; wrap the baby in a dry and clean towel.

Aftercare

- Apply powder over the skin folds (optional).
- Keep the cord open and dry.
- Dress the baby as early as possible. Wrap him/her in blanket to prevent chills.
- Comb the hair.
- Hand over the baby to mother for feeding.
- Take articles to the utility room. Disinfect the towels and basin. Clean, dry, and replace in their proper place.
- Wash hands.
- Record the procedure in the nurse's record with date and time.

Highlights

> - Baby bath is given to maintain hygiene of the baby to prevent colonization of harmful organisms.
> - Types of baby bath are sponging, tub bath, lap bath, and oil bath.
> - Baby should not be bathed within an hour after feed because moving may cause vomit.
>
> **Some considerations in baby bath are:**
> - Fitting baths into families schedule.
> - Preventing heat loss before starting the procedure.
> - Preservation of the skin acid mantle.
> - Preventing the skin trauma.
> - Care of the cord.
> - Ensure that before giving the bath the infant's temperature should be normal.
> - Vigorous cleaning of vernix is not recommended.
> - Babies <2,500 g are not to be given bath.

KANGAROO MOTHER CARE

Definition

Kangaroo mother care (KMC) is a special way of caring low-birth-weight (LBW) infant by skin-to-skin contact.

Components

- Skin-to-skin contact: Direct, continuous, and prolonged skin-to-skin contact is provided between the mother and the baby to promote thermal control.
- Exclusive breastfeeding: Skin-to-skin contact promotes lactation and feeding interaction with exclusive breastfeeding for adequate nutrition and to improve desired weight gain.

Uses

- Maintains thermoregulation and metabolism
- Enhances sensory stimulation
  - Skin-to-skin contact (tactile)
  - Listen to mother's voice (auditory)
  - Breastfeed (taste)
  - Mother's body odor (olfaction)
  - Eye-to-eye contact with the mother (vision)
- Less prone to apnea.
- Protects against nosocomial infections
- Better weight gain
- Facilitates psychological bond between mother and baby
- One of the best methods for transporting small (stable) babies
- Increases the opportunities for parenting (father and mother)
- Does not require additional staff compared to incubator
- Less expensive

Prerequisites

- Reclining chairs/bed with adjustable backrest or pillow or ordinary chair
- Mother's clothing: Light dress with front open/gown, shawl, KMC bags (**Figs. 1.13A and B**), etc.
- Baby's clothing: Front open sleeveless shirt, cap, socks, nappy, and mittens

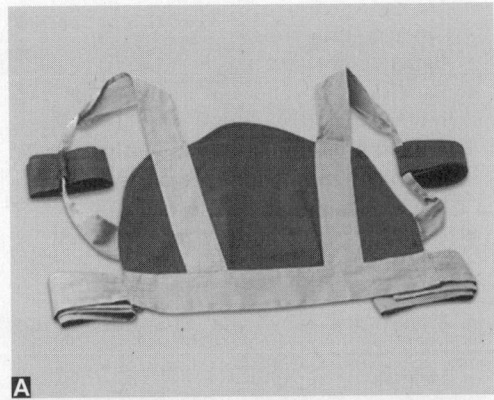
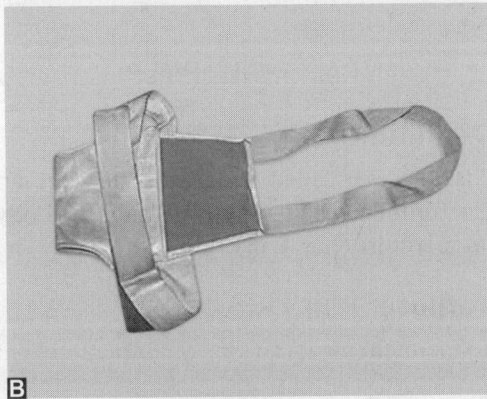

Figs. 1.13A and B: Commercial kangaroo mother care bags.

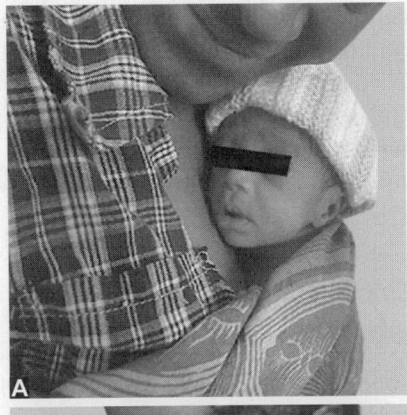
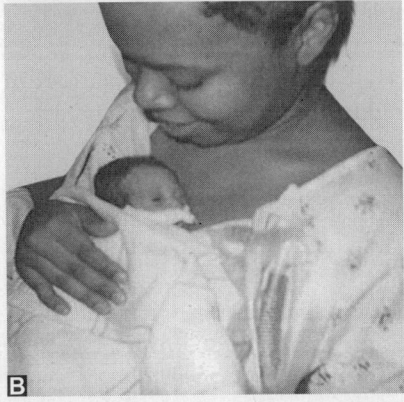

Figs. 1.14A and B: Kangaroo mother care positioning.

Eligibility Criteria

For Babies

- All stable newborn (<2,000 g) soon after birth
- Sick LBW infants: Few days after treatment
- <1,200 g with serious prematurity: Few weeks after birth and adequate treatment

For Mothers

Physically and mentally stable
Note: If mother is not able to do, other family members, especially father, of newborn can be encouraged for KMC procedure.

Preparation

- Explain the benefits of KMC to the mother and the family members and clear their doubts.
- Demonstrate the procedure to the mother gently with patience.
- Allow the mother to interact with someone who is already practicing KMC for her baby.

Procedure

- Place the baby between the mother's breasts in an upright position (**Figs. 1.14A and B**).
- Turn the baby's head to one side and in a slightly extended position, which helps to keep the airway open and allow eye-to-eye contact.

- Baby's hip should be flexed and abducted in a frog-like position. The arms should be flexed and placed on mother's chest.
- Baby's abdomen should be placed at the level of mother's epigastrium.
- Support the baby with a sling or binder or especially prepared KMC bag.
- Baby's neck position should be neither too flexed nor too extended.

Nurse's Responsibility

- Monitor the baby's vital parameters at the initial stage.
- Maintain patent airway.
- Assist the mother in breastfeeding by holding the baby near to the breast.

Duration of Kangaroo Mother Care

- Initial stage: At least for 1 hour.
- Gradually can be increased up to 24 hours/day.
- KMC can be continued until the baby gains weight around 2,500 g or reaches 40 weeks of postconception age.
- KMC can be discontinued if the baby starts wriggling to show discomfort or pulls limbs out, cries and fusses every time, when the mother tries to put the baby into skin contact.
- When mother and baby are comfortable, KMC can be continued as long as possible at health facility or home.
- Mother can provide skin-to-skin contact occasionally after the baby bath and during cold nights.

Highlights ●●●●

- ✦ Kangaroo mother care (KMC) is a special way of caring low-birth-weight infant by skin-to-skin contact.
- ✦ The components of KMC include skin-to-skin contact and exclusive breastfeeding.

The uses of KMC are:
- ✦ Maintains thermoregulation and metabolism.
- ✦ Enhances sensory stimulation.
- ✦ Protects against nosocomial infections.
- ✦ Better weight gain.
- ✦ Facilitates psychological bond between mother and baby.
- ✦ If mother is not able to do, other family members, especially father, of newborn can be encouraged for KMC procedure.
- ✦ Duration of KMC: Initial stage—at least for 1 hour, gradually can be increased up to 24 hours/day.
- ✦ Monitor the baby's vital parameters at the initial stage.
- ✦ Maintain patent airway.

RADIANT WARMER

Definition

It is otherwise called open care system. It is an electronic device used to maintain the body temperature **(Fig. 1.15)**.

Purpose

To maintain newborn's body temperature.

Parts of Radiant Warmer (Open Care System)

- Bassinet—for placing the neonate
- Quartz rods—to provide radiant heat

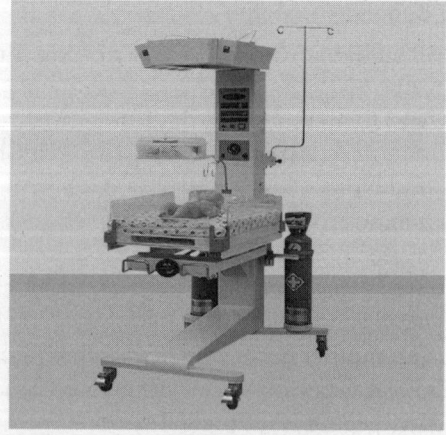

Fig. 1.15: Radiant warmer.

- Skin probe—when attached to the baby's skin senses skin temperature
- Control panel
- Heater output display
- Heater output control knobs
- Temperature selection panel
- Temperature selection knobs
- Temperature display
- Mode selection

Preparation

- Educate the parents the importance of maintaining the body temperature.
- Discuss measures that will be used to maintain the newborn in a thermal neutral environment.

Procedure

- Perform hand hygiene.
- Connect the unit to the mains and switch it on.
- Select manual mode. Select heater output to 100% for some time to allow quick prewarming of the bassinet covered with linen.
- Select servo mode. Select the desired temperature of baby as 36.5°C.
- Place the baby on bassinet.
- Connect skin probe to the baby's abdomen with the sticking tape.
- If you want the manual mode to be used, select the desired heater output.
- In the manual mode, record baby's axillary temperature.
- Check sensor probe regularly so as to ensure that it is in place.
- Ensure that skin probe is free of contact with bed.
- Cover probe with a reflective cover pad, if available (foil covered foam adhesive pad).

General Instructions

- Do not use warmer in cold room environment. It best works when the room temperature is above 20°C.
- Keeping the warmer where there is lot of air currents reduces its efficiency.
- The warmer must be prewarmed around 20 minutes before the arrival of the baby or till the temperature is reached with <50% of total heat output.
- While using the manual mode in a warmer without a temperature display, record the baby's temperature regularly, preferably q2 hourly.
- The manual mode is used for initial preparations of bed for the baby or when rapid warming of a severely hypothermic temperature at 30 minutes and then 2 hourly.
- Respond to alarm immediately. Identify the fault and rectify it.

Application of Skin Probes

Do's

- Prepare the skin using an alcohol/spirit swab to ensure good adhesion to the skin.
- Use of cling wrap (transparent polythene used for covering fruits or vegetables for storage) over the baby, tied across the panel warmer, has shown to reduce insensible water losses and result in better thermal control for very low birth weight (VLBW) (<1.5 kg) babies.

Don'ts

- Do not apply to bruised skin.
- Do not apply clear plastic dressing over probe.
- Do not use finger nails to remove skin surface probes.
- Do not reuse disposable probes.

Chapter 1: Newborn Care

Care of Radiant Warmer

- Surfaces of warmer should be cleaned daily with an antiseptic solution, such as glutaraldehyde.
- Spirit or other organic solvents must not be used to clean the glass side panels or display panel.
- For disinfection of probe isopropyl alcohol should be used.
- Every 7 days, after shifting of the baby to another cot, the equipment should be cleaned thoroughly, first by light detergent solution and then by antiseptic solution.
- The control and power units should be calibrated q4–6 months.

Advantages

- Easy accessibility
- Easy to connect the tubes of ventilated baby and do the procedures
- Better monitoring especially if the baby has respiratory distress
- Less risk of infection as compared to closed incubator
- Can be used as resuscitation trolley in the labor room

Disadvantage

More insensible water loss

Nurse's Responsibility

- Axillary temperature must be recorded and documented as per nursery policy and compare this with depicted display temperature.
- If the baby is having fever, examine the baby carefully.
- A baby who is overheated due to radiant warmer will have his skin flushed and also his sole/palms will be warm to touch in addition to warm abdomen.
- Fever due to any illness will result in warm abdomen to touch but palms/soles will be cold to touch. In addition, clinical examination reveals features that point toward sepsis in the baby.
- Offer the parents the option of skin-to-skin contact if infant is stable.

Highlights ● ● ●

- ✦ Radiant warmer is an electronic device used to maintain the body temperature.
- ✦ Prewarming of the bassinet covered with linen needed before placing the baby.
- ✦ Connect skin probe to the baby's abdomen with the sticking tape.
- ✦ In the manual mode, record baby's axillary temperature.
- ✦ Check sensor probe regularly so as to ensure that it is in place.
- ✦ Respond to alarm immediately. Identify the fault and rectify it.
- ✦ Surfaces of warmer should be cleaned daily with an antiseptic solution, such as glutaraldehyde.
- ✦ A baby who is overheated due to radiant warmer will have his skin flushed and also his sole/palms will be warm to touch in addition to warm abdomen.
- ✦ Fever due to any illness will result in warm abdomen to touch but palms/soles will be cold to touch. In addition, clinical examination reveals features that point toward sepsis in the baby.

PHOTOTHERAPY

Definition

Phototherapy consists of the application of fluorescent light to the infant's exposed skin; light promotes bilirubin excretion by photoisomerization, which alters the structure of bilirubin to soluble form (lumirubin) for easier excretion.

Articles Needed

- Overhead phototherapy lights
- Eye shields

- Disposable diapers
- Towel or disposable waterproof pad
- Bilirubin light meter
- Baby weighing scale
- Isolette temperature monitor
- Thermometer
- Input/output (I/O) chart
- For fiberoptic phototherapy: Fiberoptic blanket
- Blanket, disposable sheath, or covering pad

Indications

Phototherapy will be initiated when the bilirubin level is more than the threshold limit as follows:
- *Term neonates*
  - First day of life: >5 mg/dL
  - Second day of life: >8 mg/dL
  - After 48 hours: >15–22 mg/dL
- *Preterm babies:* Generally initiated sooner and at lower levels

Preparation of Child and Parents

- *Physical preparation*
  - Collect history from parents to determine possibility of ABO/Rh incompatibility.
  - Check the blood values of newborn.
  - Check weight.
  - Do a brief physical assessment to determine the level of hydration, consciousness, signs of jaundice, etc.
- *Psychological preparation*
  Explain the family members regarding:
  - Reason for phototherapy
  - Covering the child's eyes during the procedure
  - Possible side effects
  - Importance of checking diaper q hour and meticulous skin care

General Considerations

- Verify the intensity of phototherapy.
- Infants receiving phototherapy treatment are weighed daily.
- Serum bilirubin levels are checked as per protocol.
- Plan activity such as feeding or bathing the infant so that family members may fully participate in the child's care.

Procedure

Sl. no.	Steps	Rationale
1.	Gather the necessary articles	Promotes efficient time management and provides organized approach
2.	Perform hand hygiene	Reduces transmission of microorganisms
3.	Set up bassinet/isolette	
4.	Set up fluorescent over lights ■ Distance: open bassinet—4 inches from infant ■ Isolette: 15–18 inches (halogen lamps emit more heat than fluorescent bulbs; therefore increase the risk of burn, do not position it close to infant)	The distance between the light source and the infant affects how well the light penetrates the skin and is absorbed by the bilirubin
5.	Turn the light unit on using a light meter, verify whether the level of irradiance is appropriate to the manufacturer's recommendation for the system (min: 10–12 µW/cm²/nm)	Intensity of lights may decrease over time. Lights of less intensity may be infective or may require longer length of exposure to achieve the desired therapeutic effect
6.	Perform hand hygiene	To decrease the transmission of microorganism

Contd...

Contd...

Sl. no.	Steps	Rationale
7.	Undress the infant, leaving the diaper in place to cover the genitals	Undressing increases the amount of skin area exposed. The diaper protects the gonads against chromatic radiant damage from the phototherapy
8.	Cover the eyes completely with protective shields. Ensure that nares are open. Remove shields every 2 hours	Eyes are closed to prevent corneal excoriation and retinal damage
9.	Place the infant in bassinet or isolette turn the infant every 2 hours, assessing skin integrity, hydration, temperature, and neurological status	Ongoing assessment can detect problems early and prevent dehydration of skin

Mechanism of Action

Its action is through three modes:
1. Geometric photoisomerization of unconjugated bilirubin resulting in a more soluble form of bilirubin.
2. Converting bilirubin to lumirubin through structural isomerization, which can be excreted into the bile without the need for further hepatic conjugation.
3. Oxidation mechanism resulting in colorless by-products and excreted by liver and kidney without need for conjugation.

Complications

- Increase in environmental and body temperature
- Retinal damage
- Bronze baby syndrome (brownish black discoloration of skin, urine, and serum)
- Electric shock
- Effects on endocrine and sexual maturation (priapism)
- Dehydration and electrolyte disturbance (hypocalcemia)
- Loose greenish stools
- Increased metabolic rate
- Skin rashes, excoriation, and breakdown
- Rebound effect (subsequent increase in the serum bilirubin level after discontinuation of phototherapy)

Nurse's Responsibility

- Reassure the parents regarding their baby's progress and benefits and risks of procedure.
- Support the mother for successful and frequent breastfeeding during the therapy.
- Assess the parent's level of understanding in clarification of this process.
- On each nursing shift, the eyes are checked for evidence of discharge, excessive pressure on the lids, or corneal irritation.
- Eye shields are removed during feeding, which provides the opportunity for visual and other sensory stimulation.
- During breastfeeding switch off the phototherapy unit.
- Babies who are in open crib must have a protective glass shield between them and the light source to minimize the amount of undesirable ultraviolet (UV) light reaching their skin and to protect them from accidental bulb breakage.
- Maintaining the baby in a flexed position with rolled blankets along the sides of the body helps to maintain heat and provide comfort.
- Maintain thermoregulation.
- Adequate fluid intake should be provided either orally or intravenously. Vasodilatation increases the insensible water loss and there is excess stool loss from occasional

diarrhea (urine specific gravity should be <1.015).
- Ensure that the baby passes adequate urine (6–8 times/day).
- Weight is taken at least once a day.
- Ensure that serum bilirubin levels are obtained as per protocol. The diminishing icterus does not reflect the serum bilirubin concentration.
- Discontinue phototherapy when serum bilirubin returns to safe value as per protocol.
- Monitor clinically for rebound bilirubin rise within 24 hours after stopping phototherapy.
- Turn infant on abdomen for short period of time and will cease priapism.
- Accurate charting of the following:
  - Type of fluorescent light/manufacturer
  - Number of lamps
  - Distance between surface of lamp and neonate
  - Use of phototherapy in combination with incubator or open bassinet
  - Photometer measurement of light intensity
  - Occurrence of side effects
  - Length of time the bulb has been used
    Note: The effectiveness of light decreases after 800 hours of use. Thus the bulbs should be changed at the correct time.
  - Maintain vital signs, feeding chart, weight chart, and serum bilirubin chart.

Highlights ● ● ●

✦ Phototherapy consists of the application of fluorescent light to the infant's exposed skin; light promotes bilirubin excretion by photoisomerization, which alters the structure of bilirubin to soluble form (lumirubin) for easier excretion.
✦ Phototherapy will be initiated when the bilirubin level is more than the threshold limit.
✦ Infants receiving phototherapy treatment are weighed daily.
✦ Serum bilirubin levels are checked as per protocol.
✦ Plan activity, such as feeding or bathing the infant so that family members may fully participate in the child's care.
✦ Eye shields are removed during feeding, which provides the opportunity for visual and other sensory stimulation.
✦ During breastfeeding switch off the phototherapy unit.
✦ Maintain thermoregulation.
✦ Adequate fluid intake should be provided either orally or intravenously.
✦ Discontinue phototherapy when serum bilirubin returns to safe value as per protocol.
✦ Monitor clinically for rebound bilirubin rise within 24 hours after stopping phototherapy.
✦ Turn infant on abdomen for short period of time and will cease priapism.

INCUBATOR

Definition

An incubator (isolette) is an apparatus designed to maintain the environment suitable for a neonate. It is used for preterm babies and some full-term babies who are ill.

Incubator may be described as bassinets enclosed in plastic, with climate-control equipment designed to keep the babies warm and limit their exposure to germs.

Functions

- Oxygenation through oxygen supplementation by oxy hood or nasal cannula or even continuous positive airway pressure (CPAP) or mechanical ventilation.
- Observation: Modern incubator care involves sophisticated measurement of temperature, respiration, cardiac function, oxygenation, and brain activity.
- Protection from cold temperature, infection, noise, draughts, and excess handling.

- Provision of nutrients through IV catheters.
- Administration of medications.
- Maintaining fluid balance by providing fluid and keeping a high air humidity to prevent a great loss from skin and respiratory evaporation.

Types

1. *Transport incubator:* It is an incubator in a transportable format and is used when a sick or premature baby is moved, for example, from one hospital to another. It usually has a miniature ventilator, cardiorespiratory monitor, IV pump, pulse oximeter, and oxygen supply built into its frame.
2. *Servo controlled incubator:* (1) Single-wall incubator and (2) double-walled incubator.

Parts of Incubator

- A rigid box-like enclosure in which an infant may be kept in a controlled environment.
- AC (alternating current)-powered heater.
- A fan to circulate the warm air.
- A container for water to add humidity.
- A control valve through which oxygen may be added.
- Access port for nursing care (**Fig. 1.16**).
- Servo control to help regulate incubator air temperature.

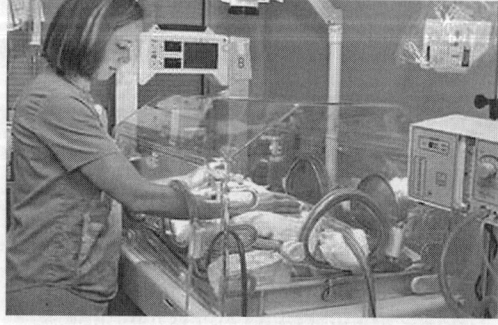

Fig. 1.16: Care of newborn in incubator.

Nurse's Responsibility

- The incubator should always be prewarmed before placing the newborn in it.
- The infant should be clothed and warmly wrapped in blankets when removed from the warm environment of the incubator for feeding or cuddling.
- Cover the head of the baby both when inside and outside to prevent heat loss.
- Frequent monitoring of baby's temperature is needed.
- Adjust the temperature of the incubator by setting the upper and lower limits of desired circulating air temperature range.
- The servo control is usually set to a desired skin temperature between 36 and 36.5°C.
- If the baby's body temperature drops, the warming device is triggered to increase heat output.
- Watch for accidental detachment of sensor probe from baby's skin that may leads to false registration of infant's skin temperature to rise and overheat the infant.
- The port holes of the incubator should not be opened frequently because frequent opening may cause convective heat loss when newborns are exposed to increase airflow velocity and turbulence. Plan the nursing care in such a way that it will not disturb the babies and prevent unnecessary exposure to outside air.
- Never leave the baby unattended when access door or hand ports or canopy is open to avoid any risk of an infant falling out of an incubator.
- When using KMC along with incubator care, the temperature of the baby must be monitored constantly.
- Always disconnect power supply before cleaning and disinfecting the incubator.
- Follow the hospital protocol for disinfecting.

- To avoid any risk of infection, clean and disinfect incubator and accessories before any use.
- The water for humidification should be changed frequently.
- Identify and correct the alarm situations to avoid patient injury.

Highlights ●●●●

- ✦ Incubator may be described as bassinets enclosed in plastic, with climate-control equipment designed to keep them warm and limit their exposure to germs.
- ✦ The main purposes are oxygen supplementation, observation, and protection from cold temperature.
- ✦ There are two types: transport incubator and servo controlled incubator.
- ✦ The incubator should always be prewarmed before placing the newborn in it.
- ✦ The infant should be clothed and warmly wrapped in blankets when removed from the warm environment of the incubator for feeding or cuddling.
- ✦ Adjust the temperature of the incubator by setting the upper and lower limits of desired circulating air temperature range.
- ✦ When using kangaroo mother care along with incubator care, the temperature of the baby must be monitored constantly.
- ✦ The port holes of the incubator should not be opened frequently because frequent opening may cause convective heat loss when newborns are exposed to increase airflow velocity and turbulence.

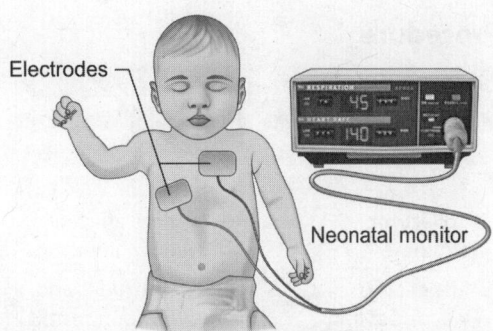

Fig. 1.17: Apnea monitor.

APNEA MONITOR

Definition

An impedance-type device that monitors both the respiratory and heart rates of an infant and sounds an alarm alerting caregiver of a possible need to perform CPR in the event of either apnea or a marked increase or decrease in heart rate.

Purpose

To check the heart and respiratory rates of the baby to make sure that he/she is breathing properly.

Indication

Infants <12 months of age with documented apnea or who have known risk factors of life-threatening apnea according to the following indication:

Diagnosis of pertussis with positive culture.

Equipment Needed

- Apnea monitor
- Two electrode patches
- Apnea monitor leads (**Fig. 1.17**)
- Apnea monitor log (optional)

Preparation of Child and Parents

- Review the child's chart to determine the reason for apnea monitoring.
- Examine the skin to ensure that there is no powder, perspiration.
- Explain the parents the reason for keeping the infant on monitor.

Parts of Apnea Monitor

It has two parts—(1) a belt with sensory wires that a baby wears around the chest and (2) monitoring unit with alarm.

Procedure

Steps	Rationale
1. Perform hand hygiene	To decrease transmission of microorganisms
2. Collect the equipment	To promote efficient time management
3. Inspect the electrodes and leads for proper functioning	Faulty electrodes and wires will not transmit the information needed to monitor the cardiorespiratory status
4. Place the monitor away from the walls and on firm surface	The monitor will work efficiently on steady surface
5. Place the infant on supine position	Reduces the risk of SIDS
6. Turn the apnea monitor (preset of apnea/alarm lapse will be done by vendor or respiratory therapist)	
7. Place the white lead to the patient's right chest above the nipple and black lead on left side. The inserts of the lead wire should point from the hands	Placing the wires away from mouth and hands of infant will decrease the chance that infant will disconnect or become entangled in head
8. Connect the lead wire into apnea monitor and then it on as per manufacturer's instruction	Each monitor has unique features according to its manufacturer
9. Remove all the equipment from contact with the child's skin for at least 10–15 min/day. During this time meticulous skin care should be given	To keep the skin remain intact and prevent breakage of skin

(SIDS: sudden infant death syndrome)

Nurse's Responsibilities

- Response to an apnea monitor must be immediate and thorough.
- If alarm sounds assess the chest movement activity.

Highlights ●●●●

- ✦ Apnea monitor is used to check the heart rate and respiratory rate of the baby to make sure that he/she is breathing properly.
- ✦ It is indicated in infants <12 months of age with documented apnea or who have known risk factors of life-threatening apnea.
- ✦ It has two parts—(1) a belt with sensory wires that a baby wears around the chest and (2) monitoring unit with alarm.
- ✦ Response to an apnea monitor must be immediate and thorough.

MEMORY EXERCISE

1. **The initial steps of neonatal resuscitation include all, *except*:**
   a. Suctioning of mouth and nose
   b. Drying the newborn
   c. External cardiac massage
   d. Flicking the newborn

2. **The Apgar score 5/10 at 5 minutes after birth indicates:**
   a. Mild distress
   b. Moderate distress
   c. Severe distress
   d. No distress

3. **Ideal time for giving baby bath:**
   a. Immediately after feeding
   b. Within 1 hour of feeding
   c. Whenever time permits
   d. Before the second feeding

4. **The assessment that focuses on reactivity of newborn in the first 24 hours:**
   a. Gestational assessment
   b. Transitional assessment
   c. Neurological assessment
   d. Physical assessment

5. **The benefits of KMC are all, *except:***
    a. Cord care
    b. Thermal control
    c. Breastfeeding
    d. Early discharge

6. **Bronze baby syndrome is due to phototherapy given in case of:**
    a. Conjugated hyperbilirubinemia
    b. Sepsis
    c. Prematurity
    d. Long duration

7. **The heater output in servo mode of radiant warmer is controlled by:**
    a. Machine
    b. Baby
    c. Both a and b
    d. None

8. **The correct order of checking vital signs in newborn:**
    a. Heart rate, respiration, temperature
    b. Temperature, respiration, heart rate
    c. Temperature, heart rate, respiration
    d. Respiration, temperature, heart rate

CHAPTER 2

Assessment Procedures

LEARNING OBJECTIVES

Upon the completion of this chapter, the learners will be able to:
- Define the basic terms.
- Recognize the needs and concerns of child and parents in admission and assessment procedures.
- Prepare the child and family for various assessments.
- Collect comprehensive history.
- Document the observations made in nurse's record accurately.

Keywords: admission, health assessment, developmental milestones, health, instruments, records and reports

ADMISSION PROCEDURE

Definition
Admission to hospital involves staying at a hospital for at least one night or more.

Types of Admission
- General inpatient units
- Emergency and urgent care departments
- Pediatric intensive care units
- Outpatient or special procedure units
- Rehabilitation unit or hospital

Indications for Admission to Isolation Room
- Very sick children who need complete rest and calm environment
- Immunocompromised children, for example, children with cancer
- Children with communicable diseases
- Children who need respiratory or contact isolation

Equipment Needed
- Bed, crib, isolette, warmer, or bassinet
- Blankets, linens, bath towel, and wash clothes
- Toiletry items
- Jar with drinking water and glass
- Diapers and wipe (if needed)
- Bedpan and urinal
- Identification band for child
- Scissors
- Measuring tape
- Weighing machine

- Thermometer
- Sphygmomanometer
- Stethoscope
- Pulse oximeter (if needed)
- Patient admission documentation forms

Preparation of Child for Hospitalization

- Read stories about experience with hospital or surgery. Talk about going to the hospital and what it will be like coming home.
- Be honest and encourage child to ask questions.
- Visit the hospital areas and go through the preadmission tour if time permits.
- Plan support to the child via your presence, telephone calls, and special items brought from home.
- Encourage the child to draw pictures to express how he or she is feeling.
- Include siblings in preparation.

Nurse's Responsibility in Admission Procedure

- Establish a trusting, caring relationship with the child and family.
- Smile, introduce yourself, and give your title.
- Explain the child and family members what will happen and what is expected of them.
- Ask the family and the child what names they prefer to be called by.
- Maintain eye contact at the appropriate level.
- Communicate with children at age-appropriate levels.
- Involve an orientation to the hospital unit.
- Briefly explain policies and routines and the personnel who involved in the care of the child.
- Obtain information about the child's history, routines, and reason for admission.
- Obtain baseline vital signs, height, and weight and perform a physical assessment.
- Recognize the needs of the family and child during interview process.
- A small bag can be brought to the hospital that contains child's clothes (hospital policy); slippers; hobby materials; and personal care items such as comb, brush, and tooth paste.

Procedure

- Perform hand hygiene.
- Assemble all the necessary equipment.
- Check the room equipment for proper functioning (e.g., light, fan, and tap).
- Prepare bed by adjusting to lowest horizontal position with top sheet and perform complete assessment of the child, which includes vital signs, height, weight, physical examination, and growth and developmental assessment.
- Explore the needs and desires of the caregivers regarding their comfort and their involvement in the direct care of their child.
- Collect specimens, such as blood and urine as ordered and send it for laboratory analysis.
- Depending upon the condition of the child, an orientation can be given to the unit stressing the areas of importance and greatest relevance (e.g., play room, toilet facility, and pantry).
- Assist the child in maintaining personal hygiene and changing to hospital dress (hospital policy).
- Administer any medication if ordered.
- Explain the policies and protocols of hospital to the parents.

Highlights

> - Admission to hospital involves staying at a hospital for at least one night or more.
> - Types of admission are general inpatient units, emergency and urgent care departments, pediatric intensive care units, outpatient or special procedure units, and rehabilitation unit or hospital.
> - Communicate with children at age-appropriate levels.
> - Involve an orientation to the hospital unit.
> - Briefly explain policies and routines and the personnel who involved in the care of the child.
> - Obtain information about the child's history, routines, and reason for admission.
> - Obtain baseline vital signs, height, and weight and perform a physical assessment.
> - Recognize the needs of the family and child during interview process.
> - Be honest and encourage child to ask questions.

HISTORY TAKING

Introduction

The health history provides the nurse with an overall picture of what the child has experienced, highlighting the areas of concern.

Prerequisites

- The consultation room or patient's room should be well lighted, comfortable, and quiet and decorated with toys and pictures to allay the anxiety of the child.
- There should be chairs for parents (informants) and the nurse and a bed or examining table for the child.
- Materials to record the history data (either a computer or chart paper and pen).

Approaching the Parent or Caregiver

- Greet the parent or caregiver by name.
- Maintain a friendly, warm, unhurried, informal, and relaxed attitude throughout the interaction with the family.
- Assess the quality of parent–child and parent–parent interactions while recording history.
- Use open-ended questions and avoid making judgmental comments.
- Show respect by remaining approachable.

Approaching the Child

- The nurse can wear variety of professional outfits, for example, colorful uniforms, tops rather than all white uniforms to avoid anxiety of the child.
- Infants and young children should be offered soft toy or a rattle to establish rapport while taking history.
- Make physical contact with the child in a nonthreatening way at first. Briefly cuddling the newborn before returning it to the caregiver, warmly shaking the hands of old children and teens, and laying your hand on head or arms of toddlers and preschoolers will convey a gentle demeanor.
- Maintain eye-to-eye contact.

Performing Health History

Basic Information/Identifying Information

Informant (mother, father, relative, child, etc.), name, age (preferably date of birth), and sex of the patient should be enquired. Parent's name age, address, telephone number, income, occupation, education, and religion should be recorded. The history may be unreliable due to informant's poor memory, intelligent, or education. The origin and ethnic background of the family is important in some genetic diseases. For example, glucose-6-phosphate dehydrogenase deficiency is common among Parsis and north Indians whereas sickle cell disease is seen in tribal population.

Presenting Complaints/Chief Complaints

The chief complaint is the specific reason for the child's visit to the hospital. The chief complaints for which the patient has been brought to the hospital should be recorded in chronological order according to the sequence of events, for example, fever for 5 days, headache 3 days, vomiting 3 days, convulsions 1 day, and loss of consciousness 2 hours.

History of Present Illness

The history of present illness is a narrative of the chief complaints from its earlier onset through its progression to the present. Its four major components are (1) the details of onset, (2) a complete interval history, (3) the present status, and (4) the reason for seeking help now (**Table 2.1**).

The informant should be encouraged to give details of sequence of events during the course of illness without the help of leading questions. The mode of onset, course of illness, and details of treatment already received must be recorded. The symptoms referable to various body systems should be reviewed. Detailed information pertaining to various symptoms manifested by the patients should be elicited, for example, pain, duration, frequency, timing, site and severity, character, radiation, precipitating, aggravating and relieving factors, and associated symptoms.

History of Past Illness

Ask for past history of common childhood diseases. Ask specifically about cold, earache, allergic manifestations, etc. In addition to illness, ask about injuries that required medical interventions, operations, and any other reason for hospitalization, including the date. Ask about commonly known allergic disorders, such as asthma, unusual reactions to drugs, food, latex products, and reaction to other contact agents, such as poisonous plants, household products, animals, or fabrics.

Table 2.1: Components of history of present illness.

Components	Examples
Time of onset	- Paroxysmal nocturnal dyspnea - Evening rise of temperature
Mode of onset	- Acute: Wet beriberi - Subacute: Endocarditis - Insidious: Nephrotic syndrome - Chronic: Tuberculosis
Progression/course of illness	- Condition becomes better (diarrhea) - Condition becomes worse (diabetes ketoacidosis) - Static condition (cerebral palsy)
Duration of illness	- More than a week: Typhoid fever - Short duration: Acute gastroenteritis - Lasts for long duration: Cough due to tuberculosis
Precipitating factors	Chest pain due to pleural effusion aggravated by respiratory movements
Relieving factors	Pain decreased due to positioning, fever reduced after some home remedies

Birth History/Perinatal History

The birth history covers the series of events that occurred during the birth of the incumbent child. There may be an association between present illness and these events. Hence, the nurse should enquire about the important events either from the mother or significant family members (if the mother is not present or not aware) or birth records.

The birth history includes all data concerning:
- The mother's health during pregnancy
- The labor and delivery
- The newborn conditions immediately after birth

Maternal diseases or medications during pregnancy (especially during first trimester), presentation, mode and place of delivery, first cry after the birth, feeding difficulties during neonatal period, birth weight, gestation, etc. should be recorded (**Table 2.2**).

Developmental History

In children suspected to have delayed development or central nervous system (CNS) disorder, a detailed developmental screening should be done. Precise timing of social smile; head control; rolling over; sitting; standing; walking; self-feeding and dressing; bladder and bowel control; speech; weight at 6 months, 1 year, and 2 years of age; approximate length at ages of 1–4 years; dentition; etc. to be enquired. Use specific and detailed questions when enquiring about each developmental milestone.

Family Pedigree

Family pedigree should be enquired and genetic diagram should be constructed (**Fig. 2.1**). History of contact with possible infections, childhood infections, and diseases should be sought. The contact may be in the family, neighborhood, or school. History of similar ailments in the family member should be asked when genetic, infective, or allergic disorders are strongly suspected. Ask for history of consanguineous marriage among parents (**Table 2.3**). In case a particular disease is manifesting only among male siblings, it is suggestive of X-linked inheritance.

Social History

Enquire about occupation, education, and income of parents. If mother is working who looks after the child at home when she is away or is the child in a crèche. Ask whether the family is nuclear or joint and whether grandparents are staying with the family or not. Calculate the per capita income by dividing total income of the family by the number of family members. Housing conditions, sewage disposal, and water source should be

Table 2.2: The important components of birth history.	
Components	Significance
Birth order	The child who born after two or three live children is prone to develop malnutrition; especially when there is no or less gap between the consequent pregnancies
Multiple pregnancy	The second twin is more prone for hypoxia, hypoglycemia, and birth trauma. These factors may result in brain damage
Mode of delivery	Natural birth/cesarean section
Place of delivery	Hospital/home/other
Person who conducted the delivery	Qualified doctor or nurse/trained dai/untrained person
Gestational age	Preterm/term/post-term (prematurity disposes the child to certain disorders such as patent ductus arteriosus (PDA)
Birth weight	Appropriate/small/large for gestational age
Birth asphyxia	Cried/did not cry soon after birth; if not, then details of resuscitation
Bluish discoloration of body	While crying or feeding
Breathing difficulties	
Apgar score at 1, 5, and 10 minutes	

Chapter 2: Assessment Procedures

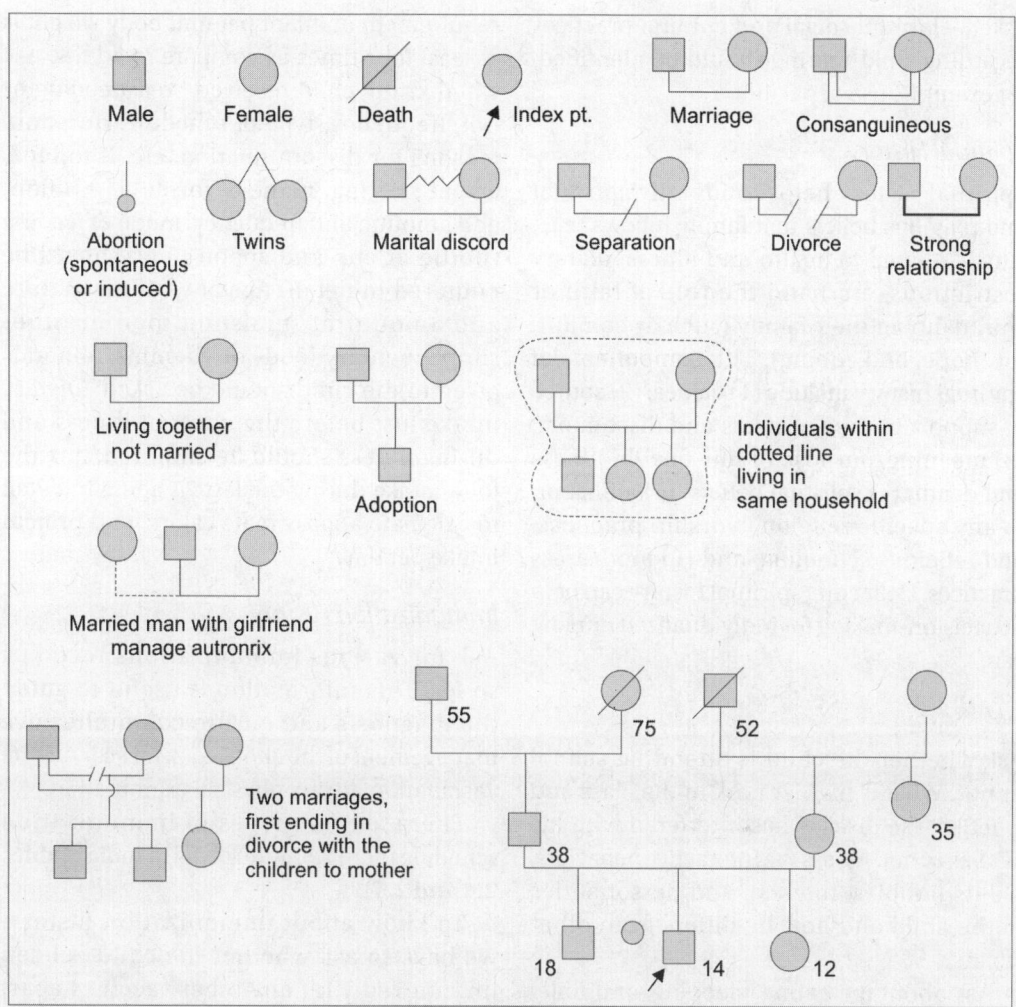

Fig. 2.1: Family pedigree chart.

Table 2.3: Degree of consanguinity.		
Degree of consanguinity	Examples	Common genetic makeup
I degree (incest)	Brother and sister/parent–child	50% genetic material is in common. Probability of expression of autosomal-recessive conditions is maximal
II degree	Half siblings/uncle–niece/aunt–nephew	25% genetic material in common
III degree	First cousins/half uncle–niece/half aunt–nephew	12.5% genetic material
IV degree	Marriage between distant relatives	6.25% or less genetic material in common. Minimal risk of consanguinity

asked. Harmful social and cultural practices regarding child-rearing should be identified, for example, use of pacifier.

Spiritual History

Spiritual history helps to identify spiritual and religious beliefs that family follows (e.g., rituals related to health and illness, dietary restrictions, etc.) and the role of faith or spirituality in their family (such as comfort, joy, hope, and coping). The components of spiritual history include (1) values; (2) source of support in time of stress and discomfort; (3) meaning/purpose of life, health, illness and death; (4) spiritual beliefs; (5) affiliation to any specific religion, worship practices, and religious schooling; and (6) food/dress practices. Collecting spiritual history can help in decision-making for individualized nursing care.

Habits

Ask whether the child is attending school or not. What is his/her rank in the class and whether the disease has interfered with his studies or not. Assess the interactive behaviors, habits hobbies, interest, and personalities of the child and how he differs from other siblings.

Ask about the eating, sleeping, and toilet habits of the child. Adolescent children should be encouraged to talk regarding their worries, anxiety, psychosexual difficulties, and substance abuse tendencies. Ask whether any pet animals are kept in the home. Enquiry should be made regarding smoking, intake of alcohol, and drug abuse by parents, which can adversely affect the family dynamics and child-rearing practices.

Feeding History

History of dietary intake is of special importance in children because they need food for growth and development. The energy or caloric requirement of infant per unit body weight is at least four times as compare to adults. Ask whether the child received breastfeeding or not, frequency, type of schedule, duration, reasons for discontinuation, etc. If top fed, age at starting, name of formula, dilution, and amount, and frequency, mode of feeding (bottle or cup and spoon), etc. should be enquired in detail. Age at weaning, nature and amount of semisolid food or other supplementary foods or vitamins/minerals given to the child should be asked. Dietary intake just before the onset of illness and during illness should be enquired. Ask the food intake during the last 24 hours in detail to calculate approximate caloric and protein intake per day.

Immunization History

Ask for various immunizations received so for. This information is useful to guide the diagnosis and ensure comprehensive management of the child. Look for scar of BCG vaccination during physical examination.

There are two types of immunization schedules commonly followed in India (**Tables 2.4 and 2.5**).

To know about immunization history, we have to ask whether the child is been immunized with any other vaccines apart from immunization schedule especially in the epidemic areas of certain communicable disease.

MISSION INDRADHANUSH

This program was launched by the Ministry of Health and Family welfare, Government of India on December 25, 2014.

Aim

To ensure that all children and pregnant women are fully immunized with vaccine-preventable diseases.

Table 2.4: National immunization schedule.

Age	Name of vaccine
Birth	Bacillus Calmette Guerin (BCG), Oral Polio Vaccine (OPV)-0 dose, hepatitis B birth dose
6 weeks	OPV-1, Pentavalent-1, Rotavirus Vaccine (RVV)-1, Fractional dose of Inactivated Polio Vaccine (fIPV)-1, Pneumococcal Conjugate Vaccine (PCV)-1*
10 weeks	OPV-2, Pentavalent-2, RVV-2
14 weeks	OPV-3, Pentavalent-3, Fipv-2, RVV-3, PCV-2*
9 months to 12 months	Measles and Rubella (MR)-1, JE**, PCV-Booster*, Vitamin A (1 lakh IU)-1st dose
16–24 months	MR-2, JE-2**, Diphtheria, Pertusis and Tetanus (DPT)-Booster-1, OPV-Booster, Vitamin A 2nd dose (2 lakh IU)****
5–6 years	DPT-Booster-2
10 years	Tetanus and adult diphtheria (Td)
16 years	Td
Pregnant mothers	Td-1, Td-2 or Td-Booster***

Source: Ministry of Health and Family Welfare, Government of India, 2020
*PCV in selected states/districts; Bihar, Himachal Pradesh, Madhya Pradesh, Uttar Pradesh (selected districts) and Rajasthan; in Haryana as state initiative.
**JE in endemic districts only.
***one dose if previously vaccinated within 3 years.
****Vitamin A should be given thereafter once in 6 months up to 5 years.

Table 2.5: Indian Academy of Pediatric (IAP) vaccination schedule.

Age	Name of vaccine
Birth	BCG, OPV-0, Hep B-1
6 weeks	DTwP1/DTap1, IPV-1, Hep B-2, Hib-1, PCV-1, Rotavirus-1
10 weeks	DTwP2/DTap2, IPV-2, Hep B-3, Hib-2, PCV-2, Rotavirus-2
14 weeks	DTwP3/DTap3, IPV-3, Hep B-4, Hib-3, PCV-3, Rotavirus-3
6 months	Influenza vaccine (flu vaccine)
6 months onwards	Typhoid conjugate vaccine (TCV)
9 months	MMR1/MR
12 months	Hepatitis A 1, Japanese Encephalitis(JE) [for endemic areas]
15 months	MMR2, Varicella 1, PCV booster
16 to 18 months	DTwP/DTap 1st booster, IPV 1st booster, Hib 1st booster
18 months	Hepatitis A 2
4 to 6 years	DTwP/DTap 2nd booster; MMR3+Varicella 2
9 to 12 years	Tdap/Td HPV 2 doses for girls (minimum 6 months interval between 2 doses)

Source: Indian Academy of Pediatrics, 2019.

Scope

The name depicts seven colors of rainbow, which targets vaccinating all children against the following seven vaccine-preventable diseases:
- Diphtheria
- Pertussis
- Tetanus
- Tuberculosis
- Polio
- Hepatitis B
- Measles

In high-risk states, Japanese encephalitis (JE) and *Haemophilus influenzae* type B (Hib).

Intensified Mission Indradhanush

This is launched in October 2017; weeklong immunization drives from seventh of each month.

Highlights

- The health history provides an overall picture of what the child has experienced, highlighting the areas of concern.
- Patient's room should be well lighted, comfortable, and quiet and decorated with toys and pictures to allay the anxiety of the child.
- Maintain a friendly, warm, unhurried, informal, and relaxed attitude throughout the interaction with the family.
- Assess the quality of parent–child and parent–parent interactions while recording history.
- Use open-ended questions and avoid making judgmental comments.
- Make physical contact with the child in a nonthreatening way at first.
- The components of history are basic information/identifying information, presenting complaints/chief complaints, history of present illness, history of past illness, birth history/perinatal history, developmental history, family pedigree, social history, spiritual history, habits, feeding history, and immunization history.
- Ask whether the child is been immunized with any other vaccines apart from immunization schedule especially in the epidemic areas of certain communicable disease.
- Mission Indradhanush is initiated to ensure that all children and pregnant women are fully immunized with vaccine-preventable diseases.

VITAL SIGNS

Definition

Vital signs or cardinal signs are the important signs that indicate the status of the body's vital functions. Temperature, pulse, respiration, and blood pressure (BP) are called vital signs.

Purposes

- To find out the general condition of the child
- To get idea about possible diseases
- To take decision regarding treatment of child
- To identify the progress of child's recovery

Assessment of Vital Signs

Temperature

Sites for checking temperature: (1) oral, (2) axillary, (3) tympanic, and (4) rectal.

Types of thermometer

1. Glass thermometer **(Fig. 2.2)**

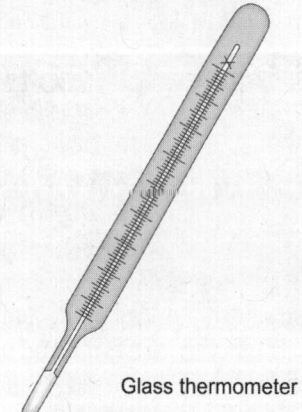

Fig. 2.2: Glass thermometer.

2. Digital thermometer **(Fig. 2.3)**

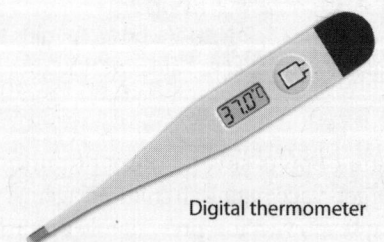

Fig. 2.3: Digital thermometer.

3. Disposable or single-use plastic thermometer strips (chemical dot thermometer) **(Fig. 2.4)**

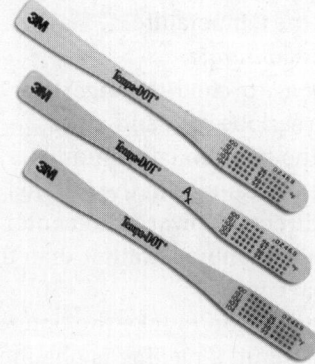

Fig. 2.4: Single use thermometers.

4. Infrared thermometer **(Fig. 2.5)**

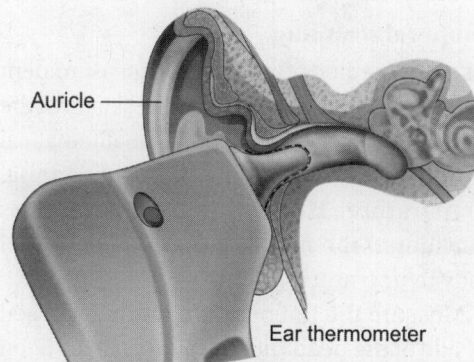

Fig. 2.5: Infrared thermometers.

Equipment needed

A clean tray containing:
- Thermometer
- A bottle containing antiseptic solution
- A bottle containing plain water
- A small bowl containing dry cotton swabs
- A small bowl containing wet cotton swabs
- Kidney tray or paper bag
- TPR chart or pen and paper
- Wrist watch with seconds

Preparation
- Explain the procedure to the mother and child as appropriate.
- Depending on the site/route of checking, assess for the following:
  - *Oral*—feeding, age, oral problems, level of consciousness, and understanding
  - *Rectal*—diarrhea, imperforated anus, etc.

Procedure

Oral route (above 6 years)
- Wash hands.
- Shake the thermometer down to bring the reading below 35°C.
- Clean the thermometer with dry swab from bulb to stem in circulatory motion.
- Keep the thermometer under the patient's tongue, to the right or left of the pocket at the base of the tongue.
- Tell the child to close his/her lips but not the teeth around the thermometer.
- Leave the thermometer in place for at least 2 minutes.
- Take out the thermometer and read the temperature.
- Wipe the thermometer with wet swab or wash it in soapy lukewarm water and rinse it in cold water, dry it, and store it.
- Wash your hands and record the temperature.

Axillary temperature
- To take an axillary temperature, the thermometer is kept under the patient's arm.
- Wash your hands.
- Prepare the thermometer just as you would to take an oral temperature.
- Keep the thermometer under the child's arm in the axilla.
- Hold the child's arm tight against the chest and leave the thermometer in place for 5 minutes.
- Take out the thermometer and read the temperature and clean and store the thermometer.
- Wash hands and record the temperature.

Checking axillary temperature using digital thermometer
- Wash hands.
- Take the digital thermometer out of its holder.
- Insert the tip of thermometer into single-use plastic cover or clean the tip with soap and warm water (or clean with alcohol wipes).
- Switch on and place the tip of thermometer in the center of armpit.
- Tuck the child's arm closely against the body.
- Leave the thermometer in place until beep sound appears and temperature reading appears in the window of thermometer.
- Note the readings.
- Clean the tip with alcohol wipe (dispose the tip cover if used).
- Put the thermometer back to the holder.

Rectal temperature
Rectal temperature is considered the most accurate. They are usually taken only with infants and children who cannot yet hold a thermometer in their mouth without breaking it.
- Wash hands.
- Place the child on side line or prone position or on mother's lap.
- Prepare the thermometer as explained earlier.
- Apply some water-soluble lubricant on a tissue or gauze piece and then on to the first 2.5 cm of the thermometer from bulb.
- Ask the child to take a deep breath (if older enough) and keep the thermometer into the anus from 1.5 to 4 cm, depending on the child's age and size.
- Do not force the thermometer.
- Hold the thermometer in place for 2 minutes.
- Remove the thermometer, wipe it with a tissue or dry cotton swab, and discard the tissue.
- Read the mercury level.
- Wash and rinse the thermometer, wipe it with disinfectant, dry it, and store it.
- Wash hands.
- Record the temperature.

Tympanic membrane
- Note the age of child if younger than 3 years, pull the earlobe back and down.
- Insert the tympanic thermometer gently into the ear canal with the infrared sensor beam directed toward the center of the tympanic membrane rather than the side of the ear canal.
- Push the button to take the temperature and hold until a reading is obtained. The length of time required for the temperature to register varies per manufacturer but only a few seconds at most.

Temporal scanning
It is a new method of temperature measurement that uses infrared scanning on the skin over the temporal artery combined with a mathematical computation to determine the child's arterial temperature. The arterial temperature is considered the most accurate reflection of body temperature.
- Measure the temperature on the exposed side of the head (not the side that has been lying on a pillow or covered by a hat).
- Slide the sensor tip externally in a horizontal line across the child's forehead, midway between the eyebrows and hairline and ending at the temporal artery.
- Hold it in position until the device registers the temperature reading, which usually requires one second (**Fig. 2.6**).
- Accuracy may be affected by excessive sweating.

Nurse's responsibility in checking temperature
- Take an oral or tympanic temperature for children older than 6 years.

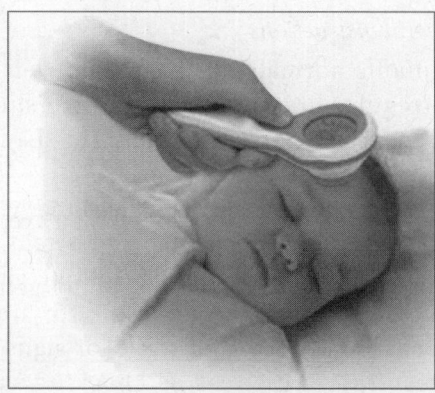

Fig. 2.6: Temporal scanning.

- Take a tympanic, axillary, or rectal temperature for children who are younger than 6 years, disoriented, unconscious, or in severe respiratory distress.
- Do not take a rectal temperature if a child has had any immune or hemolytic disorder, rectal surgery, or diarrhea.
- Do not take a tympanic temperature if a child has had ear surgery or has ventilation tubes or infection.
- Use axillary method only if other methods are not possible.
- Regardless of method you use, remain with the child to ensure safety.
- Hold the temperature probe in place for required time. Do not use glass and mercury thermometers if possible.

Pulse

Sites for checking pulse

- For children <2 years: Apical pulse—the point of maximum intensity (PMI), the point on the chest wall where the heartbeat is heard, most distinctly, is just above and outside the left nipple of the infant at the third or fourth intercostal space. The PMI moves to a more medial and slightly lower area until 7 years of age, when it is heard best at the fourth or fifth intercostal space at the midclavicular line.
- Apical pulse rate should also be taken if the child has a cardiac problem, such as an irregular heart rate or a congenital heart defect, as well as before administering certain medications, such as digoxin.
- For children >2 years: Radial pulse. Other sites are:
  - Carotid pulse (unconscious child)
  - Brachial pulse
  - Femoral pulse
  - Popliteal pulse
  - Posterior tibialis pulse
  - Dorsalis pedis pulse

Preparation

- Explain the procedure to the parent and the child as appropriate.
- Allow the child to examine or handle the stethoscope to become familiar with equipment.
- Make the child to be calm and quite.
- Give any play material for distraction.

Equipment needed

- A stethoscope (pediatric size)
- Wrist watch with seconds or pulsometer
- Alcohol wipes for cleaning ear piece and chest piece
- Paper and pen

Procedure

- Wash hands.
- Clean the chest piece and ear piece with alcohol wipes.
- Turn the chest piece to on mode; check for audibility.
- Keep the diaphragm on the site explained above and once you hear the heartbeat start to count from 0, 1, 2, 3, 4, till the completion of 1 minute.
- In older children palpate the radial pulse for a full minute.

- Note any irregularities in strength or rhythm.
- Document the method used to obtain pulse measurement as well as any activity of the child during the assessment and any action taken.

General instructions
- Assess the heart rate while the child is resting or sleeping.
- The heart rate in infants is much faster than in adults, it also varies in infants and children who are anxious, fearful, or crying. For an accurate heart rate, wait for several seconds until the heart rate slows, then count for one full minute.
- As the child grows, the heart rate slows and the range of normal value narrows.
- The radial pulse is difficult to palpate accurately in children <2 years of age because the blood vessels lie close to the skin surface and are easily obliterated.

Respiration

Preparation of client
- Explain the procedure to the parents and the child as appropriate.
- Assess the respiration when the child is resting or sitting quietly.

Procedure
- Wash hands.
- Ask the caregiver/parents to hold the child on lap or keep in lying position.
- Count for respiratory rate for a full minute.
- Infant's respirations are primarily diaphragmatic so count the abdominal movements.
- After 1 year of age count the thoracic movements.
- Document the rate, activity of the child, any deviations from normal and any action taken.

General instructions
- Infants normally display an uneven or irregular breathing pattern with short pauses between some breaths. This may be accentuated when they are ill.
- Take respirations before taking other vital signs, as you will be unable to obtain an accurate respiratory rate if a child is crying.
- If you cannot obtain a respiratory rate because of crying, observe for signs of respiratory distress by checking skin color, pallor, and the presence of breath sounds. Signs of respiratory distress include xiphoid retraction, dilation of nostrils, and expiratory grunt.
- Assess the respiration when the child is resting or sitting quietly, since the respiratory rate often changes when infants or young children cry, are fed, or become more active.

Blood Pressure

Equipment needed
- Pediatric stethoscope
- BP cuff (appropriate size for child)
- Doppler or electronic monitor (if available) or sphygmomanometer
- Paper and pen

Preparation
- Explain the procedure to the parent and the child as appropriate.
- Allow the child to handle the equipment when appropriate. Encourage preschool or school-age child to use equipment to take BP on a doll or stuffed animal.
- Use terminology appropriate to child's age.

Sites for checking blood pressure
- *Upper arm:* 2 cm above antecubital fossa, auscultation area—brachial artery
- *Lower arm/forearm:* 2 cm above wrist, auscultation area—radial artery

- *Thigh:* 2 cm above popliteal fossa, auscultation area—popliteal artery
- *Calf/ankle:* 2 cm above ankle, auscultation area—posterior tibialis and dorsalis pedis artery

Procedure
- Wash hands.
- Place the correct size cuff on infant's or child's bare arm.
- Inflate the cuff until the radial pulse disappears or about 30 mm Hg above expected systolic reading.
- Place the stethoscope light over the artery and slowly release air until pulse is heard.
- Record reading as in adults.
- Record the BP on paper to be transferred to permanent document.

Doppler or electronic monitor
- Obtain the monitor, dual air hose, and proper cuff size.
- Plug in monitor (unless battery operated) and attach dual hose if necessary.
- Attach appropriate-size BP cuff and wrap around child's limb.
- Turn on power switch and record the reading.

General instructions
- When choosing a cuff, measure the width of the cuff against the width of the child's arm.
- The cuff should cover approximately two-third of the upper arm.
- The bladder of the cuff should be long enough to encircle the arm without overlapping.
- Be sure to use the same size of cuff each time.
- The cuff size will vary with the child's age and size.
  - The cuff bladder width should be at least 40% of the circumference of the upper arm at its midpoint (**Table 2.6**).
  - The cuff bladder length should cover 80–100% of the circumference of the upper arm (**Fig. 2.7**).

Table 2.6: The size of cuff for pediatric age-groups.

Age	Width (cm)	Length (cm)	Max. arm circumference (cm)
Newborn	4	8	10
Infant	6	12	15
Child	9	18	22
Adolescent	10	24	26

- To measure BP using the upper arm, place the limb at the level of the heart, place the cuff around the upper arm, and auscultate at the brachial artery.
- When obtaining BP in the lower arm again position the limb at the level of heart, place the cuff above the wrist, and auscultate the radial artery.
- For measurement in thigh, place the cuff above the knee and auscultate the popliteal artery.
- To obtain BP on calf or ankle, place the cuff above the malleoli or at the midcalf and auscultate the posterior tibialis or dorsalis pedis artery.
- Systolic pressure in children is read at the moment you hear the first Korotkoff sounds as you lower the manometer pressure. The point at which the sound disappears is the diastolic pressure.

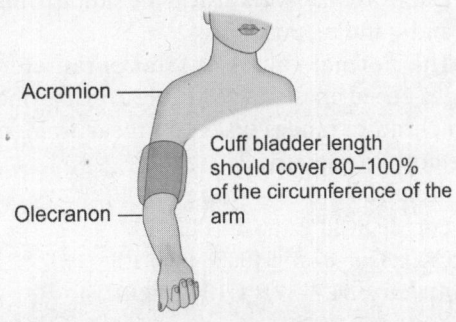

Fig 2.7: Cuff bladder.

Table 2.7: Normal values of vital signs.

Age	Pulse (minute)	Respiration (minute)	Systolic BP	Diastolic BP
Newborn	140–160	30–60	50–70	–
Infant	120–160	30–40	60–100	35–55
Toddler	80–130	20–40	70–100	45–65
Preschooler	70–110	20–30	90–110	50–70
School age	75–120	16–22	95–120	60–80
Adolescent	70–100	15–20	94–140	62–87

(BP: blood pressure)

- The systolic BP sometimes can be heard to a measurement of zero, so document the reading as systolic pressure *P* for pulse.
- Due to the small arm vessels in infants and young children, it may be very difficult to hear the Korotkoff sounds by auscultation.
- In children older than 1 year, the systolic pressure in the thigh tends to be 10–40 mm Hg higher than in the arm.
- Systolic BP will increase if the child is crying or anxious. So measure the BP when the child is quiet and relaxed.
- If the reading is lower in the leg than in the arm, always consider coarctation of aorta or interference with circulation to the lower extremities.
  Also pay attention to the pulse pressure, unusually wide (>50 mm Hg) or narrow (>10 mm Hg) pulse pressure readings suggest a congenital heart defect.
- Infants and children presenting with cardiac complaints should have BP assessed in all four extremities and also in the sitting, lying, and standing positions.

The normal values of vital parameters varies based on their age **(Table 2.7)**. Normal temperature ranges based on measurement methods in pediatrics:
- *Rectal:* 36.6–38°C (97.9–100.4°F)
- *Ear:* 35.8–38°C (96.4–100.4°F)
- *Oral:* 35.5–37.5°C (95.9–99.5°F)
- *Axillary:* 34.7–37.3°C (94.5–99.1°F)

Highlights

- Sites for checking temperature are (1) oral, (2) axillary, (3) tympanic, and (4) rectal.
- Insert the tympanic thermometer gently into the ear canal with the infrared sensor beam directed toward the center of the tympanic membrane rather than the side of the ear canal.
- Do not take a tympanic temperature if a child has had ear surgery or has ventilation tubes or infection.
- Temporal scanning is a new method of temperature measurement that uses infrared scanning on the skin over the temporal artery combined with a mathematical computation to determine the child's arterial temperature.
- Assess the heart rate while the child is resting or sleeping.
- The heart rate in infants is much faster than in adults, it also varies in infants and children who are anxious, fearful, or crying.
- For an accurate heart rate, wait for several seconds until the heart rate slows, then count for one full minute.
- Take respirations before taking other vital signs, as you will be unable to obtain an accurate respiratory rate if a child is crying.
- When choosing a cuff of sphygmomanometer, measure the width of the cuff against the width of the child's arm.
- The cuff bladder width should be at least 40% of the circumference of the upper arm at its midpoint.
- The cuff bladder length should cover 80–100% of the circumference of the upper arm.

ANTHROPOMETRIC MEASUREMENTS

Definition

Anthropometry refers to study of measurement of human part, such as height, weight, head circumference (HC), chest circumference, and mid-arm circumference.

Weighing the Infant or Child

Purposes

- To calculate the dosage for medications
- To calculate the nutritional requirements
- To identify loss/gain of weight
- To assess the child's actual weight and find out the degree of malnutrition
- To monitor the growth

Indications

- All children below 1 year of age (routine)
- Children who have diarrhea and vomiting
- Child with edema, for example, nephrotic syndrome and cardiac problems
- Child with malnutrition
- Child who is seeking medical assistance (outpatient/inpatient)

Equipment needed

- Weighing scale appropriate for child's age and ability to sit or stand
- Disposable paper covering for scale
- Paper and pen to record the weight
- Cleaning solution and equipment according to institutional policy

Preparation

- Check if the scale/measuring devices used are appropriate for age and safety of the child.
- Check if the scales are measuring and weighing in kilogram.
  Note: All weighing machines should be serviced annually.
- Prepare the child by giving age-appropriate explanation and where necessary use distraction.
- Consider the child's gender, culture, and privacy.
- If child is frighten and uncooperative and making accurate measurement is impossible, postpone measuring until the child is relatively calm.
- Remove the nappies, shoes, or slippers.
- Infant's should ideally be weighed nude and weighed on baby scales until the age of 2 years.
- Children over 2 years should be weighed in light clothing without shoes on standing or sitting on scales.

Disable children unable to sit or stand should be weighed in light clothing on a hoist scale if available. If not available the weight can be calculated by weighting the parent and the child together and then parent separately.

Types of weighing scale

- Conventional beam balance scale
- Hanging scale (in community setting)
- Ground scale
- Electronic weighing machine

Procedure

- Explain the procedure to child and caregiver.
- Wash hands.
- Place the scale on a flat even surface.
- Clean the scale with swabs (hospital policy).
- Place the paper on scale.
- Balance scale to reading of "0."
- Weigh the infants with no clothing, older child in underwear or lightweight gown.
- The child must be kept completely on the scale and the weight fully borne (**Fig. 2.8**).
- Always hold one hand within inch of the child for safety.
- Note the reading on the scale.
- Pick up the child or have older child step off scale.
- Remove and discard paper cover.
- Record the weight on paper to be transferred to permanent document.

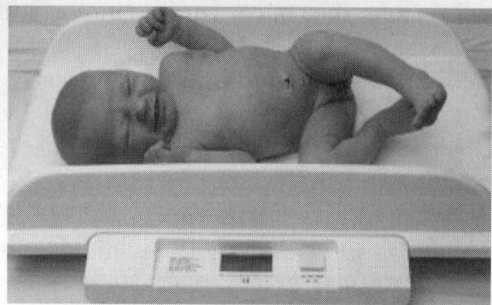

Fig. 2.8: Checking weight using electronic weighing machine.

- Clean the scale according to the hospital policy.
- Report weight as appropriate.

Nurse's responsibility

- For infants and children who continue to be inpatients, weight should be measured at least weekly.
- More frequent monitoring may be indicated depending on the age or clinical condition, for example, neonates, cardiac, renal patients, and critically ill patients.
- Weigh the hospitalized child at the same time using same scale, same amount of clothing each time child is weighed.
- All measurements should be plotted on growth chart and reviewed by the medical team in order to determine the need for further assessment or intervention.
- Weight must be recorded in medical, nursing, and drug charts where appropriate the patient held record.
- In the outpatient clinic, the measurements should be directly entered the child's medical notes.
- It is good practice to compare the measurements to the previous recording as this could detect any possible error in measurement or acute change in medical condition.
- For any reasons clothing has not been removed or a child weighed with additional equipment, for example, splint and cast, this must be recorded in nurse's chart.

Formulas for calculating expected weight

1. Weight at 3–12 months: $\dfrac{\text{Age in months} + 9}{2}$
2. Weight at 1–6 years: Age in years $\times 2 + 8$
3. Weight at 7–12 years: $\dfrac{\text{Age in years} \times 7 - 5}{2}$

On an average, the ideal birth weight is 3.25 kg. The newborn losses up to 10% of his weight during first week, it is however regained by the age of 10 days. After this, weight gain occurs at a rate of 25–30 g a day for the first 3 months and 40 g a month during the rest of the first year of life. The infant doubles his birth weight by the age of 5 months and trebles it by 1 year. He increases it 4 times by 2 years, 5 times by 3 years, 6 times by 5 years, and 10 times by 10 years.

Postprocedure care

- The child should be redressed and left comfortable.
- After use, the measuring equipment should be cleaned with detergent and hot water followed by an alcohol impregnated wipe.
- Perform hand hygiene.
- If the equipment is contaminated with blood, it should be cleaned with soap and water followed by the hypochlorite solution.
- Record the child's weight with date and time.

Measuring Height

For children under 2 years, it is advisable to measure the recumbent length while the child lies supine with legs fully extended at hips and knees and feet at right angles to legs.

In older children, standing height is measured by making the child stand against a vertical scale or wall.

Equipment needed

- Infantometer (for <2 years old)
- A vertical scale fixed against the wall
- Scale or pointer
- Pen and paper

Types of measuring devices/scales (standing height)
- Holtan stadiometer
- Magnimeter
- Seca height measure
- Length: Infantometer

Preparation
- The length board should be placed on a flat, stable surface such as table.
- Explain the procedure to the mother and the child as appropriate.
- Remove shoes and thick sports socks in the case of older children.

Procedure

1. *Measuring length*
   - Cover the length board with a thin cloth or soft paper for hygiene and for the baby's comfort.
   - Explain the mother that she will need to place the baby on the length board herself and then help to hold the baby's head in place while you take the measurement.
   - Show her where to stand when placing the baby down, that is, opposite to you, on the side of the length board away from the tape (**Fig. 2.9**).
   - Also show her to place the baby's head (against fixed head board) so that she can move quickly and surely without distressing the baby.
   - Ask her to lay the child on his back with his head against the fixed head board, compressing the hair.
   - Quickly position the head so that an imaginary vertical line from the ear canal to the lower border of the eye socket is perpendicular to the board.
   - Ask the mother to move behind the head board and hold the head in this position.
   - Check if the child lies straight along the board and does not change the position. Shoulder should touch the board, and the spine should not be arched.
   - Hold down the child's legs with one hand and move the foot board with other.
   - Read the length accurately.
   - Remove the baby from board and hand over to mother.
   - Record it on paper.

2. *Measuring height*
   - Child stands with feet together and shoulders back. Ideally the heels, buttocks, shoulders, and back of head should touch the back plate/wall.
   - Place the head board gently on top of the head and position the head as follows: The child should look straight ahead with the lower border of the bony orbit (eye sockets) and the auditory canal in the same horizontal line. This is called the "Frankfurt plane" (**Fig. 2.10**).
     » Ask the child to take a deep breath while supporting the head in the correct position and applying gentle upward pressure.
     » Ensure the heels remain on the ground.
     » Ask the child to breathe out and relax and record the measurement.
     » Read the height to the last complete millimeter; do not round up or down.
     » Plot height on appropriate centile chart. Use simple dot to mark the height.

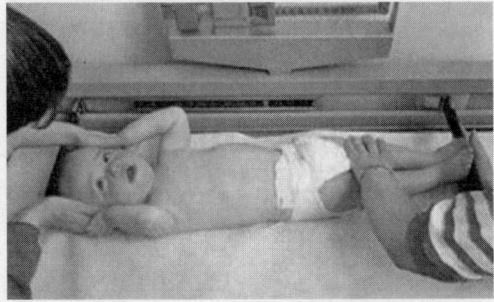

Fig. 2.9: Measuring length of an infant.

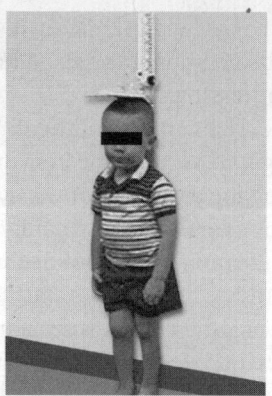

Fig. 2.10: Measuring height.

Formulas for calculating expected height
- 2–12 years (cm): Age (years) × 6 + 77
- 2–12 years (in.): Age (years) × 21/2 + 30

On an average, the ideal length of a full-term infant at birth is 50 cm. It rises to 60 cm at 3 months, 70 cm at 9 months, 75 cm at 1 year, 85 cm at 2 years, 95 cm at 3 years, and 100 cm at 4 years. Thereafter, the child gains little over 5 cm every year until the onset of puberty.

Weight for height
It is calculated by dividing actual weight by weight corresponding to the height and then multiplying the quotient by 100. A value below 90.5% indicates malnutrition and above 120% over weight/obesity.

$$\frac{\text{Actual weight}}{\text{Weight corresponding to height}} \times 100$$

Degree of Malnutrition

Formula for calculating degree of malnutrition

$$\frac{\text{Actual weight}}{\text{Expected weight}} \times 100$$

Classification of degree of malnutrition
There are different types of classifications used by the health-care personnel around the world to calculate degree of malnutrition. Commonly used classifications are as follows:

1. *IAP classification based on weight for age:*
   - 81–100%: Normal
   - 71–80%: Grade I
   - 61–70%: Grade II
   - 51–60%: Grade III
   - <50%: Grade IV

Note: The alphabet K is postfixed in presence of edema.

2. *WHO classification*:

Nutritional status	Body weight (percentage standard) for weight	Edema	Deficit in weight for height
Under weight	80–60	0	Minimal
Nutritional dwarfism	<60	0	Minimal
Marasmus	<60	0	++
Kwashiorkor	80–60	+/++	+/++
Marasmic kwashiorkor	<60	+	++

3. *Welcome trust classification*: It is based on deficit in body weight for age and presence or absence of edema.
   - 60–80% of expected weight for age with edema: Kwashiorkor
   - 60–80% without edema: Undernutrition
   - <60% without edema: Marasmus
   - <60% with edema: Marasmic kwashiorkor

4. *Waterlow classification*:
   a. Weight for height

Classification	Weight for height (percentage of expected)
Normal	>90
Mild wasting	80–90
Moderate wasting	70–79
Severe wasting	<70

b. Height for age

Classification	Height for age (percentage of expected)
Normal	>95
First-degree stunting	90–95
Second-degree stunting	85–89
Third-degree stunting	<85

Head Circumference

Head circumference or occipitofrontal circumference (OFC) is the maximum circumference of the head.

Indications
- For children up to 3 years of age and for any child with a head size that is in question.
- The OFC reflects intracranial volume pressure, which is a significant finding.

Factors affecting head circumference
- Brain development
- Intracranial pressure
- Hydrocephalus
- Brain tumor
- Some congenital defects, such as microcephaly

Equipment needed
- A flexible nonstretchable measuring tape
- Paper and pencil to record the measurement

Preparation
- Explain the procedure to the mother.
- Ask the mother to hold the baby or keep the baby in supine position on bed.

Procedure
- Wash hands.
- Clean the tape with alcoholic wipe (depending on hospital policy).
- The tape should be passed around the head, positioned just above the eyebrow ridges, above the ears, and around the occipital prominence at the back of the head.
- The tape should be pulled snugly to compress hair and the measurement recorded to the nearest 0.1 cm (**Fig. 2.11**).
- As equal to HC, shape of the head is important too.
  - A boat-shaped head suggests the scaphocephaly.
  - Asymmetrical: Plagiocephaly
  - Flattened occiput—may be a feature of Down's syndrome
  - Frontal and/or parietal bossing or box-like head is suggestive of rickets

Normal values
- At birth: 35 cm
- 3 months: 40 cm
- 6 months: 43 cm
- 1 year: 45 cm
- 2 years: 48 cm
- 7 years: 50 cm
- 12 years: 52 cm

Chest Circumference

Procedure
- For measuring chest circumference, place the tape at the level of the nipple in a plane at right angle to the spine (**Fig. 2.12**).
- Record the measurement in mid respiration.

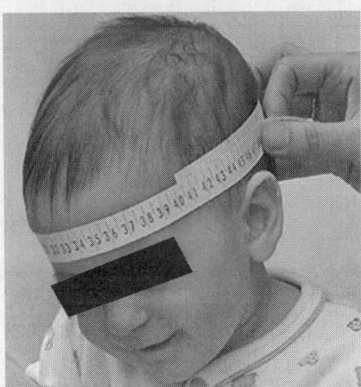

Fig. 2.11: Head circumference.

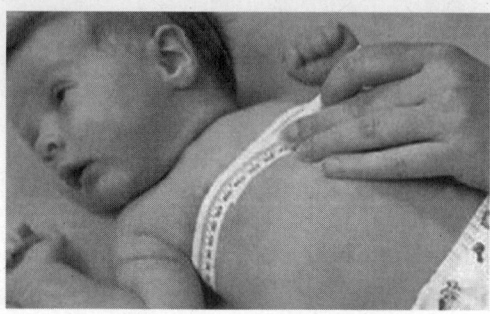

Fig. 2.12: Chest circumference.

General instructions
- As rapid head growth occurs during the first 2 years of life, HC should be measured monthly in infants who continue to be inpatients.
- Generally speaking, if brain does not develop normally, as in mental retardation, the head size is likely to be small. Occasionally, however, the small size of the head may be secondary to premature union of the skull structures, the so-called craniosynostosis or craniostenosis.
- Large head may be the result of hydrocephalus, rickets, chondrodystrophy or syphilis, or familial macrocephaly, which is harmless.

Head/chest circumference ratio
- At birth, HC is larger than chest circumference by about 2 cm.
- By 6–12 months, both are equal.
- After first year, chest circumference tends to increase by 2.5 cm.
- By the age of 5 years, it is more or less 5 cm greater in size than HC.

Mid-arm Circumference
Mid-arm circumference (MAC) is measured midway between the point of the shoulder (acromion) and olecranon process.

Procedure
- Let the arm hang naturally by the side of the body.
- Then place the tape firmly without compressing the tissues around the upper arm at a point midway between tip of the acromion process and olecranon process (**Fig. 2.13**).
- Read the measurement.

General instructions
- The maximum circumference of the upper arm measured when the arm is hanging by the side of the body.
- MAC is said to remain constant between 16.25 and 16.75 cm.
- Any child in this age-group with a circumference below 80% (about 12.5 cm) of the reference international standard is said to be considered suffering from malnutrition (**Table 2.8**).

Shakir's tape method
It is simple and age-independent tool for assessing malnutrition. This special tape has colored zones: red, yellow, and green, corresponding to the readings of MAC (**Table 2.9**).

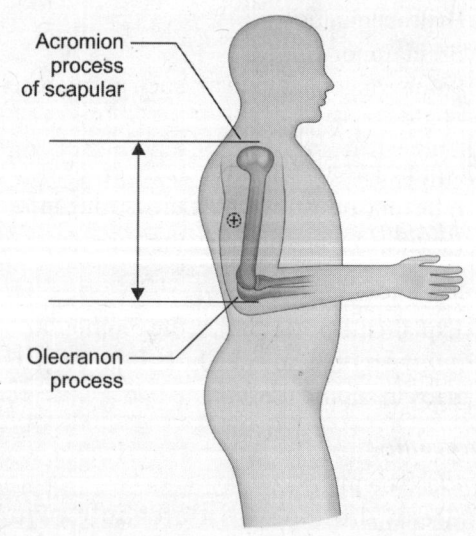

Fig. 2.13: Assessment of mid-arm circumference.

Table 2.8: Normal values.

Age	Mid-arm circumference (cm)	
	Male	Female
Birth	12.2	12.0
1 year	12.6	12.5
3 years	13.6	13.3
6 years	14.9	14.8
9 years	16.5	16.5
12 years	17.4	18.2
15 years	20.3	20.6

Table 2.9: Inference based on Shakir's tape method.

MAC (in cm)	Color of tape	Inference
>13.5	Green	Normal
12.5–13.5	Yellow	Borderline
<12.5	Red	Waste

(MAC: mid-arm circumference)

Bangle test

It is usually done in children below 5 years of age. The child's arm is inserted into a bangle with an inner diameter of 4 cm. If the bangle crosses the elbow, then we can consider that MAC is decreased. This test can be applied when there are no other resources available for measuring MAC. However, it is not an accurate test.

Skinfold Thickness

Of various skinfolds, triceps skinfold is the most popular.

Equipment needed

Lange's or Harpenden skinfold calipers.

Procedure for measuring triceps skinfold thickness

Hold a fold of skin between thumb and index finger and measure the midarm over triceps area on the left side (**Fig. 2.14**).

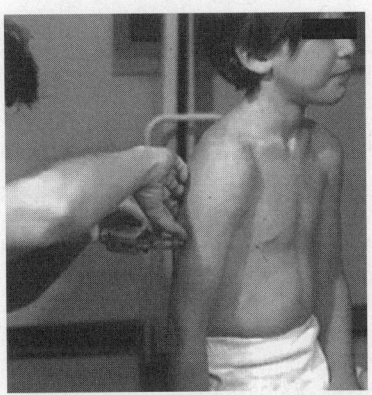

Fig. 2.14: Triceps skinfold thickness.

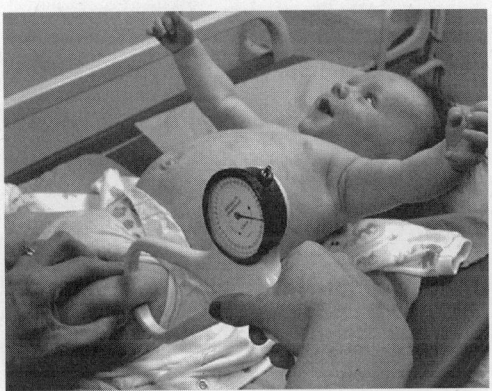

Fig. 2.15: Quadriceps skinfold thickness.

Quadriceps skinfold thickness

Hold the fold of skin in the midpoint of the anterior surface of the thigh, midway between patella and the inguinal fold (**Fig. 2.15**).

Highlights

- Anthropometry refers to study of measurement of human part, such as height, weight, head circumference (HC), chest circumference, and mid-arm circumference.
- Infants should ideally be weighed nude and weighed on baby scales until the age of 2 years.

- Children over 2 years should be weighed in light clothing without shoes on standing or sitting on scales.
- For any reasons clothing has not been removed or a child weighed with additional equipment, for example, splint and cast, this must be recorded in nurse's chart.
- When measuring height, the child should look straight ahead with the lower border of the bony orbit (eye sockets) and the auditory canal in the same horizontal line. This is called the "Frankfurt plane."
- HC or occipitofrontal circumference (OFC) is the maximum circumference of the head.
- Mid-arm circumference is measured midway between the point of the shoulder (acromion) and olecranon process.
- Abdominal girth is the measurement of the distance around the abdomen at a specific point.

ABDOMINAL GIRTH

Definition

Abdominal girth is the measurement of the distance around the abdomen at a specific point.

Indications

- Children who have the presence of or risk factors of abdominal distension, for example, cirrhosis of liver and nephrotic syndrome.
- To assess the general fat deposition as a gross measure of weight gain in obese children.

Equipment Needed

- Paper measuring tape marked in centimeters
- Ballpoint pen or marker
- Stethoscope

Preparation

- Explain the procedure to the child and the family, including the rationale for performing the procedure and frequency.
- Explain to the child that small pen marks will be made on the abdomen.
- Assure the child that these marks are not permanent and will wash off.
- If age appropriate, allow the child to look at and touch the measuring tape to be used.
- Let the child measure the examiner's wrist or other object. Give the child time to ask questions immediately before the procedure.

Procedure

- Determine previous abdominal measurements.
- Wash hands.
- Auscultate bowel sounds with stethoscope before measuring the abdominal girth.
- The preferred position is supine with child's knees flexed or for an infant, hold legs flexed at the knees and hips.
- Remove or move aside clothing that interferes with the ability to apply the measuring tape around the abdomen.
- Do not measure over the clothing.
- Visualize the child's abdomen to evaluate for symmetry contour, peristalsis, and abnormalities, such as distension or a mass.
- Place the palm under child's waist and slide tape through under your own hand.
- If serial measurements are to be made, mark the exact area on either side of umbilicus of top edge and bottom edge of tape with a pen marker.
- Place the tape snugly across the umbilicus but not clinching the waist line.
- Ensure that the measuring tape is placed underneath the child lying flat for an accurate measurement.
- Measure the recording nearest full millimeter level (**Fig. 2.16**).

Chapter 2: Assessment Procedures

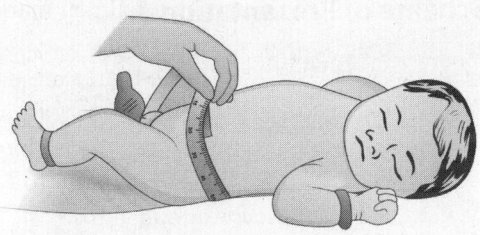

Fig. 2.16: Measuring abdominal girth.

Postprocedure Care

- Evaluate previous assessments and note any changes in abdomen, including girth, firmness, color, and bowel sounds.
- Record abdominal girth, date and time of measurement, and factors pertinent to abdominal assessment.
- Document any abdominal pain reported by child or assessed during girth measurement.
- Inform physician or nurse practitioner of any significant changes.

General Instructions

- Measure girth with the child in the same position each time.
- If serial measurements are to be made, mark exact area on either side of umbilicus of top edge and bottom edge of tape with a pen marker.
- Measure girth directly above the umbilicus in infants with umbilical arterial or venous catheters.
- If serial measurements are to be completed and the child is uncomfortable with movement, the tape may be left in place under the child for the next measurement.
- Ensure that the tape is lying flat under the child.
- If the child wears diapers, check the tape for soiling by urine or stool at every diaper change.

PHYSICAL EXAMINATION

Definition

Physical examination is a thorough inspection or a detailed study of the entire body or some part of the body to determine the general physical or mental conditions of the body.

Equipment Needed

A clean tray containing:
- Pediatric stethoscope
- Pen light
- Percussion hammer
- Tape measure
- Weighing machine
- Spatula
- Stadiometer
- Laryngoscope
- Tuning fork
- Wrist watch
- Pair of gloves
- Otoscope
- Nasal speculum
- Tongue depressor
- Ophthalmoscope
- Vital signs tray
- Cotton balls in a bowl
- Play materials
- Development assessment tools

Setting

The setting for doing physical examination should be:
- Well-lighted, warm, colorful, and comfortable room.
- Warm hands.
- Toys, pictures, and cartoons should be kept to allay apprehension of the child.
- Avoid deep yellow/blue curtains for proper evaluation of jaundice and cyanosis.

Approach

- The approach of the nurse should be gentleness, confidence, sympathy, patience, tact, compassion concern, kind look, and love for children.
- Sneaky observation of the child, offering small bright object or candy.
- Approach the child with a smile.
- Adopt a play attitude and follow an unstructured approach.
- The undressing of the child should be limited.
- Relatively traumatic examinations, such as percussion throat examination should be done in the end.
- The older child may be explained about the procedure.

Positions

Positioning during physical assessment is based on the age of child if:
- 0–3 months of age: Examination table
- 3 months to 1 year of age: Mother's lap
- 1–3 years of age: Standing or mother's lap
- >3 years old: Examination table

Sequence of Examination

- The examination pattern should be unstructured.
- Auscultation may be done in the beginning in an infant suspected to have cardiac problems because conventional sequence would lead to crying.
- This should be followed by inspection, palpation, percussion, recording of vital signs, elicitation of deep tendon reflexes, ear, nose and throat (ENT) examination, and examination of the painful site should be done last.

Scheme of Presentation

Body part	Presentation
General appearance	Attitude, posture, appearance, cry, comfortable, gravely sick, toxic, restless, dyspneic, orthopneic, level of consciousness, evidence of meningeal irritation
Body build—nutrition	Body frame, muscle mass, subcutaneous fat, anemia, cyanosis, jaundice, edema and lymphadenopathy
Anthropometry	Weight, height (or length <2 years), mid-arm circumference, upper segment to lower segment body ratio and degree of malnutrition
Vital signs	Temperature, pulse, respiration, blood pressure
Spine	Spinal deformity, kyphosis, lordosis, scoliosis, swelling, tenderness, and range of movements
Head and face	Head size, shape, bossing, fontanels, sutures, Macewen's sign, characteristic facies, facial dysmorphism, and abnormalities in the eyes, ears, nose, mouth, chin, etc.
ENT	Orodental hygiene, teeth, gums, tongue, tonsils, buccal mucosa, examination of ears, nose, and throat
Eyes	Ptosis, corneal opacity, bitot spots, cataract, glaucoma, white reflex, strabismus, and fundus examination
Neck	Hairline, webbing, IVP, arterial and venous pulsations, thyroid gland, trachea, cysts, fistulae, lymph glands, etc.
Skin and appendages	
Nails	Clubbing, flattening or koilonychias, color, translucent bands, splinter hemorrhages

Contd...

Contd...

Body part	Presentation
Skin	Color, texture, turgor and elasticity, skin rash, nodules, purpura, ecchymoses, pigmentation, pyoderma, eczema, neuroectodermal dysplasia, nevi, xanthoma, spider angioma, and palmar erythema
Hair	Distribution, color, texture, brittleness, eyebrows, eyelashes, hirsutism
Evidence of deficiency states	Evidences of dehydration, PEM, deficiencies of vitamins, minerals and trace elements
Bones and joints	Deformities of long bones, thorax, spine, hands and feet, evidences of arthritis, bony tenderness, rickets, etc.
Genitals and sexual maturity stages	Are genitals normal or ambiguous Sexual maturity stage: Normal, retarded, or advanced (precocious)
Developmental examination	Is development normal? Globally retarded or retarded in a specific field, developmental age and developmental quotient

(PEM: protein energy malnutrition; IVP: intravenous pyelogram; ENT: ear, nose and throat)

General Appearance

It is a cumulative, subjective impression of the child's physical appearance, state of nutrition, behavior, personality, interactions with parents and nurse, posture, development, and speech.

- Note the facies (facial expression and appearance) for pain, happy, discontented, frightened, mentally deficient, or acutely ill.
- Observe the posture and position and types of body movements. For example, the child with hearing or vision loss may characteristically tilt the head in an awkward position to hear or see better. Low self-esteem child may assume a slumped, carelessness, and apathetic pose.
- Note the child's hygiene in terms of cleanliness, unusual body odor, the condition of hair, nails, teeth, and feet and clothing.
- Nutritional status or body built should be observed, for example, slender and tall, well-built, well-defined musculature, poor muscle tone, and bony prominence.
- Assess for the child's behavior, such as child's personality, activity level, and reaction to stress, requests, frustration, interaction with others, degree of alertness, and response to stimuli. Note the attention span, eye contact, reaction to nurse/family members.
- Record an overall estimate of child's speech, development, motor skills, coordination, and recent area of achievement. For example, for 18-month-old child, motor development advanced for age; climbs, runs, jumps, and manipulates small objects with ease, beginning to name many objects; uses two-word phrases and enjoys talking to self and others.

Skin

Assess for color, texture, temperature, moisture, and turgor.

Methods involved: inspection and palpation.

Inspection

- Normal color of skin
  - White race: Light skinned vary from milky white and rose to a deeply hued pink.
  - Dark-skinned children: Various brown, red, yellow, olive green, and bluish tones in their skin; have hyperpigmented areolas, genitals, and linea nigra.
  - Asians: Yellow tone (wheatish).
  - Assess for any abnormal coloration of skin (**Table 2.10**).
- Inspect the entire body for nevi and vascular and other lesions. Note their location, size, distribution, characteristics, and color (**Table 2.11**).
- Note the presence of hyperpigmented nevi (Mongolian spots), which appears as blue

Table 2.10: Variation in color and their causes.

Sl. no.	Variations in color and their causes	Appearance in light skin	Appearance in dark skin
1.	Cyanosis: Bluish discoloration, reflects hypoxia	Bluish tinge, especially in peripheral conjunctiva, nail beds, earlobes, lips, oral membranes, soles and palms	Ashen gray lips and tongue
2.	Pallor: Paleness/decreased pinkness due to anemia, shock, fever or syncope	Loss of rosy glow in skin, especially face	Ashen gray appearance, in black skin. More yellowish brown in brown skin
3.	Erythema: Redness due to increased blood flow, exposure to cold, localized infection, hyperthermia, allergy, increased number of red blood cells (RBCs)	Redness easily seen anywhere on body	Much more difficult to assess, rely on palpation for warmth or edema
4.	Ecchymoses: Large diffuse area usually black and blue caused by hemorrhage of blood into the skin	Purplish to yellow green areas; may be seen anywhere on skin	Very difficult to see, unless in mouth or conjunctiva
5.	Small size (ecchymoses); distinct, pinpoint hemorrhages 2 mm or less in size; can denote some type of blood disorders	Purplish pinpoint mass easily seen on buttocks, abdomen, and inner surface of arms or legs	Usually invisible except in oral mucosa and conjunctiva
6.	Jaundice: Yellowish discoloration of skin caused by bile pigments	Yellowish staining seen on eyes, skin, finger nails, soles, palms, and oral mucosa	Most reliably assessed in sclera, hard palate, palms, and soles
7.	Lack of color in skin hair and eyes is related to albinism	–	–

Table 2.11: Vascular lesions and their significance.

Sl. no.	Description	Significance
1.	Salmon nevi: Light pink macules usually on eyelids, nasal bridge, back of neck (stork bite)	Usually fade over time, but may never go away completely. No complications
2.	Strawberry nevus: Raised reddish papule made of blood vessels (hemangiomas)	Present at or develop after birth; recede over time, usually by age of 9 years. No complications

Contd...

Contd...

Sl. no.	Description	Significance
3.	Nevus flammeus: Dark purple red flat patches grow with the child (port-wine stain)	May be associated with Sturge–Weber's syndrome. May be disfiguring; may be removed with laser therapy
4.	Purpura: Larger purple macules	Bleeding under the skin, occur with bleeding disorders, meningococcemia
5.	Ecchymoses	Injury
6.	Petechiae	Bleeding disorders, meningococcemia

or gray, variably and irregularly shaped macules.
- Inspect for rashes and note the types of lesions, distribution, drying, scabbing, and any drainage.
- In adolescents the skin examination may reveal open or closed comedones (pimples or blackheads) across the face, chest, and back. Teens may sport tattoos, brandings, or various body piercings; inspect these areas for signs of infection.
• Document the presence of any lacerations, abrasions, or burns. Note the distribution of injury and whether it seems consistent with the mechanism described in the health history.

Palpation
• Palpate the skin for temperature, moisture, texture, turgor, and edema. Use back of your hand to assess the skin's temperature, comparing the right side of the body to left and upper to lower. Note any difference in temperature.
• Determine the tissue turgor or elasticity in the skin, by grasping the skin on the abdomen between the thumb and index finger, pulling it taut, and quickly releasing it. Elastic tissue immediately assumes its normal position without residual marks or creases. In case of poor skin turgor, it remains suspended or tented for a few seconds before slowly falling back on the abdomen.
• When edema is present, palpate the area to determine its extent.
• Palpate for any lumps or protrusions to determine the size, firmness, or tenderness.

Accessory structures
• Inspect the hair for color, texture, quality, distribution, and elasticity.
  - Normal: Lustrous, silky, strong, and elastic hair
  - Poor nutrition: Stringy, dull, brittle, dry, friable, and depigmented
• Record any bald or thinning spots.
• Inspect the hair and nails for general cleanliness. Also examine for lesions, scaliness, and evidence of infestations, such as lice or ticks, signs of trauma, for example, scars and mass.
• In adolescents and preadolescents, look for growth of secondary hair.
• Inspect the nails for color, shape, texture, and quality. Normally the nails are pink, convex, smooth, and hard but flexible. The edges are usually white and extend over the fingers.
• Creases: The palms normally show three flexion creases. In some situations, such as Down's syndrome, the two distal horizontal creases are fused to form a single horizontal crease (transpalmar crease).

Head

Inspection
• Examine the head and face for shape and symmetry.
  - Some infants have a slight flattening of the back of the head since the recommended sleeping pattern is supine.

- Observe the infant's head shape by looking down on it from above. Observe whether the head appears centered on the neck or tilts to one side.
  - Pull the infant from supine position into sitting to determine the extent of head lag.
  - To determine in older infants and children, ask the child to turn the head in different directions, either by simple commands or by following a colorful objects.
- Observe the infant's face when crying, smiling, or babbling for symmetry of muscle movement.
  - In older children, ask to puff out their cheeks, make kisses, look surprised, and stick out their tongue.

Palpation

- Palpate the skull for patent sutures, fontanels, fractures, and swellings.
  - Normally the posterior fontanel closes by 6–8 weeks and anterior fontanel closes by 18 months. The fontanel should be neither depressed nor taut and bulging, though it is not uncommon to see it pulsate or briefly bulge if the baby cries.
  - Dehydration can cause the fontanel to be shrunken; increased intracranial pressure and overhydration can cause them to bulge.
- Palpate the sutures for overriding or open and lumps or other deformities.
- Use the fingertips to palpate for occipital, postauricular, preauricular, submental, and submandibular lymph nodes, noting their size, mobility, and consistency.

Neck

Inspection

Inspect for symmetry. The infant's neck is short; by 4 years of age the child's neck should be similar to adult size. Webbing or excessive neck skinfold may be associated with Turner's syndrome, and lax neck skin may occur in Down's syndrome.

Manipulation

Assess the flexibility through full range of motion.
- Pain or resistance to range of motion may indicate meningeal irritation.
- Do not assess neck mobility in trauma victim.

Palpation

- Palpate the cervical and clavicular lymph nodes with the distal part of the fingers using gentle but firm pressure in a circular motion. Tilt the head slightly upward to allow better access.
- Assess for swelling, mobility, temperature, and tenderness.
- Enlarged cervical lymph nodes frequently occur in association with upper respiratory tract infection (URTI)
- and otitis media.
- Palpate the trachea; the thyroid is usually palpable only in older children.

Eyes

External structures

Inspection
- Inspect the lids for proper placement on the eye. When the eye is open, the upper lid should fall near the upper iris. When the eyes are closed, the lids should completely cover the cornea and sclera.
- Observe the eyes for symmetry and spacing, even distribution of eyelashes and eyelids, and presence of epicanthal folds.
- Note the child's ability to blink.
- The eyes should look symmetrical and both should be facing forward in the midline when the child is looking directly ahead.
- The iris should be perfectly round and sclera should be clear. Tiny black marks in the sclera of highly pigmented people are normal.

- The cornea should be uniformly transparent.
- Inspect the inner and outer canthus and conjunctiva for inflammation, discharge, or swelling.
- Using a small pen light, inspect the function and clarity of the pupil by putting your nondominant hand on the child's forehead and moving the light toward and away from each eye. This will elicit the blink reflex. Next observe whether the pupil contracts with the light and expands when the light is removed. Make the same motion with a small toy or object and direct the child to look at it. The eyes demonstrate accommodation, or focusing at different distances, if the pupil constricts as the object moves closer. Normal findings on examination of the pupils may be recorded as PERRLA, which stands for pupils are equal, round, and reactive to light and accommodation.
  - Absence of pupillary reflexive action after age of 3 weeks may indicate blindness.
  - Intermittent strabismus (crossing of the eyes) is normal up to 6 months. Persistent strabismus at any age or intermittent strabismus after 6 months of age should be evaluated by a pediatric ophthalmologist.
  - Normal color of iris is usually established by 6 months.
- Assess eye muscle strength using two tests:
  1. *Hirschberg test*: Bring the pen light to the middle of your face and direct the child to look at it. The small dot of the reflected light seen in the iris should be symmetrically placed in each eye.
  2. *Cover test*: Cover one of the child's eyes and instruct to focus on an interesting object. The eye should not waver. While the child is still focusing with the first eye, remove the cover from the second. Observe the uncovered eye for movement. Report any movement or drift.
- To test peripheral vision, have the child focus on a specific point or object directly in front. Bring a finger or small object from beyond the range of vision into the area of the peripheral vision. When the child sees the object from the side, while still focusing on the object or point in front, the child should say "stop."

Internal structure
- Use ophthalmoscope to inspect the internal eye structures. Observe the glow of the pupil, which appears red (creamy colored in children with very dark eye color). Inspect the optic disk, macula, fovea, and blood vessels.
  - Absence of red reflex may indicate the presence of cataracts.
- Assessment of the internal structures of the eye is best accomplished by an advanced practitioner with experience in this type of assessment.

Testing visual acuity
- The child should stand 10 ft from chart with their heels at the 10-ft line. Test the right eye first by covering the left. Children who wear glasses should be screened with them on. Tell the child to keep both eyes open during examination. Use Snellen's chart for testing. If the child fails to read the current line, move up to the chart until a line is found that the child can pass. Then begin moving down the chart until the child fails to read. To pass the child should correctly identify 4–6 symbols on the line. Repeat the procedure covering the right eye.
- For children unable to read the letters and numbers use tumbling E or HOTV tests (preschool children).
  1. *Tumbling E:* The capital letter E pointing in four directions **(Fig. 2.17)**.

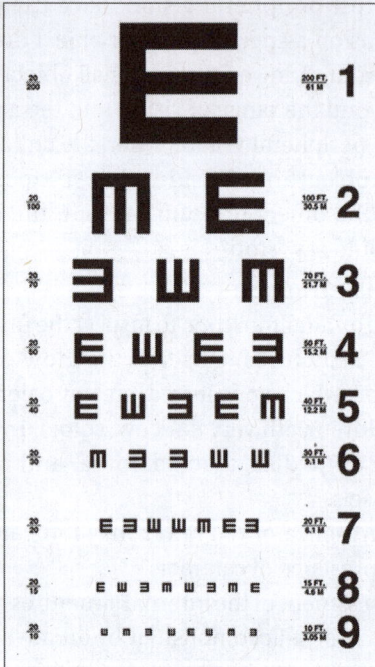

Fig. 2.17: Tumbling E chart.

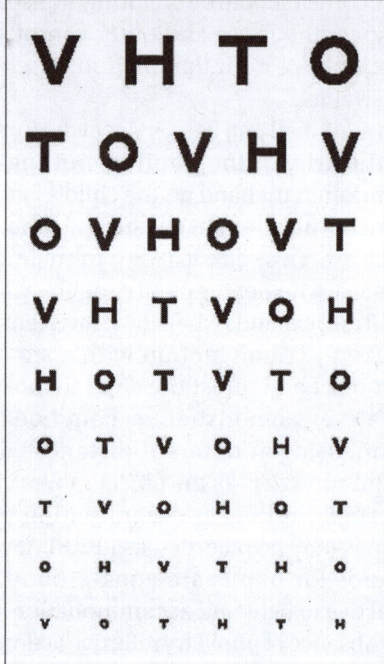

Fig. 2.18: HOTV chart.

2. *HOTV chart*: It consists of a wall chart composed of letters H, O, T, and V (**Fig. 2.18**). The child is given a board containing a large H, O, and T. The examiners point to a letter on the wall chart and the child matches the correct letter on the board held in his hand.

3. *Allen card test*: It uses common figures to test the child's vision. The examiners walk slowly flipping through the cards and presenting different pictures as the child correctly calls out. When the child misses the figure, the examiner moves forward to confirm that the child is able to identify at that point (**Fig. 2.19**). The figures in the card should be 20/30 in size.

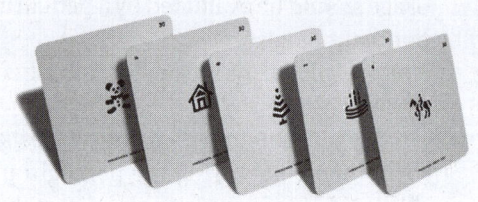

Fig. 2.19: Allen cards.

4. *LH symbol or Lea cards*: It is a spiral bound set of flash cards. It contains large pictures of a house, apple, circle, and square. It contains the symbol size and visual acuity value for a 10-ft testing distance (**Fig. 2.20**).

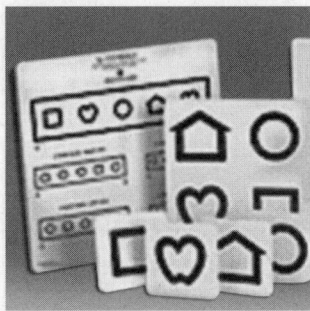

Fig. 2.20: LH symbol cards.

In infants
- Checking for light perception by shining a light into the eyes and noting responses, such as pupillary constriction and blinking.
- Another test is to fix on and follow a target. Hold the infant upright while moving your face slowly from side to side.

Color vision

The tests available for color vision include the Ishihara test and the Hardy–Rand–Ritter test. Each consists of cards on which is printed a color field composed of spots of a certain confusion color. Against the field are a number of symbols similarly printed in dots but of a color likely to be confused with field color by the person with color vision impairment. As a result, the figure or letter is invisible to an affected individual but is clearly seen by a person with normal vision.

Ears

External structures
- Assess the placement of the external ears on the head. They should be symmetrical and placed no lower than the eyes. The pinna should deviate not >10° from an imaginary line that is perpendicular to a line drawn between the outer canthus of the eye and the top of the ear.
- Low-set ears may be associated with genetic abnormalities or syndrome. Note the protrusion or flattening of the ears, note the presence of pits or skin tags in the periauricular area. Observe the exterior ear canal.
- A waxy cerumen that is soft and an orangish brown color is normally found lubricating and protecting the external ear canal and should be left in place or washed gently away. Note for any drainage, pull on the auricle and palpate the mastoid process, neither of which should result in pain in healthy child.

Internal ear
- Position the child, restrain if necessary. Gently pull down on the earlobe of the infant and up on the outer edge of the pinna in older children to straighten the ear canal. Insert the appropriate-size speculum into the ear canal to visualize the canal and tympanic membrane. It should be pink, have tiny hairs, and free from scratches, drainage, foreign bodies, and edema.
- The tympanic membrane should appear pearly pink or gray and should be translucent, allowing visualization of the bony land marks. Compress the pneumatic insufflatory bulb to provide a puff of air, this causes motion of the tympanic membrane, tympanic membrane immobility, holes or perforation and the presence of tympanostomy tubes, scaring or vesicles should be assessed.
- Hearing acuity of the older children can be assessed by tuning fork test to find out the type of hearing loss (**Table 2.12**).

Nose

External structure

Compare the placement and alignment by drawing an imaginary vertical line from center point between the eyes down to the notch of the upper lip. The nose should lie exactly

Table 2.12: Tuning fork test for assessing hearing acuity.

Condition	Rinne's test	Weber's test
Normal	Air conduction is better than bone conduction	Vibrations heard similarly on both sides
Sensorineural hearing loss	Both air conduction and bone conduction are decreased	Vibration heard better on normal side
Conduction hearing loss	Bone conduction is better than air conduction	Vibration is better on affected side

symmetric. Note for any deviation to one side, and asymmetry in size. Observe the alae nasi for any sign of flaring, which indicates respiratory difficulty.

Internal structures

Inspect the anterior vestibule by pushing the tip upward, tilting the head backward with the help of flashlight. Note the color of mucosal lining (red), swelling, discharge, dryness, or bleeding. Inspect the septum, which divides the vestibules equally. Note any deviation. Test the older child's sense of smell by having the child close the eyes and identify a familiar scent such as peppermint or coffee. Palpate the sinuses for tenderness.

Mouth and Throat

Lips: It should be moist, soft, smooth, and pink, symmetric when relaxed or tensed.

Oral cavity: Ask the child to open the mouth wide; to move the tongue in different directions for full visualization, and to say "ahh," which depresses the tongue for full view of the back of the mouth (tonsils, uvula, and oropharynx). The oral cavity should be pink, moist, and healthy. Observe the movement of tongue when the child cries, or babbles. Ask the older child to touch the tongue to roof of the mouth and then stick out the tongue and move it from side to side.

Teeth: Inspect for number in each dental arch, for hygiene and for occlusion or bite. Inspect for plaque, dental caries, and fluorosis.

Gum: Inspect for color, bleeding.

Palate: The arch should be dome shaped. Inspect for intactness. A narrow, flat roof or a high, arched palate affects the placement of the tongue and can cause feeding and speech problems.

Chest

Inspection

- Observe for size, shape, symmetry, movement, breast development, and the bony landmarks formed by the ribs and sternum.
  - *Size:* Measure the size by using measuring tape at the level of nipples.
  - *Shape:* Circular during infancy. As the child grows the anteroposterior diameter to be less than the lateral diameter.
  - *Movement:* Bilaterally symmetrical and coordinated with breathing. During inspiration, the chest rises and expands, the diaphragm descents and the costal angle increases. During expiration, the chest falls and decreases in size, the diaphragm rises and the costal angle narrows.
  - *In younger children:* Respiration is principally diaphragmatic or abdominal.
  - *In older children:* Respiration is chiefly thoracic.
- Observe the position of the nipples (slightly lateral to the midclavicular line between the 4th and 5th ribs).
- Record early or late breast development. In adolescent girls, palpate the breast for evidence of any masses or hard nodules.

Lungs

Inspection: Observe for respiratory movements; evaluate respiratory rate, rhythm, depth, and quality.

Palpation: Evaluate respiratory movements by placing each hand flat against the back or chest with thumbs in midline along the lower costal margin of the lungs. During respiration, your hands will move with the chest wall. Palpate for the presence of tactile fremitus with palms or fingertips while the infant is crying or the older child says "99."

Percussion: The anterior lung is percussed from apex to base, usually with the child in the supine or sitting position. Each side is percussed in sequence to compare the sounds. Note the resonance over lung fields. Hyperresonance may be present in conditions such as asthma.

Auscultation: Use pediatric stethoscope for auscultating infant or child. Place the infant in a sitting position or propping in a parent's lap. Breath sounds will be loud, clear with adequate aeration throughout all lung fields.

Compare findings of right and left side. Note the adventitious breath sounds, such as wheezes or crackles, document their locations and whether they are present on inspiration or expiration or both.

Classification of breath sounds

1. *Vesicular:* Entire surface except upper intrascapular area and beneath manubrium. Inspiration is louder, longer, and higher pitched than expiration. Sound is soft, swishing noise.
2. *Bronchovesicular:* Heard over manubrium and in upper intrascapular regions when trachea and bronchi bifurcate. Inspiration is higher pitched.
3. *Bronchial:* Heard only over trachea near suprasternal notch. Inspiratory phase is short, whereas expiratory phase is long.

Heart

Inspection: Note the presence of pallor, cyanosis, mottling, or edema, which may indicate a cardiovascular problem.
- Inspect the anterior chest wall from an angle comparing both sides of the rib cage with each other.
- Observe for the apical impulse. Note clubbing of the fingertips, distension of neck veins.

Palpation: Using fingertips palpate the chest for lifts and heaves or thrills, which are not normal. Palpate for apical pulse.
- Check the pulses and compare the upper body to lower part, as well as left versus right, noting strength and quality. Note the warmth of the distal extremities.
- Assess capillary filling time, by pressing the skin lightly on a central site, such as forehead or a peripheral site, such as nail beds and quickly release it. The time it takes for blanched area to return to its original color is the capillary refill time (normal <3 seconds).

Auscultation

Auscultate the heart sound with at least two positions: sitting and reclining. Auscultate the heart rate in the area of PMI. Develop a systematic approach to auscultation of the heart.

- Listen over all four valvular areas anteriorly. Note S1, S2, extra heart sounds, or murmurs.
- S1 is usually loudest at the mitral and tricuspid areas and increases in intensity with fever, exercise, and anemia.
- S2 is usually intense at aortic and pulmonic areas.
- S3 may be heard in some healthy children and is normal.
- S4 is usually considered abnormal and occurs with cardiac disease.
- Auscultate for murmurs, note the location and timing. Systolic murmur occurs in association with S1, a diastolic murmur in

association with S2. Sinus arrhythmia is a common and normal finding in children and adolescents.

Abdomen

Inspection

- Inspect for size, shape, and symmetry.
- Normally, in infant and toddler the abdomen is rounded and protruded due to immature musculature.
- The skin should be uniformly taut without wrinkles or creases.
- Superficial veins are usually visible in light skinned, thin infants but distended veins are abnormal finding.
- Examine the umbilicus for size, hygiene, and evidence of any abnormalities, such as hernias. Observe the movement of the abdomen and peristaltic waves.

Auscultation

- Listen for bowel sounds, such as metallic clicks and gurgles.
- Their frequency per minute should be recorded (e.g., 5 sounds/min). It may be stimulated by stroking the abdominal surface with a finger nail.
- Report absence of bowel sounds or hyperperistalsis.

Palpation

- *Superficial:* Lightly place your hand against the skin and feel each quadrant, noting any areas of tenderness, muscle tone, and superficial lesions, such as cysts.
- *Deep:* It is used for palpating organs and large blood vessels and for detecting masses and tenderness that were not discovered during superficial palpation. Place one hand on top of the other and palpate from the lower quadrants to the upper. The edge of the liver may be felt at the right costal margin. The descending colon may be felt in the left lower quadrant as a small column and the bladder as a soft balloon below the umbilicus. The kidneys are rarely palpable. The abdomen should be soft and nontender. Palpate the inguinal area, the costal margins, and tympany over the remainder of the abdomen. A full bladder may yield dullness to percussion.

Genitalia and Anus

- Provide privacy; keep the child covered as much as possible.
- In adolescents, it should be examined at last.

Male

- Inspect the penis and scrotum for size, color, skin integrity, and obvious masses.
- Note the external appearance of the glans and shaft of the penis, the prepuce and the urethral meatus. Examine for signs of swelling, skin lesions, inflammation, etc.
- The urethral meatus is carefully examined for location and evidence of discharge.
- Hair distribution is also noted.
- Note the location and size of the scrotum. It should hang freely from the perineum behind the penis, and the left scrotum normally hangs lower than the right. The skin is loose and highly rugated. In adolescents, it will be deeply pigmented.
- Palpate for identification of the testes, epididymis, and inguinal hernia. The testes are felt as small, ovoid bodies about 1.5- to 2-cm long.
- Prevent cremasteric reflex by warming hands.

Female genitalia

- Examine for size and location of the structures of the vulva. Determine the presence and distribution of pubic hair.
- Inspect the labia majora and minora for size, color, and skin integrity. Redness or swelling may occur with infection, sexual abuse, or

masturbation. Lesions indicate sexually transmitted diseases (STDs)
- Gently spread the labia to inspect the clitoris, urethral meatus, and vaginal opening for edema or redness.
- Observe for any vaginal discharge. A small amount of clear mucus-like discharge is normal. Palpate the Bartholin glands and ducts for cysts.

Anus
- Inspect for fissures, rash, hemorrhoids, prolapse, or skin tags. It should appear moist and hairless.
- Gently stroke the anal area to elicit anal reflex. Inspect anal sphincter tone by inserting a gloved finger lubricated with water-soluble jelly just inside the anal sphincter. Note the general firmness of the buttocks and symmetry of the gluteal folds.

Back
- Note the general curvature of the spine in resting posture. The spine should be flexible, with good muscle tone and no rigidity.
- Assess the back and hip and shoulder height for symmetry. Examine the preadolescent and adolescent for development of scoliosis.
- Note mobility of the vertebral column by having child bend forward and side to side. Inspect for discoloration, tufts of hair, or dimples. Movement of cervical spine should be effortless.

Extremities
- Inspect each extremity for symmetry of length and size; refer any deviation for orthopedic evaluation.
- Count the fingers and toes to notice polydactyl (extra digit) or syndactyly (fusion of digits).
- Inspect for temperature and color.
- Assess the shape of bones. The infant's feet and legs appear bowed and secondary to in utero positioning but can be straightened through passive exercise. Bowing of legs is common in toddler. When it persists past the time, it is termed genu varum (bow legs).
- Genu valgum (knock knees) is usually present until the child is 7 years old.
- Observe the child walking, noting any difficulty with leg position or balance.
- Note the normal flat foot in the toddler and young child. The arch develops as the child grows and the muscles become less lax.
- Check the mobility of the joints by performing range of motion. Determine the upper extremity strength by having the child push up or down against the examiner's outstretched hand and lower extremity by having the child push against the examiner's hands with the soles of the forefoot.
- Inability to straighten the foot to midline may indicate club foot.
- Palpate the joints for heat, tenderness, and swelling.

Highlights ●●●●

- Physical examination is a thorough inspection or a detailed study of the entire body or some part of the body to determine the general physical or mental conditions of the body.
- The setting for doing physical examination should be well-lighted, warm, colorful, and comfortable room.
- Auscultation may be done in the beginning in an infant suspected to have cardiac problems because conventional sequence would lead to crying.
- This should be followed by inspection, palpation, percussion, recording of vital signs, and elicitation of deep tendon reflexes.
- ENT examination and examination of the painful site should be done last.
- General appearance is a cumulative, subjective impression of the child's physical appearance, state of nutrition, behavior, personality, interactions with parents and nurse, posture, development, and speech.

DEVELOPMENTAL ASSESSMENT

Principles
- *Systematic approach:* Complete each area of development at a time.
- *Simple language:* Use simple and clear language that can be understandable by the child.
- *A fun activity:* Make assessment as a fun giving and motivating activity.
- *Quality of skill:* The assessment should focus on how best the child can perform the activity for a particular age, not just able to do or not.
- *Assistance:* Developmental skills can be observed directly or can take assistance from the caregivers.

General Guidelines for Developmental Assessment
- *Easy to difficult:* Start from the activity that the child can do with less effort.
- *Progression:* Workup gradually until the child can no longer perform the task.
- *Gross motor at end:* Always try to assess the gross motor milestones at the last; otherwise child may not cooperate.
- *Positioning:* Keep the child in optimal position to enhance cooperation during assessment. Children <2 years can be kept on caregiver's lap, for 2–3 years old we can use small chairs and table/cot/floor for older children.

Types of Developmental Assessment
1. *Formal assessment:* It is carried out by trained personnel using age-specific standardized development assessment tools.
2. *Informal assessment:* It is carried out by health-care personnel (doctors and nurses) and students by comparing book picture with patient picture.

Methods
1. Gesell development evaluation—for gross motor, fine motor, social, adaptive, and language behavior
2. Amiel-Tison method—muscle tone, neuro and sensory responses, and neurobehavioral assessment
3. Vinel and Ravel's social maturity scale social and adaptive mental development
4. Bayley Scales of infant development (motor and mental)
5. Brazelton neonatal behavioral scales
6. Vojta technique—postural reactions and central coordination
7. Binet–Kamath and Weshler Intelligence Scale
8. Denver Developmental Screening Test (DDST)

In the Community Setup
1. Baroda Developmental Screening Test (BDST)
2. Trivandrum Developmental Screening Chart (TDSC)
3. Word side screening system (WSST)
4. Draw a Man Test (for preschool children)

Equipment Needed
A clean tray containing:
- Torch
- Red ring of 6.5-cm diameter
- Red ball of 5.0 cm
- Ten 2–5-cm-sized colorful cubes
- Jingle bell
- Rattle
- Cup with a handle
- Bunch of keys
- Pellets or beads
- Picture books

- Paper and crayons
- Percussion hammer

Indications

- Follow-up of high-risk neonates for early detection of cerebral palsy and mental retardation
- Complete evaluation of children with developmental, chromosomal, and neurological disorders
- To differentiate children with retardation in specific fields of development

Developmental History

Accurate history of developmental milestones is often difficult to obtain due to poor observation and educational status of the mother.

The milestones should be asked in chronological order in a simple and lucid manner.

- Ask the mother how the development of the index child (sick child) when compared to his siblings.
- Ask whether the child interacts and plays with other children of his age or likes the company of younger children.
- The effort should be made to identify whether the child is fully retarded or backward (delayed) only in an individual or specific field, for example, delayed speech in deaf child and delayed walking in a child with congenital dislocation of hip.
- In older children, consider the school performance, proficiency in games, motor dexterity, and social behavior.

Developmental Milestones

The child is placed in different postures and positions depending upon his chronological age and assessed for developmental responses. *Note:* In preterm babies, corrected age (conception age) should be used as the chronological age.

Ventral Suspension

Suspend the infant in a prone position by supporting the abdomen of the baby on his palm. The extension of neck and flexion of the extremities observed.

Age	Response
Newborn	Head hangs completely and back is rounded
4 weeks	Head momentarily lifted up, elbows flexed
6 weeks	Head held momentarily in the same plane as rest of the body
8 weeks	Head maintained in the same plane and momentarily lifted beyond this
12 weeks	Head maintained well beyond the plane of the rest of the body

Prone Position

The infant is placed on the examination table in a prone position and watched for the position of head, arms, pelvis, and legs.

Age	Response
Newborn	Head is kept to one side, pelvis raised; knees are drawn up under the abdomen
4–6 weeks	Hips and knees are partially extended, can lift chin off the couch momentarily
8 weeks	Head maintained in the midline with chin lifted off the couch
12 weeks	Pelvis kept flat on the couch, arms are stretched out in full extension
16 weeks	Chest is maintained off the couch, arms are stretched out in full extension
20 weeks	The body weight is supported on forearms
24 weeks	Weight is supported on hands, and baby rolls from prone to supine Indian babies first learn to roll from supine to prone because they are usually not nursed in prone position

Supine Posture and Sitting

The infant is placed supine on the couch and pulled to sitting position by lifting at the forearms (traction response).

Age	Response
Newborn	Complete head lag
4 weeks	Head maintained in plane of the body momentarily when baby is held in a sitting position back is rounded. Chin may be lifted momentarily
12 weeks	Head held up when supported in a sitting position but it tends to bob forward
16 weeks	When pulled up, there is slight head lag during the beginning and then head is flexed beyond the plane of the body. When held in sitting position and baby is swayed, the head wobbles
20 weeks	No head lag, head is stable without wobbling and back is straight
24 weeks	When about to be pulled up, lifts head off the couch in anticipation. Can sit supported in a palm or high chair
28 weeks	Can sit on the floor with hands forward for support
32 weeks	Can sit momentarily on the floor without support
36 weeks	Sits steadily without support and can lean forward and recover his balance
40 weeks	Can sit up from supine position. Can turn sideways and twist around to pick up an object

Vertical Supine, Standing, and Walking

Age	Response
Newborn	Walking reflex during first 2–3 weeks
8 weeks	Can hold head up more than momentarily

Contd...

Age	Response
24 weeks	Puts almost all weight of the body on the legs
28 weeks	Bounces with pleasure
36 weeks	Pulls self to stand, can stand with support
44 weeks	Lifts one foot while standing
48 weeks	Walks two hands held or holding the furniture
1 year	Walks few steps independently
15 months	Creeps stairs, can kneel without support
18 months	Can crawl up and down the stairs without help, pulls a wheel toy
2 years	Walks up and down the stairs with 2 ft on each step, walks backward on imitation, picks up objects from floor without falling, runs, can kick a ball
2.5 years	Can walk tip toes, jumps on both feet
3 years	Goes upstairs with one foot on each step, jumps off the bottom step
4 years	Comes downstairs with one foot each step, can skip on one foot
5 years	Skips on both feet

Fine Motor, Adaptive, and Social Responses (Manipulations)

Age	Response
Newborn	Grasp reflex
4 weeks	Hands mostly closed
8 weeks	Hand kept open more often
12 weeks	Hands mostly open, grasp reflex disappears, plays with a rattle when it is placed in the hand

Contd...

Contd...

Age	Response
16 weeks	Tries to reach objects but overshoots, hands come together during play
20 weeks	Goes for objects and gets them usually with bidextrous approach, puts objects into mouth, plays with toes
24 weeks	Drops one object when another is given, holds rattle, picks up a cube with crude palmar grasp
28 weeks	Unidextrous approach to objects, transfers object from one hand to other, feeds self with a biscuit, bangs object with each other or on the tabletop, retains one cube when another is offered
40 weeks	Pincer grasp to pick up a pellet
1 year	Gives toy to examiner, puts one object after another into the basket, mouthing is much reduced
15 months	Self-feeds with a cup, builds tower of 2–3 cubes, holds 2 cubes in one hand
18 months	Can self-feed with a spoon, makes tower of 3–4 cubes
2 years	Makes tower of 6–7 cubes, can turn door knob, puts on and take off socks, shoes, and pants
2.5 years	Can hold pencil in hand to scribble lines
3 years	Makes tower of 9–10 cubes; can dress and undress, manage button, and draw a circle

Social, Mental, and Language Development

Age	Response
4 weeks	Watches mother intently when she speaks to him. Follow a dangling object up to 90°, quietens on sound of bell
6 weeks	Social smile follows moving person
8 weeks	Fixes and focuses gaze, eye-to-eye contact, vocalizes

Contd...

Contd...

Age	Response
12 weeks	Hand regard, recognizes mother, can follow an object up to 180°, babbles when spoken to, sequels with pleasure and gets excited on seeing a toy
16 weeks	Demonstrates excitement when food is being prepared, laughs loud, turns head toward sound of bell/rattle
20 weeks	Smiles at mirror image, dry during daytime if toilet-trained
24 weeks	No more hand regard, shows displeasure when toy is taken away, demonstrates likes and dislikes, when an object is dropped he looks for it searchingly, dry by night
28 weeks	Imitates actions and sounds, enjoys "pee-a-boo" games, responds to name, pats mirror image, and says monosyllables such as "ba," "ma," "da" Imitates sounds, responds to "no," produces disyllables such as "mama," "dada" "ba-ba"
32 weeks	Pulls clothes of mother to attract attention, waves bye-bye, repeats performance that is laughed at
40 weeks	Gives toy to examiner, interested in picture book, shakes head for "no," says two to three words with meaning
1 year	Jargon speech, indicates the need for potty and parts are wet
2 years	Repeats what is said, uses the words "I," "me," "you" lisping and some stuttering are common. Can point to three parts of a doll
3 years	Normal speech, knows his name, attends to toilet needs except for wiping, can dress and undress

Interpretation of Developmental Findings

- The global developmental delay in all the spheres is suggestive of mental retardation.
- Isolated delay in gross motor development may occur due to poor physical growth due to protein energy malnutrition.

- Lack of environmental stimulation and poor interaction by parents may adversely affect neuromotor development.
- Delay in an isolated sphere of motor development like walking may be due to congenital dislocation of hips.
- Isolated delay in the development of speech is most commonly due to deafness.
- Children with autistic spectrum disorder must be differentiated from children with mental retardation. This disorder is four times more common in boys than girls.

Highlights ● ● ● ●

+ The developmental assessment should focus on how best the child can perform the activity for a particular age.
+ Developmental assessment can be formal assessment which are carried out by trained personnel using age-specific standardized development assessment tools or informal assessment that are carried out by healthcare personnel (doctors, nurses) and students by comparing book picture with patient picture.
+ The global developmental delay in all the spheres is suggestive of mental retardation.
+ Isolated delay in gross motor development may occur due to poor physical growth due to protein energy malnutrition.
+ Lack of environmental stimulation and poor interaction by parents may adversely affect neuromotor development.

NEUROLOGICAL EXAMINATION

Indications

- Brain injury
- Intracranial bleeding
- Intracranial tumors
- Neurologic conditions, for example, meningitis and encephalitis
- After cranial surgery

Components of Assessment

1. Level of consciousness (orientation and cognition)
2. Pupillary signs (size, reactivity to light, quality of reaction)
3. Motor tone and strength (hand grasp, pronator drift, leg movement, motor strength of extremities)

Equipment Needed

A clean tray containing:
- Measuring tape
- Pen light
- Reflex hammer
- Blunt tip needle
- Cotton swab
- Children's play materials (e.g., crayons, paper, blocks, colorful pictures, books, ball, and play dolls)
- Common scents (e.g., orange, vanilla, and jasmine) vision chart
- Flavors (salt, sugar, lemon)
- Tongue blade
- "O" shaped cereal

Preliminary Assessment

- Assess the child's previous neurologic, general health, nutritional, and developmental history.
- Assess the understanding of child's family regarding his/her current health status.

Preparation

- Explain the procedure and the purpose of neurologic examination to the child and the family.
- Review results of child's last neurologic assessment to provide baseline data.
- Review child's medical diagnosis, developmental, and health history to determine whether any neurologic changes may be consistent with current health problems or medical history.

Procedure

- Perform hand hygiene
- Observe the child at rest, noting behavior, and mood; response to surroundings and movements.
- Assess level of consciousness, noting stimulus needed to elicit arousal, quality of response to stimuli, and length of response time.
- Measure the HC
- Inspect the child's cranial shape for symmetry and palpate fontanels to assess whether they are open, note if sunken or bulging.
- Inspect child's skin, noting neurocutaneous findings, such as sacral dimples, spine curvature, and hemangiomas.

Reflex Assessment

1. *Biceps:* Flex the child's forearm, place your thumb over child's antecubital space, and tap with reflex hammer.
   Response: slight flexion at the arm when the tendon is tapped
2. *Triceps:* Abduct the child's arm and support forearm with your hand or hold child's wrist over his/her chest to flex arm at elbow. Tap directly above elbow.
   Response: partial extension
3. *Brachioradialis tendon:* Place the child's arm and hand in relaxed position with arm flexed and palm down. Tap the radius about 1 in. above the wrist.
   Response: Flexion of forearm and upward turn of the palm.
4. *Patellar:* With the child sitting on edge of table or bed with legs dangling, use reflex hammer to tap front outer aspect of child's knee, midline, and just below patella.
   Response: slight extension
5. *Achilles' tendon:* Assist the child to a seated position on the edge of a table or bed. The child's legs should dangle freely over the edge. Support child's foot at 90° angle and use reflex hammer to tap back of child's heel. If child is in supine position, flex one leg at knee and hip supporting the lower position of that leg on the opposite shin. Lightly support foot in your hand in dorsiflexion and tap Achilles' tendon.
   Response: Plantar flexion
6. *Babinski:* Strike the outer sole of the child's foot from heel to toes with the handle of reflex hammer and note movement of toes.
   Response: In children older than 2 years of age, the toes should flex downward. Upward movement of the big toe with other toes fanning outward is called Babinski sign.
7. *Kernig's sign:* With child lying supine, lift child's leg with flexion at knee and hip. Note any pain or resistance.
8. *Brudzinski's sign:* An involuntary flexion of the hip and knees when neck is passively flexed (positive in meningitis).
9. *Anal reflex:* Gently stroke the perianal skin, the child will contract the anal sphincter.
10. *Abdominal reflex:* With child lying supine, stroke abdominal skin in all four quadrants by moving handle of reflex hammer from the side toward the midline. The umbilicus should move toward the stroking in children >6 months.
11. *Cremasteric reflex:* Gently stroke inner aspect of a male child's thigh; the testis of the side of the stroked thigh should retract into inguinal canal.

Assessment of Level of Consciousness

The level of consciousness of the child will be assessed by using Glasgow Coma Scale (**Table 2.13**).

Muscle Strength

- Assess the grip strength, individual muscle strength and assessment findings are generally graded from 0 to 5.

Chapter 2: Assessment Procedures

Table 2.13: Glasgow Coma Scale.

Activity	Best response	Score
Eyes open	Spontaneous	4
	To speech	3
	To pain	2
	None	1
Motor	>1 year	
	Follow commands	6
	Localizes pain	5
	Withdraws to pain	4
	Abnormal flexion	3
	Abnormal extension	2
	None	1
	<1 year	
	Normal spontaneous movement	6
	Withdraws to touch	5
	Withdraws to pain	4
	Abnormal flexion	3
	Abnormal extension	2
	None	1
Verbal	>1 year	
	Oriented	5
	Confused	4
	Inappropriate words	3
	Nonspecific sounds	2
	None	1
	<1 year	
	Coos, babbles	5
	Irritable cry, consolable	4
	Cries to pain, persistent cry	3
	Moans to pain, restless	2
	None	1

0- No movement
1- Trace muscle contraction
2- Active movement
3- Active movement against gravity
4- Active movement against gravity + resistance
5- Normal power of movement

- Ask the child to squeeze your fingers.
- Ask the child to make muscles by bending arms at elbows with palms facing body and resist your attempt to straighten arm to assess biceps strength.
- *Triceps:* Ask the child to extend arms and resist your attempt to flex or bend arm.
- *Quadriceps:* While child is seated with legs dangling over edge of bed or table, ask the child to extend each leg straight and resist your attempt to bend leg.
- *Gastrocnemius muscle:* Ask the child to press the sole of foot against your hand.
- *Tibial-radialis strength:* Ask the child to bend toes up toward his/her face while you place your hand on top of foot.
- *To detect spasticity:* Passively move the child's extremities, noting tone ease of movement (it should be smooth and flexible).
- Lift smaller children under armpits and note child's ability to lock shoulders and prevent slip through.
- Ask the child to sit on stool or chair and rise to standing position, keeping arms crossed in front of chest.
- Ask the child to draw a picture and build a tower of blocks (to assess motor dexterity).
- Ask the child to pick up a small object, such as a piece of cereal observing finger and hand movements bilaterally.
- With arm lifted away from body, ask the child to quickly press thumb and index finger together and apart repeatedly and then have the child use thumb to alternatively touch each finger of same hand. Observe movements of one hand and then other.

Cerebella Assessment (Balance and Coordination)

- Ask the child to walk, run, hop, skip, and walk heel to toe.

- Technique to elicit actions includes rolling a ball along the floor and asking a young child to go get it or having a child to run and try to catch his or her parent.
- Ask the child to use index finger to touch his/her nose alternatively touching your index finger in various locations near child's body, noting tremor or postpointing.
- To assess the Romberg's sign, ask the child to stand with feet together, arms at sides, and eyes closed, like a soldier (should not fall over).

Cranial Nerve Assessment

I cranial nerve
Ask the child to identify some common odorous material (e.g., orange, chocolates) with his/her eyes closed.

II cranial nerve:
- *Acuity of vision:* >3 years— the vision can be screened by use of Snellen's charts. In infants—checking blinking response to bright light, turning of head toward diffuse light, or following red moving ball or ring. The visual acuity in term newborn baby is around 6/45 and it gradually matures to an adult level of 6/6 by the age of 6–7 years.
- *Field of vision:* >3 years—an object suspended from a thread is gradually brought from the periphery toward the eye and child is asked to indicate when the object is visualized.
- *Color vision:* >3 years—by showing different color objects.

III, IV, and VI cranial nerves
Look for squint, movements of eye balls, diplopia, and nystagmus. The child is asked to look at the examiner's fingers that are moved slowly horizontally in either direction and vertically up and down.

Infant: doll's eye movement phenomenon is used to test the ocular movements.

V cranial nerve
- *Infant:* Note strength of infant's suck of pacifier, examiner's thumb, or bottle.
- *Children:* Assess the strength of bite and ability to discern light touch on face.

VII cranial nerve
Note symmetry of facial expressions.
- *Infant:* Monitor during spontaneous cries or smile.
- *Older child:* Ask the child to whistle or blow. Ask him to blow out his cheeks with air under pressure and test the tension on both sides by taping each cheek with finger. Assess taste by asking to discern certain common tastes (salt, sugar).

VIII cranial nerve
- Enquire any hearing defect, tinnitus, vertigo, and dizziness. Ask for response of the child to noise of jet plane, banging of door, music, calling of his name, etc. Use Weber's or Rinne's test.
- *Infants:* Assess for startle response, blinking of eyes, sudden change or cessation of activity, turning of head toward the sound stimuli of a bell, whistle, squeaky toy, etc.

IX and X cranial nerve
Ask the child to identify different tastes on the back of the tongue and tell the child to swallow. A tongue blade may be used to elicit the gag reflex.

XI cranial nerve
Ask the child to turn his/her head from side to side against mild resistance, or to shrug the shoulders.

XII cranial nerve
Ask the child to stick out his/her tongue and instruct him/her to speak.

Highlights ●●●●

- The components of neurological assessment: (1) level of consciousness (orientation and cognition), (2) pupillary signs (size, reactivity to light, quality of reaction), and (3) motor tone and strength (hand grasp, pronator drift, leg movement, motor strength of extremities).
- Review child's medical diagnosis, developmental and health history to determine whether any neurologic changes may be consistent with current health problems or medical history.
- The level of consciousness of the child will be assessed by using Glasgow Coma Scale.

DOCUMENTATION

Definition

Documentation is defined as written evidence of the interactions between and among health professionals, clients, their families and health care organizations.

Purposes of Records

- Records are means of communication in health care
- In assessing, diagnosing, and identifying problems, plan, and implement of care
- Essential for evaluation of nursing intervention
- Progress of child health status
- To foster continuity in nursing care and avoid duplication
- Serve as a legal document
- Can be extensively used for pediatric research and education
- Can be used for nursing audit and quality assurance
- For reimbursement of health insurance
- Serve as a permanent record of client information and care

Types of Nurses Records and Reports in Pediatric Unit

- Admission
- Transfer (e.g., unit to unit)
- Discharge
- Treatment or procedure (e.g., procedure requiring consent or unusual treatment)
- Change in patient's or family's condition
- Patient incident (e.g., medication error)
- Patient or caregiver education

Formats for Documentation of Nursing Care

1. APIE format
   - A—*assessment*: Subjective and objective data of the child, circumstances, conversations, patient/family education needs, etc.
   - P—*planning*: Includes nursing plans, and family goals for treatment
   - I—*implementation*: The type of care provided (name of the procedure, time, date, observations made, etc.)
   - E—*evaluation*: Outcome of the procedure; does the problem solved or need met
2. SOAPIER format
   - S—subjective data
   - O—objective data
   - A—assessment
   - P—plan of nursing care
   - I—implementation of specific nursing intervention
   - E—evaluation of child's response
   - R—revision of care
3. PIE charting
   - P—problem of child
   - I—implementation of care
   - E—evaluation of child's response to the care
4. DAR charting
   - D—data (information about child condition)

- A—action (nursing intervention)
- R—response (response of the child to intervention)
5. CBE (charting by exception): Recording only abnormal and significant findings and avoiding lengthy information.

Types of Reports

1. *Summary/handoff report:* Shift report, while transferring a child to another health-care facility
2. *Walking round reports:* Report occurs during health-care team rounds
3. *Incidence or occurrence reports:* Reporting the unusual occurrence, for example, medication error and accidents in ward

Nursing Considerations in Documentation of Special Circumstances

1. *Documentation of vaccination*: The following information to be documented in the medical record:
   - Day, month, and year of administration.
   - Manufacturer and lot number of vaccines.
   - Name, address, and title of the person administering the vaccine.
   - Additional data to record are the site and route of administration.
   - Evidence that the parent or legal guardian gave informed consent before the immunization was administered.
   - Any adverse reaction after the administration of vaccine is reported to the vaccine adverse event reporting system.
2. *Documentation of child abuse:*
   - History of injury
     » Date, time, and place of occurrence
     » Sequence of events with recorded with times
     » Presence of witnesses, especially person caring for child at time of incident
     » Time lapse between occurrence of injury and ignition of treatment
     » Interview with child when appropriate, including verbal quotations and information from drawing or other play activities
     » Interview with parent, witness, or other significant persons, including verbal quotations
     » Description of parent–child interaction (verbal interaction, eye contact, touching, parental concern)
     » Name, age, and condition of other children in home (if possible)
   - *Physical examination*
     » Location, size, shape, and color of bruise; approximate location, size, and shape on drawing of body outline
     » Distinguishing characteristics, such as a bruise in the shape of a hand, round burn (possibly caused by cigarette)
     » Symmetry or asymmetry of injury; presence of others injuries
     » Degree of pain; any bone tenderness
     » Evidence of past injuries; general state of health and hygiene
     » Developmental level of child; perform screening text (*see* "Developmental Assessment" section)
3. *Documenting a telephonic report:*
   - Provide clear, accurate, and concise information:
     » When call was made?
     » Who made the call?
     » To whom information was given
     » What information was given?
     » What information was received?

Guidelines for Documentation

- All children who are admitted for health care requires documentation.

- A minimum of two unique patient identifiers must be used to verify patients (e.g., child full name, date of birth, and medical record number).
- Only hospital-approved abbreviations and symbols are to be used in records.
- Allergies must be documented immediately in the health record.
- Entries must be made as close as possible to the time of the occurrence of the event being documented.
- The nurse who enters the information must have direct personal knowledge of the information being recorded.

Highlights ● ● ●

✦ Documentation is defined as written evidence of the interactions between and among health professionals, clients, their families, and healthcare organizations.
✦ There are different types of formats used in various hospitals for documenting nursing care. The following are the common formats used widely:
  a. APIE format
  b. SOAPIER format
  c. PIE charting
  d. DAR charting
  e. CBE (charting by exception).
✦ The nurse who enters the information must have direct personal knowledge of the information being recorded.
✦ Entries must be made as close as possible to the time of the occurrence of the event being documented.

MEMORY EXERCISE

1. The average pulse rate of an adolescent is:
   a. 60–100 bpm
   b. 60–120 bpm
   c. 75–110 bpm
   d. 80–120 bpm
2. An 8-year-old child gives history of a strict vegetarian diet followed in family. The pediatric nurse should be alert for signs of:
   a. Vitamin B1 deficiency
   b. Vitamin B2 deficiency
   c. Folic acid deficiency
   d. Vitamin B12 deficiency
3. At which age the child should be referred to a pediatrician if he/she has not begun to walk?
   a. 9 months
   b. 12 months
   c. 15 months
   d. 18 months
4. Around what age the child will be able to build a tower of three building blocks?
   a. 12 months
   b. 18 months
   c. 9 months
   d. 21 months
5. The expected weight of 5-year-old child is:
   a. 17 kg
   b. 18 kg
   c. 16 kg
   d. 19 kg

CHAPTER 3

Assisting in Diagnostic Procedures

LEARNING OBJECTIVES

Upon the completion of this chapter, the learners will be able to:
- Recall basic terms of diagnostic procedures.
- List the indications for various diagnostic procedures in pediatric setup.
- Arrange equipment and supplies need for diagnostic procedures.
- Explain the parents and children about need for particular procedures.
- Collect blood, urine, and stool samples for investigation.
- Assist in performing diagnostic procedures.

Keywords: venipuncture, specimen, collection, diagnosis, analysis, cerebrospinal fluid, cardiac cycle, positioning, atraumatic care, heel stick, catheterization, heart.

COLLECTION OF BLOOD SAMPLE (VENIPUNCTURE)

Definition
The puncture of a vein typically to withdraw blood for investigations or to administer medications through vein.

Indications
- To test the levels of blood glucose and electrolytes
- To determine complete blood count
- To find the cause of infection: to identify the microorganism (blood culture)
- To determine the patient's hemodynamic status before undergoing special procedures
- To diagnose diseases, such as malaria and HIV

Equipment Needed
- Antiseptic solution
- Pair of sterile gloves
- Blood collection tubes [Ethylenediaminetetraacetic acid (EDTA) and plain tubes **Table 3.1**)]
- Pen light
- Butterfly needle (23 ga)
- 5-mL syringe with needle
- Gauze pieces/cotton balls in a bowl
- Tourniquet
- EMLA cream (atraumatic care)
- Laboratory requisition form
- Towel/clean paper/mackintosh

Preparation
- Check if the laboratory form matches the patient's identity.

Table 3.1: Types of blood collection tubes.

Sl. no.	Color of the tube	Agent present	Purpose
1.	Blue-top tube	Sodium citrate (Na citrate)	This tube is primarily used for coagulation studies (PT and PTT). Complete filling of this tube is essential to obtain accurate results
2.	Lavender-top tube	EDTA	Its primary use is for the CBC and individual components of the CBC. The larger (6 mL) tube is used for blood bank procedures
3.	Red-top tube	Plain	Used for many chemistry tests, drug levels, and blood bank procedures
4.	Navy blue-top tube (two types)	One with K2 EDTA and one with no anticoagulant	Used primarily for trace metal analysis
5.	Serum separator tube	Clot activator and serum gel separator	Used for many chemistry tests. It cannot be used for certain drug levels or any blood bank procedures
6.	Green-top tube	Sodium heparin or lithium heparin	Used for plasma determinations
7.	Gray-top tube	Potassium oxalate	Used primarily for glucose tolerance testing
8.	Yellow-top tube	CPDA	Used for blood grouping determinations and cell preservations

(EDTA: ethylenediaminetetraacetic acid; PT: prothrombin time; PTT: partial thromboplastin time; CBC: complete blood count; CPDA: citrate-phosphate-dextrose solution with adenine)

- Successful venipuncture ideally requires advanced notice.
- The use of anesthetic gels and creams (e.g., EMLA cream) is vital to minimize pain and distress during procedure, and these must be applied in advance.
- If the procedure is urgent, then ethyl chloride spray is very useful.
- Depending on the age and level of understanding, as much as possible explain the procedure to the child and parents. Parents must be offered the choice of whether to be involved in the procedure.
- Use distraction techniques during the procedure.

Positioning

- *Older children:* Sitting or lying down
- *Younger children:* Need for supportive holding and restraint
- *For babies up to 9 months:* Swaddle them to include the three limbs being not used
- *For children who can sit on a parent's lap:* Cuddle them by putting the arm that you are using under the cuddler's arm (**Fig. 3.1**)

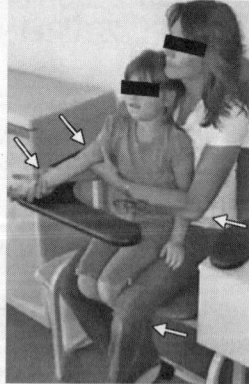

Fig. 3.1: Positioning pediatric clients during venipuncture.

Site for Venipuncture

- Dorsum of hand
- Antecubital fossa (**Figs. 3.2A to C**)
- Scalp vein (neonates)
- Veins of ankle region

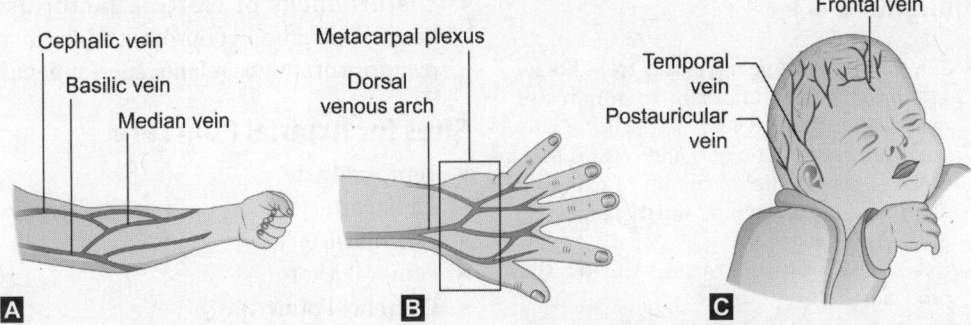

Figs. 3.2A to C: Sites for venipuncture in pediatric clients: (A) Antecubital fossa, (B) Dorsum hand, and (C) Scalp veins.

Procedure

- Perform hand hygiene and don gloves.
- Select the appropriate vein for blood collection.
- Immobilize the child.
- Do skin preparation.
- Put the tourniquet on the patient about 2-finger widths above the venipuncture site.
- Use a thumb to draw the skin tight about 2-finger widths below the puncture site.
- Puncture the skin 3–5 mm distal to the vein; this site allows good access without pushing the vein away.
- If the needle enters alongside the vein rather than into it, withdraw the needle slightly without removing it completely, and angle it into the vessel.
- Carefully collect the blood, not moving the needle in the vein.
- After the required amount of blood has been collected, release the tourniquet.
- Place dry gauze piece over the venipuncture site and slowly withdraw the needle.
- Ask the parent to continue applying mild pressure.

Postprocedure Care

- Dispose the needle in a sharps container.
- Put on adhesive bandage on the patient if necessary.
- Label the tube with the patient's ID number and date.
- Send the specimen bottles with proper requisition form immediately as possible.
- Properly dispose of all contaminated supplies.
- Remove gloves and perform hand hygiene.

General Instructions

- Ask the parents to rhythmically tighten and release the child's wrist to ensure adequate flow of blood.
- Keep the child warm, which may increase the rate of blood flow by as much as sevenfold and in the case of infants, by swaddling in a blanket.
- Warm the area to be punctured with warm cloth to help dilate the blood vessels.
- Use a transilluminator or pen light to display the dorsal hand veins and the veins of antecubital fossa.
- Avoid 25-G needles because this may be associated with an increased risk of hemolysis.
- Place dry gauze piece over the venipuncture site and slowly withdraw the needle.
- Ask the parent to continue applying mild pressure.

Highlights

- The puncture of a vein typically to withdraw blood for investigations or to administer medications through vein.
- The use of anesthetic gels and creams (e.g., EMLA cream) is vital to minimize pain and distress during procedure, and these must be applied in advance.
- Use distraction techniques during the procedure.
- The common sites for venipuncture are (1) antecubital fossa, (2) dorsum hand, and (3) scalp veins.
- Puncture the skin 3–5 mm distal to the vein, this site allows good access without pushing the vein away.
- Keep the child warm, which may increase the rate of blood flow by as much as sevenfold and in the case of infants, by swaddling in a blanket.
- Warm the area to be punctured with warm cloth to help dilate the blood vessels.
- Avoid 25-G needles because this may be associated with an increased risk of hemolysis.

ARTERIAL PUNCTURE

Definition

An arterial puncture is an invasive procedure that is performed to obtain a sample of arterial blood for analysis.

Indications

- Arterial blood gas (ABG) analysis
- Invasive blood pressure monitoring
- Oxygen saturation and pH
- Patient's acid–base state
- For accurate diagnosis of respiratory failure

Contraindications

- Bleeding disorders, for example, platelet count below normal
- Disturbances of clotting factor as in hemophilia and hypoprothrombinemia or overdose of anticoagulants, such as heparin.

Sites for Arterial Puncture

- Temporal artery
- Radial artery
- Brachial artery
- Femoral artery
- Deep heel puncture
- Indwelling arterial catheters

Equipment

A sterile tray containing:
- Heparinized syringe with 21- to 23-G needle
- Sterile swabs in a bowl
- Heparinized collection tubes betadine
- Spirit
- Kidney tray
- Pair of gloves
- Light source

Preparation

- Adequate circulation should be assessed before arterial puncture by observing capillary refill or performing Allen's test (**Fig. 3.3**).
- Comfort the child before doing the procedure. Because crying, fear, and agitation also affect blood gas values.
- Explain the procedure to the parents.
- Apply local anesthesia (EMLA cream) well before the procedure to minimize the pain.
- No matter how or by whom specimen is collected, children fear loss of blood. They mistakenly believe that blood taken from their body is threat to their lives. Explaining that their body continuously produces blood provides them to measure of reassurance regarding this aspect of stress proving procedure.

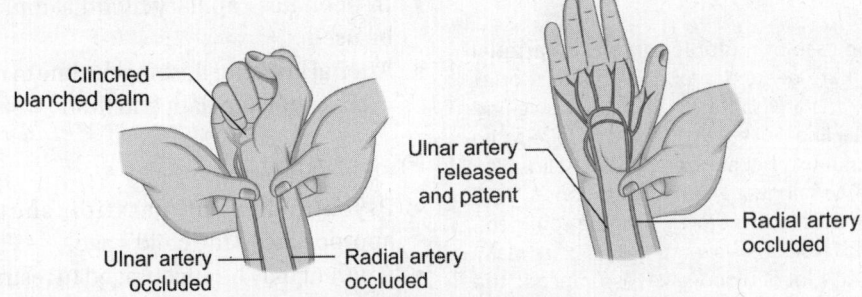

Fig. 3.3: Performing Allen's test.

Procedure

- Perform hand hygiene and don gloves.
- Prepare the site aseptically, employing spirit, iodine, and spirit in that order.
- In the case of a radial puncture, the wrist is kept extended and the radial artery palpated and left hand fingers kept on it.
- Then the bevel facing upward, the needle is inserted little superior to the proximal skin crease inclined at an angle of 45° to the artery. At this stage the needle should be gradually withdrawn as gentle suction is maintained.
- If blood fails to flow into the syringe, another attempt should be made by pushing the needle again in either direction without withdrawing it from the skin.
- Once the sample of blood has been collected, the puncture site should be kept pressed for 5 minutes or more to safeguard against bleeding.

Postprocedure Care

- The syringe/tube containing blood sample is sealed and preserved in ice.
- It must be carried to the laboratory for immediate blood gas analysis.
- Praise the child for cooperation.
- Watch for bleeding from the puncture site.

Nurse's Responsibilities

- In the case of multiple samples of arterial blood are needed over a relatively shorter time, it is advisable to place an indwelling arterial line. Such a line would require to be continuously heparinized (1 U/mL saline; 3–5 mL/h) to safeguard against thrombosis.
- When the blood is drawn, a simple comment, such as just look how red it is, you are really making a lot of blood, gives assurance to the child.
- Institute pain reduction techniques to lessen the discomfort of the procedure.

Highlights ●●●●

> ✦ An arterial puncture is an invasive procedure that is performed to obtain a sample of arterial blood for analysis.
> ✦ The common sites for arterial puncture are temporal artery, radial artery, brachial artery, femoral artery, deep heel puncture, and indwelling arterial catheters.
> ✦ Arterial puncture should not be done when child has bleeding disorders, for example, platelet count below normal or disturbances of clotting factor as in hemophilia and hypoprothrombinemia or overdose of anticoagulants, such as heparin.
> ✦ Adequate circulation should be assessed before arterial puncture by observing capillary refill or performing Allen's test.

Contd...

Contd...

- In the case of multiple samples of arterial blood are needed over a relatively shorter time, it is advisable to place an indwelling arterial line. Such a line would require to be continuously heparinized (1 U/mL saline; 3–5 mL/h) to safeguard against thrombosis.
- When the blood is drawn, a simple comment, such as just look how red it is, you are really making a lot of blood, gives assurance to the child.
- Institute pain reduction techniques to lessen the discomfort of the procedure.

BLOOD GAS ANALYSIS

Definition
Blood gas analysis also called ABG analysis is a procedure to measure the partial pressure of oxygen and carbon dioxide gases and the pH (hydrogen ion concentration) in arterial blood.

Purposes
- To diagnose and evaluate respiratory diseases and conditions.
- To evaluate metabolic conditions that cause abnormal blood pH, for example, diabetic ketoacidosis.
- To monitor children on O_2 therapy, for example, premature infants.
- To monitor the levels of arterial CO_2 and O_2 in children with artificial ventilation.

Contraindications
- Child with hemophilia
- Child with low platelet count
- Child who is on anticoagulant therapy

Sites
- Radial artery
- Brachial artery
- Dorsalis pedis artery
- Femoral artery (only in emergency)
- In neonates capillary blood samples may be used
- Arterial line after flushing the line to remove excess anticoagulant and fluid

Preparation
- Psychological preparation should be appropriate to the child's age.
- A parent may be encouraged to restrain the child during sample collection.
- For children receiving O_2 therapy, the O_2 concentration must remain constant for 20 minutes before sample collection.
- If the test is specifically ordered without O_2, the gas may be turned off for 20 minutes before the blood sample is taken to guarantee accurate test results.

Equipment
- Anticoagulate sterile syringe with needle
- Waste syringe (for 3 mL of waste) if arterial line draw
- Patient label and laboratory collection slip
- Antiseptic solution
- Gauze pieces
- Pair of sterile gloves
- Protective eye wear and gown in the anticipation of splashing
- Container with ice deep enough to immerse syringe beyond the level of specimen

Procedure
- Perform hand hygiene and don gloves and gown.
- Perform Allen's test (both the radial and ulnar arteries should be compressed at a level approximately 1 cm proximal to the wrist joint while the patient's hand is squeezed for approximately 5 seconds then released. The palmar surface of the hand should be blanched. Release the compression on the ulnar artery. It is normal for the palmar surface to flush

within 5 seconds). Prolonged delay before flushing indicates decreased ulnar artery flow.
- The skin over the puncture site is cleaned with antiseptic solution.
- Palpate the site to stabilize the artery. Slight hyperextension of the joint can be achieved by placing a rolled up towel under the joint, this can aid in palpation and stabilization of the artery.
- Hold the syringe with the bevel of the needle upward, keeping the needle at a 25–45° angle to the artery.
- Insert the needle through the skin into the artery taking care not to puncture the posterior wall of the artery. If the artery is not entered immediately, the needle may be slightly pulled back then redirected into the artery.
- Arterial pressure should cause the blood to flow into the syringe.
- Withdraw the needle when an adequate sample has been obtained.
- Immediately place dry gauze or cotton over the puncture site and apply pressure.
- Single handedly cap the needle then remove from syringe.
- Expel any air bubbles from the sample and cap the syringe.
- Mix the sample by rolling and tilting syringe.
- Place a sterile bandage over the puncture site to keep it clean.

Technique for Obtaining Sample from Arterial Line

- Turn the stopcock off to patient.
- Remove the sterile cap from stopcock.
- Attach sterile syringe to stopcock.
- Open stopcock to syringe and intra-arterial catheter and obtain ABG sample.
- Activate flush device to clear arterial line.
- Turn stopcock off to the patient and flush side port of stopcock into sterile syringe until all blood is cleaned from stopcock.
- Close stopcock and replace sterile protective cap.
- Prepare arterial sample by holding syringe upright and remove air bubbles.
- Immediately seal syringe with cap. Roll and tilt syringe gently to ensure heparin mixing.

Aftercare

- Timely and appropriately transport the sample for analysis.
- After the blood sample has been taken, apply pressure to the site for about 10 minutes or until bleeding has stopped after which a dressing is applied.
- Make the child to be calm and quiet.
- Observe for signs of bleeding or impaired circulation at the puncture site.

General Instructions

- Follow standard precautions for prevention of exposure to blood-borne pathogens when performing arterial blood collection.
- The syringe used to collect the sample for a blood gas analysis must contain a small amount of heparin to prevent clotting of the blood.
- The air must be excluded from the syringe both before and after the sample is collected.
- If radial artery is lacking collateral ulnar circulation, it should be avoided as puncture site.
- For transportation, the syringe should be capped with a blind hub, placed on ice, and immediately sent to the laboratory for analysis to guarantee the accuracy of the results.
- If not analyzed immediately, store the sample in ice (2–4°C).
- Never attempt femoral artery puncture in neonates.

Complications
- Hematoma
- Arteriospasm
- Arterial occluding
- Bruising at the puncture site
- Impaired circulation around the puncture site
- Pain
- Infection

Normal Values
- PO_2: 75–100 mm Hg (normally decline with age)
- PCO_2: 35–45 mm Hg
- pH: 7.35–7.45
- SaO_2: 94–100%
- HCO_3^-: 22–26 mmol/L (mEq/L).

Highlights ● ● ● ●

Blood gas analysis also called arterial blood gas analysis (ABG) is a procedure to measure the partial pressure of oxygen and carbon dioxide gases and the pH (hydrogen ion concentration) in arterial blood.

The main purposes are as follows:
- To diagnose and evaluate respiratory diseases and conditions.
- To evaluate metabolic conditions that cause abnormal blood pH, for example, diabetic ketoacidosis.
- To monitor children on O_2 therapy, for example, premature infants.
- To monitor the levels of arterial CO_2 and O_2 in children with artificial ventilation.
- For children receiving O_2 therapy, the O_2 concentration must remain constant for 20 minutes before sample collection.
- If the test is specifically ordered without O_2, the gas may be turned off for 20 minutes before the blood sample is taken to guarantee accurate test results.
- The syringe used to collect the sample for a blood gas analysis must contain a small amount of heparin to prevent clotting of the blood.

Contd...

Contd...
- The air must be excluded from the syringe both before and after the sample is collected.
- If radial artery is lacking collateral ulnar circulation, it should be avoided as puncture site.
- For transportation, the syringe should be capped with a blind hub, placed on ice, and immediately sent to the laboratory for analysis to guarantee the accuracy of the results.
- If not analyzed immediately, store the sample in ice (2–4°C).

CAPILLARY BLOOD SAMPLING

Definition
It is an invasive procedure in which capillary blood is obtained by pricking the finger or heel of the patients. The specimen is then collected with a pipette, placed on a glass slide or piece of filter paper, or is absorbed by the tip of a microsampling device.

Types
1. *Heel stick:* For infants <18 months
2. *Finger stick:* For children >18 months who require specimen of <2.5 mL

Equipment
- Mechanical (automated) lancing device or lancet
- Antiseptic wipes
- 2 × 2 sterile gauze pieces
- Pair of gloves
- Specimen container or capillary tube
- Warming supplies (cloth)

Preparation
- Assess the child for signs of poor perfusion, local edema, infection at the site, and impaired blood coagulation. The presence of these findings can lead to inadequate

sampling, blood specimen contamination, increased pain, and infection.
- Avoid edematous areas because the presence of fluid can contaminate blood specimen.
- Rotate the sites of puncture to decrease complications.
- Apply topical anesthetic (e.g., lidocaine) for finger stick procedure as time allows, based on child's preference.
- Do not use lidocaine if the child is receiving methemoglobin-inducing agents, for example, sulfonamides and acetaminophen.
- Question the parents about the existence of coagulation disorders in the family history and previous signs of blood dyscrasias.
- Verify physician's order for laboratory test.
- Explain the procedure to parents and child as appropriate. Prepare the child as appropriate. Provide therapeutic play or involve the child to help with the procedure. Encourage the parents to remain with the child during the procedure.
- Discuss with the parents about comfort measures. For example, swaddling, use of sucrose pacifiers, and distraction techniques that they can use with their child.

Procedure

- Apply warming device to the area for 5–10 minutes before puncture (warm cloth <109°F or 42.8°C).
- Perform hand hygiene and don gloves.
- Remove warming device.
- Select and identify the puncture site:
  - *Heel: <18 months*
    » Lateral to an imaginary line drawn from the middle of the great toe and running parallel to the medial aspect of the heel (**Fig. 3.4**). Never puncture the back of the infant's heel because

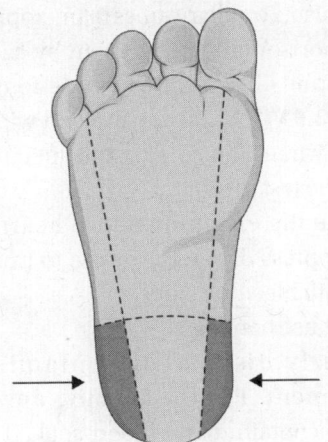

Fig. 3.4: Site of heel stick.

the calcaneus is closest to the surface in that location.
  - *Finger: >18 months*
    » The side of the third or fourth finger near the tip (**Fig. 3.5**).
- Clean the puncture site with the antiseptic and allow drying for 30 seconds. Then dry with the sterile gauze.
- If topical anesthetic has been used, remove before cleaning.
- Place extremity in dependent position while gently applying intermittent pressure to surrounding area; collect the blood in appropriate container.

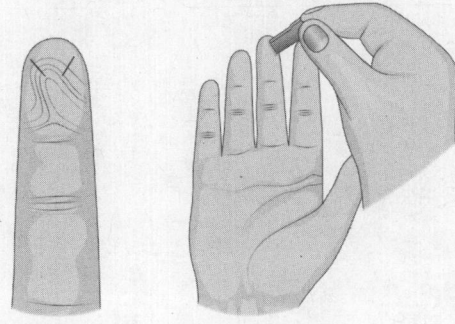

Fig. 3.5: Site for finger stick.

- When using capillary tubes or micropipettes, hold horizontally to fill them by capillary action and fill two-third to three-fourth full **(Figs. 3.6A to C)**. Cover the end with your finger when transferring the specimen to bed side test tube.
- Elevate the extremity above heart level. Gently press dry sterile gauze to puncture site until bleeding stops.
- Do not use bandages.
- Properly dispose of contaminated equipment. Put the lancing device in sharps container and blood-soaked gauze in biohazard bag.
- Remove gloves and perform hand hygiene.
- Perform bed side laboratory testing or label the specimen with child's name, I.P. No., and date and time of collection, and sign it.
- Transport specimen to laboratory in appropriate manner (e.g., ice, refrigeration).

Aftercare

- Monitor the child for signs of pain and involve parent in providing comfort measures. For example, rocking, cuddling, swaddling, talking in a quiet and soothing voice, providing pacifiers, praise, and presenting a small reward.
- Assess puncture wound daily for signs of infection, scaring, and calcified nodules, or bruising.
- Document the following: Date and time, site of puncture, specimen obtained, amount of blood loss, and child's response to procedure.
- Maintain running total of blood loss in neonate or when multiple blood samples are being obtained.

Highlights ●●●

- ✦ Capillary blood sampling is an invasive procedure in which capillary blood is obtained by pricking the finger or heel of the patients.
- ✦ Assess the child for signs of poor perfusion, local edema, infection at the site, and impaired blood coagulation.
- ✦ Apply topical anesthetic (e.g., lidocaine) for finger stick procedure as time allows.
- ✦ Swaddling, use of sucrose pacifiers and distraction techniques can minimize the pain.
- ✦ Apply warming device to the area for 5–10 minutes before puncture.
- ✦ When using capillary tubes or micropipettes, hold horizontally to fill them by capillary action and fill two-third to three-fourth full.
- ✦ Maintain running total of blood loss in neonate or when multiple blood samples are being obtained.

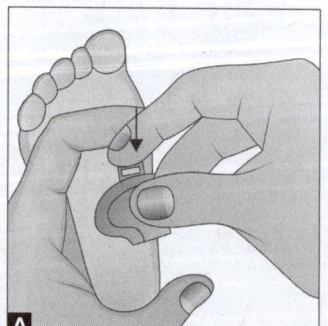
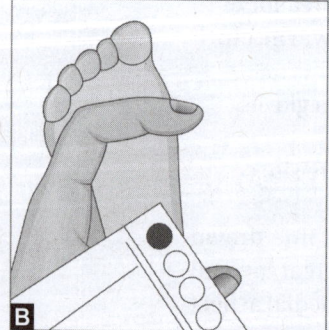
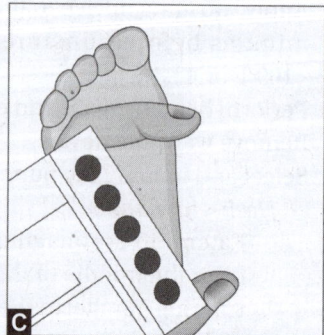

Figs. 3.6A to C: Steps in heel stick procedure: (A) Pricking the site with lancet and (B and C) Collecting blood.

URINE SPECIMEN COLLECTION

Definition
The urine specimen collection is a procedure used to obtain a sample of urine from a patient for diagnostic tests.

Purposes
- To test for any abnormalities that may be present, such as bacteria, ketones, or drugs
- Screening for urinary tract infection (UTI), renal disorders, and detection of systemic and metabolic disorders
- Evaluation of treatment

Types
1. Clean catch
2. Urine culture
3. Midstream specimen of urine

Equipment Needed

For Culture
- A sterile urine cup for older child
- A sterile urine bag for infants
- A bedpan for the child who is unable to use toilet
- Sterile swabs
- Sterile towels
- Sterile gloves
- Laboratory request form
- Disposable diaper
- Sterile bowl with distilled water
- Antiseptic solution
- Mackintosh

For Random Specimen
- Pediatric urine collection bag
- Urine specimen container
- Laboratory request form
- Disposable diapers of appropriate size
- Scissors
- Gloves
- Wash cloth
- Soap
- Water
- Towel
- Bowl
- Mackintosh

For Timed Specimen
- 24-hour pediatric urine collection bag with evacuation tubing
- 24-hour urine specimen container
- Label
- Laboratory request form
- Scissors
- Two disposable diapers of appropriate size
- Gloves
- Wash cloths
- Soap water
- Bowl
- Towel
- Sterile 4 × 4 gauze pads
- Compound benzoin fixture
- Small medicine cup
- 35-mL Luer lock syringe or urometer
- Tubing clamp
- Specimen preservative, such as formaldehyde solution
- Mackintosh

Preparation
- Explain the procedure and its reason to the child and parents.
- If the child is old enough, give adequate guidelines and allow collecting the urine sample.

Precaution
The skin of the genital area should be cleansed with a mild disinfectant to prevent contamination of the urine specimen or irritation of the delicate membranes of the area.

Procedure

Wash hands and don gloves.
- *For female child*
  - The area around the vulva is wiped and dried thoroughly with the sterile swabs and towels, working from the front to back.
  - If the child is unable to use the toilet, the bedpan is placed beneath her.
  - When the urine begins to flow, the first part is allowed to pass into the toilet or bedpan.
  - Then the sterile container is placed in position and filled with the midstream portion of the urine.
  - The reminder of the urine is then allowed to pass into the toilet or bedpan.
  - Place the lid securely on the cup.
- *For male child*
  - Retract the fore skin.
  - The area around the penis and the urethra is wiped and dried thoroughly with the sterile swab and towels working from front to back.
  - If the child is uncircumcised, the fore skin should be held back during the complete procedure to prevent the skin contaminating the sample.
  - The child then begins to pass urine into the toilet or urinal.
  - The sterile container is placed in position and filled with the midstream portion of the urine taking care that penis does not touch the sides of the container.
  - The remainder of the urine is then allowed to pass into the urinal.
  - The lid is placed securely on the cup.
- *For infants*
  - The genitals are cleansed and dried thoroughly using the sterile wipes and towels.
  - A sterile collection bag is placed over the area with the adhesive tape firmly stretched on to the baby's skin.
  - A fresh diaper is put on the child over the collecting bag and checked frequently for the child having passed urine into the bag.
  - When the specimen is obtained, it is poured into a sterile container and sent immediately for testing.
- *For the uncooperative child*
  - Give the child water or other fluids to drink.
  - Clean the external genitalia.
  - The child can be seated on the lap of the mother/nurse who should then encourage the child to urinate and collect as much as urine as possible in sterile container.

Note: Urine collected from diaper is not recommended for laboratory testing since contamination from the diaper material may affect the results.

Aftercare

- The child should be made comfortable.
- Praise the child for cooperation.
- All swabs, towels, and gloves should be disposed in appropriate container.
- The nurse should wash the hands and dry thoroughly.
- The specimen should be sent for testing as quickly as possible. Speed in testing the sample is essential in order to obtain an accurate result.

Highlights ● ● ● ●

- ✦ The urine specimen collection is a procedure used to obtain a sample of urine from a patient for diagnostic tests.
- ✦ To collect urine in babies, a sterile collection bag is placed over the area with the adhesive tape firmly stretch on to the baby's skin.
- ✦ A fresh diaper is put on the child over the collecting bag and checked frequently for the child having passed urine into the bag.

Contd...

Contd...

+ In case of uncooperative child, the child can be seated on the lap of the mother/nurse who should then encourage the child to urinate and collect as much as urine as possible in sterile container.
+ Urine collected from diaper is not recommended for laboratory testing since contamination from the diaper material may affect the results.
+ The specimen should be sent for testing as quickly as possible. Speed in testing the sample is essential in order to obtain an accurate result.

STOOL SPECIMEN COLLECTION

Definition
Stool specimen collection is the process of obtaining a sample of a patient's feces for diagnostic purposes.

Purposes
- To determine the presence of infection, bleeding, or hemorrhage
- To observe the amount, color, consistency, and presence of fats, mucus
- To identify parasitic ova and bacteria

Equipment needed
- Specimen container with label
- Spatula
- Plastic wrap to place over the toilet
- Pair of gloves
- Laboratory request form
- Toilet wipes
- Rectal swab stick (if needed)
- Diaper (in the case of newborn, infants, and young children)

Preparation
- Explain the parents and the child (as appropriate) the need for collecting stool specimen.
- Provide privacy in the case of older children.

Procedure
Put on the glove.
- *For older children*:
  - Patient can collect the specimen by passing feces into plastic wrap stretched loosely over the toilet bowl.
  - A portion of the sample is then transferred into the supplied container with the help of spatula.
- *For younger children and infants*:
  - The diaper should be lined with plastic wrap.
  - A urine bag can be attached to the child to ensure that stool specimen is not contaminated with urine.

Aftercare
- The child should be made clean and comfortable.
- All contents of kit, towels, plastic wrap, and gloves should be disposed of in appropriate containers.
- Wash your hands thoroughly.
- Speed in testing the sample is essential, in order to obtain the accurate result. Therefore, the specimen should be sent for testing as quickly as possible.
- Document the procedure: Time of specimen collection, stool color, amount, consistency and odor, the test to be performed, and the skin condition.

General Instructions
- For testing ova and parasites, specimen collection containers that contain chemical preservatives must be used.
- For culture, the best samples are of loose, fresh stool, sometimes, more than one stool will be collected for a culture.
- Swabs from a child's rectum can also be tested for viruses (occasionally).
- Testing for blood in the stool is often performed with a quick test. First stool is smeared on a card, and then few drops of a

developing solution are placed on the card. An instant color shows that blood is present in the stool.

Highlights ● ● ● ●

- Stool specimen collection is the process of obtaining a sample of a patient's feces for diagnostic purposes.
- In the case of older children, patient can collect the specimen by passing feces into plastic wrap stretched loosely over the toilet bowl. A portion of the sample is then transferred into the supplied container with the help of spatula.
- In young children and infants, the diaper should be lined with plastic wrap.
- A urine bag can be attached to the child to ensure that stool specimen is not contaminated with urine.
- For testing ova and parasites, specimen collection containers that contain chemical preservatives must be used.
- For culture, the best samples are of loose, fresh stool, sometimes, more than one stool will be collected for a culture.
- Swabs from a child's rectum also can be tested for viruses (occasionally).
- Testing for blood in the stool is often performed with a quick test.

LUMBAR PUNCTURE

Definition

Lumbar puncture (LP) or spinal tap is the technique of using a spinal needle to withdraw cerebrospinal fluid (CSF) from the spinal cord.

Indications

- *Diagnostic:* For diagnosis of malignancy and infection as well as measurement of CSF pressure
- *Therapeutic:* For intrathecal administration of chemotherapeutic agents (methotrexate, hydrocortisone, and cytarabine)
- *Research:* Measurement of drug levels

Contraindications

- Elevated intracranial pressure (ICP) is an absolute contraindication until the etiology is clarified. This is due to risk of uncal herniation from mass lesion.
- Infected over lying skin, due to potential for infection seeding.
- Severe bleeding diathesis or severe thrombocytopenia are relative contraindications due to increased risk of spinal subdural hematoma.

Personnel Required for Lumbar Punctures

- Pediatrician to perform the procedure
- Registered nurse (RN) to assist the procedure
- Doctor/nurse to observe the patient if sedated

Equipment Needed

A sterile LP tray contains:
- Drapes
- 1% lidocaine
- Appropriate needles and syringes for infiltration
- Three to four collecting tubes
- Spinal needle with stylets
- Antiseptic solution (povidone iodine or 0.5% chlorhexidine)
- Sterile gloves
- A 22-G spinal needle (or smaller) should be used to reduce the incidence of spinal headache.

Preparation

Psychological Preparation

- A full explanation of the reasons for LP, what the procedure entails, and the potential risks and complications must be given.
- An age-appropriate explanation should also be given to the child.

Chapter 3: Assisting in Diagnostic Procedures

- Ensure that the child and family understand what is involved and that any concerns or questions have been adequately addressed. This can be supported by written information sheet. Written/oral consent obtained (institutional policy).
- Option for analgesia and sedation should be discussed with the child and family appropriate to the child condition.
- Parents may wish to stay with the child during the procedure and may help to reassure the child by talking or holding a hand or head stroking. This is appropriate where the child is conscious and before and after any general anesthesia.
- Allowing a child to prepare for the procedure through the use of play is a useful part of the preparation process, for example, with dolls, soft toys/action figures, art, and stories. This is beneficial where time and child condition allows.
- For children with acute lymphoblastic leukemia, initial LP may ideally be performed under short-acting general anesthesia to ensure that the child is still. This may reduce the possibility of a traumatic LP, which could lead to transfer of peripheral blast cells into the CSF.

Physical Preparation
- Review history of prior procedure with the parents.
- If there is any question of raised ICP, a careful fundoscopic and neurological examination is required to rule out papilledema or focal neurological deficit. If there is any doubt that raised ICP exists, a CT scan and neurosurgery consultation should be obtained.
- Proper positioning of the child is most crucial to ensure the success.
- The child may be placed in a seated position with neck and spine maximally flexed, with arms resting on a bed side table (older child) or leaning over a pillow and held against a seated assistant (younger child) **(Figs. 3.7A and B)**.
- Lateral position with neck bent in full flexion and knees bent in full flexion up to chest, approximating a fetal position as much as possible.
- Drawing an imaginary line between the two posterior iliac crests will allow identification of the L4–L5 or L3–L4 interspaces.

Procedure
- While using sterile technique don sterile gloves.

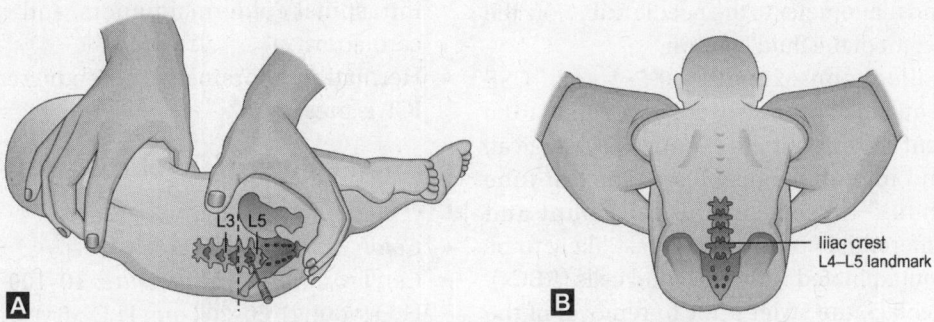

Figs. 3.7A and B: Site and positioning of child for LP: (A) Lying (C-shaped) position and (B) Sitting position. (LP: lumbar puncture)

- Clean, prepare, and drape the area.
- Infiltrate skin and deeper tissues with 1% lidocaine. When experienced at performing LPs, it may be unnecessary to use lidocaine if EMLA cream has been applied to the skin.
- Review tray setup, ensure that lids of collecting containers are unscrewed and containers are readily available.
- Review patient position and restraint.
- Identify L4–5 or L3–4 interspaces and insert the spinal needle with stylet in place, along the midline with bevel facing upward.
- Proper alignment of the needle is aided by placing the thumb of the noninserting hand on the spinous process above the interspace being used.
- Direct the needle slightly cephalad along the imaginary line toward the umbilicus and advance it slowly. Resistance may be felt as the needle penetrates the ligamentum flavum and further smaller "pop" may be felt as the needle penetrates dura. These changes are not always felt so the stylet should be frequently withdrawn to look for the presence of CSF. If none is visible, rotate the needle 90° to attempt to free the bevel of any occluding tissue. If no CSF is forthcoming, replace the stylet, advance the needle slightly, and recheck.
- If an opening ICP is required, once CSF is seen in hub, attach the three-way stopcock and manometer to the needle hub. Note the height of the fluid column.
- Collect approximately 0.5–1 cc of CSF sequentially in each of the sterile tubes to be sent for appropriate chemical, cytological, and microbiological tests. The last tube should be sent for the cell count and differential count as it is least likely to be contaminated with red blood cells (RBCs).
- Replace the stylet prior to removal of the needle as this may reduce incidence of post LP headache.
- Remove LP needle and apply pressure over the puncture site.

Postprocedure Care

- A small adhesive bandage should be placed over the puncture site.
- The patient should be kept in recumbent in semiprone position approximately for 6 hours postprocedure.
- Label the specimens before sending to laboratory.
- Check for any leakage of CSF.
- Monitor vital parameters.
- Encourage to drink extra fluids for the next 24 hours.
- If headache occurs advice for bed rest.

Complications

- Post-LP or spinal headaches: Common in teenagers
- CSF leakage
- Respiratory distress
- Traumatic tap: Localized bleeding resulting from rupture of venous plexus overlying the dura.
- Painful paresthesia due to nerve root irritation
- Rare complications: Local infections, hematoma, arachinoiditis, persistent leg paresthesias, transient cranial nerve palsies, rupture of nucleus pulposus, formation of intraspinal epidermal tumors, and vagal cardiac arrest
- Herniation of brainstem when increased ICP is present

Normal Values of Cerebrospinal Fluid

- *Color*: Crystal clear
- *Cerebrospinal fluid pressure*: 10–100 mm H_2O (young), 60–200 mm H_2O >8 years
- *Glucose*: 40–80 mg/dL (two-third of blood glucose)

- *Protein*: 15–50 mg/dL. For newborn: –150 mg/dL
- *Leukocytes:*
  - Total count (TC): <5/mL. For newborn: 20/mL.
  - Differential count (DC):
    » Lymphocytes: 60–70%
    » Monocytes: 30–50%
    » Neutrophils: None
    » Normally, there are no RBCs in the CSF unless the needle passes through the blood vessel on route to the CSF. In this case, there should be more RBCs in the first tube collected than the last tube.

Highlights

- Lumbar puncture (LP) or spinal tap is the technique of using a spinal needle to withdraw cerebrospinal fluid (CSF) from the spinal cord.
- LP is commonly done for diagnosis of malignancy and infection, measurement of CSF pressure, and for intrathecal administration of chemotherapeutic agents.
- Elevated intracranial pressure is an absolute contraindication for LP.
- Proper positioning of the child is most crucial to ensure the success.
- The child may be placed in a seated position with neck and spine maximally flexed, with arms resting on a bed side table (older child) or leaning over a pillow and held against a seated assistant (younger child).
- Drawing an imaginary line between the two posterior iliac crests will allow identification of the L4–5 or L3–4 interspaces.
- The patient should be kept in recumbent in semiprone position approximately for 6 hours post procedure.
- Normally, there are no RBCs in the CSF unless the needle passes through the blood vessel on route to the CSF.
- Encourage to drink extra fluids for the next 24 hours.
- If headache occurs advice for bed rest.

LIVER BIOPSY

Definition

Liver biopsy is the removal of a piece or small portion of tissue from the liver for diagnostic purpose.

Indications

- Indian childhood cirrhosis and other cirrhosis
- Hepatitis
- Unexplained hepatomegaly
- Tuberculosis (abdominal)

Contraindications

- Prolonged prothrombin time
- Thrombocytopenia
- Blood dyscrasias
- Extrahepatic obstructive jaundice with enlarged bladder
- Cancer of the liver
- Infection of the lower lobe of the right lung

Equipment Needed

A sterile tray containing:
- Tru-Cut needle or Vim-Silverman needle with the stylet or Menghini needle
- Sterile cotton swab with antiseptic solution
- Procaine 1%
- Syringe with needle
- Sponge holder
- Kidney tray
- Tincture benzoin
- Specimen bottles
- Pair of sterile gloves, gown, and mask
- Center hole towel

Preparation

- Explain the procedure to the parents.
- Obtain a written consent.
- Ensure that the prothrombin time is ascertained; arrange for blood.

- Monitor vital signs.
- Administer sedatives as prescribed.
- Administer injectable vitamin K.

Procedure

- Perform hand hygiene.
- Make the child to lie on the edge of the table with his hands kept behind the head.
- Clean the area with antiseptic wipes.
- Infiltrate the area with local anesthesia at the level of 10th intercostal space in the midaxillary line (right side).
- Then liver biopsy needle with the stylet is inserted through the 9th or 10th intercostal space or through subcostal approach into the liver tissue (**Fig. 3.8**).
- Then the stylet is withdrawn and the split portion is pushed inside the hollow needle.
- It is advanced further into the liver.
- At this stage, the outer needle too is advanced into the liver fully.
- Thereafter, the whole needle is rotated.
- This breaks the liver chip (that is attached to the needle) from the rest of the liver.
- The entire apparatus is withdrawn and the skin wound is sealed with Tincture benzoin.

Postprocedure Care

- Place a cotton pad over the site and turn the child on his right side.
- Place a small pillow under his costal margin and make him remain in the same position.
- Monitor vital signs every 10–15 minutes for first few hours and then half an hourly for first 24 hours.
- Watch for complication of liver biopsy.
- Send the specimen to the laboratory with request form.
- Keep the biopsy site aseptic.

Complications

- Hemorrhage
- Shock and collapse
- Bile peritonitis
- Pneumothorax
- Injury to adjacent organs

Highlights ●●●●

- ✦ Liver biopsy is the removal of a piece or small portion of tissue from the liver for diagnostic purpose.
- ✦ Ensure that the prothrombin time should be ascertained, arrange for blood before the procedure.
- ✦ Then liver biopsy needle with the stylet is inserted through the 9th or 10th intercostal space or through subcostal approach into the liver tissue.
- ✦ Immediately, after the procedure, place a cotton pad over the site and turn the child on his right side.
- ✦ Place a small pillow under his costal margin and make him remain in the same position.
- ✦ Monitor vital signs every 10–15 minutes for first few hours and then half an hourly for first 24 hours.
- ✦ Watch for complication of liver biopsy.

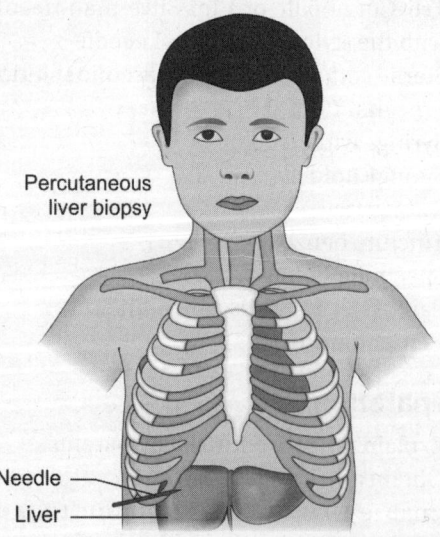

Fig. 3.8: Site for insertion of liver biopsy needle.

KIDNEY BIOPSY

Definition
Kidney biopsy is a medical procedure in which a small piece of tissue is removed from the kidney for microscopic examination.

Indications
- Children with nephrotic syndrome not responsive to usual therapy with corticosteroids
- Progressive renal failure of obscure cause
- Undiagnosed hematuria
- Conditions, such as systemic lupus erythematosus (SLE)
- For evaluation of response to the therapy and prognosis of the disease

Contraindications
- Bleeding diathesis
- Polycystic disease
- Solitary kidney
- Severe systemic hypertension
- Hydronephrosis
- Tumors of kidney or adrenals

Equipment Needed
A sterile tray containing:
- Tru-Cut or Vim-Silverman needle with stylet
- 1% procaine or xylocaine injection
- Needle with syringe
- Antiseptic solution in a bowl
- Sterile gauze pieces
- Sponge holder
- Specimen collection container
- Pair of sterile gloves
- Center hole towel

Site for Biopsy
The usual site for biopsy is 2 cm below and median to the tip of the 12th rib (lower border).

Position Used
Prone position with head turned to a side, arms abducted, and forearms by the side of the head. A pillow or rolled up towel is placed under his abdomen (**Fig. 3.9**).

Preparation of Child and Parents
- Explain the procedure, its consequences, and reason for performing to the parents and child as appropriate.
- Obtain a written consent from parents.
- Check out for the following:
  - Every child fixed for kidney biopsy must have a plain X-ray of the abdomen, ultrasound, and an intravenous pyelogram (IVP) for ascertaining the position and size of the kidneys prior to the procedure.
  - The child should be sedated prior to the procedure (as explained in "Bone Marrow Aspiration" section).
  - Position the child as explained above.

Procedure
- Perform surgical hand scrub.
- Wear gloves.

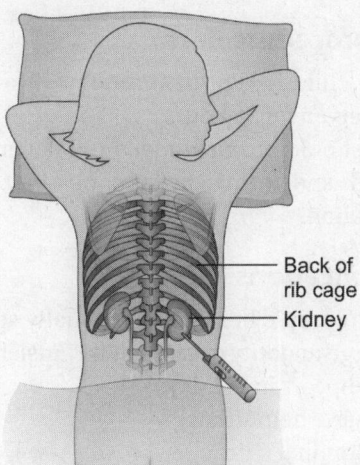

Fig. 3.9: Positioning of child and site for kidney biopsy.

- Paint the site with antiseptic solution.
- Infiltrate the site with 1% procaine injection.
- Then a 20-G long needle (about 8 cm) is inserted gradually in a sagittal plane parallel to the spine until it hits the kidney. The latter moves up and down with respiration, provided that it is in the depth to which has entered is marked and it is withdrawn.
- The track is anesthetized.
- Then, Tru-Cut or Vim-Silverman needle with stylet is introduced along the anesthetized tract, while the patient takes deep breath, till it pierces the kidney capsule.
- The position is confirmed by to and fro movement of the needle with respiration.
- The stylet is removed and the forked cutting needle is inserted to its full length.
- The child is asked to hold the breath and the other needle is pushed deeper so that it covers fully the forked needle.
- The whole apparatus is now rotated a full circle (360°), leading to cutting in of the biopsy material from the kidney.
- Finally, the apparatus is withdrawn and the puncture site is sealed with tincture benzoin.

Postprocedure Care

- The child is kept in supine position and observed for 24 hours.
- He should be encouraged to take enough fluids and normal diet after he is out of the sedation.

Complications

- Microscopic hematuria is usually seen in a large majority of cases. It is transient and disappears in 2–3 days
- Massive hemorrhage
- Abdominal pain
- Hematoma
- Intrarenal arteriovenous fistula

Highlights

✦ Kidney biopsy is a medical procedure in which a small piece of tissue is removed from the kidney for microscopic examination.
✦ The usual site for biopsy is 2 cm below and median to the tip of the 12th rib (lower border).
✦ The child should be placed in prone position with head turned to a side, arms abducted, and forearms by the side of the head. A pillow or rolled up towel is placed under his abdomen.
✦ Every child fixed for kidney biopsy must have a plain X-ray of the abdomen, ultrasound, and an IVP for ascertaining the position and size of the kidneys prior to the procedure.
✦ The child should be sedated prior to the procedure (as explained in "Bone Marrow Aspiration" section).
✦ After the procedure, the child is kept in supine position and observed for 24 hours.
✦ He should be encouraged to take enough fluids and normal diet after he is out of the sedation.

BONE MARROW ASPIRATION

Definition

It is an invasive procedure by which a marrow is obtained through a fine bore needle.

Indications

- For diagnosis of malignant cells
- To diagnose aplastic anemia and bone marrow suppression

Sites for Bone Marrow Aspiration

- *Children younger than 2 years*: A point on the anterior-medial aspect of tibia about 2.5 cm below the tibial tubercle.
- *Older children*: Posterior or anterior iliac spine

Note: Sternum is usually avoided in children because the bone is more fragile and adjacent to vital organs.

Position
- If the posterior iliac crest is used, the child is positioned prone (**Fig. 3.10**).
- Sometimes a small pillow or folded blanket is placed under the hips to facilitate obtaining the bone marrow specimen.
- In the case of anterior iliac crest, supine position is used.

Equipment Needed
A sterile tray containing:
- Pair of sterile gloves
- Trocar and cannula (pediatric size)
- 20-mL syringe
- Center hole towel
- 1% procaine or xylocaine injection
- Syringe and needle
- Povidone iodine solution in a bowl
- Sterile gauze pieces
- Pressure bandage
- Sponge holder
- Dustbin at the foot end of the procedure table
- Specimen bottles/containers/8–10 glass slides

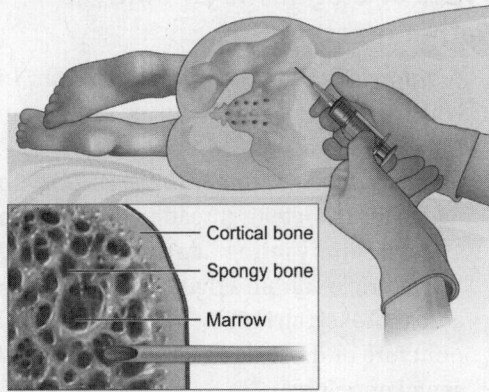

Fig. 3.10: Bone marrow aspiration (positioning and site selection—posterior iliac crest).

Preparation of Child and Parents
- Bone marrow aspiration is one of the most painful procedures. Adequate explanation should be given to parents and child as appropriate.
- Obtain a written consent.
- Sedation should be given to the child to reduce the pain and anxiety.
- Most sedation protocols combine opioid analgesics with a benzodiazepine for anxiolysis and sedation. Sedation is induced with agents, such as ketamine, propofol, and methohexital.

Procedure
- Perform surgical scrub.
- Don gloves.
- Position the child appropriate to the site selected.
- Paint the area with antiseptic wipes.
- Infiltrate the skin with procaine 1% up to the periosteum.
- Place the center hole towel over the site.
- Insert the trocar and cannula with rotating action through the skin down to the periosteum and then through the cortex into the marrow cavity.
- As soon as the needle enters the cavity, some "give" is felt and there is sudden lack of resistance.
- With the needle firmly fixed in situ, trocar is removed.
- A fleck of marrow on the tip of the trocar confirms that the needle is in the marrow cavity.
- Fit a dry 20-mL syringe to the needle.
- With strong suction for a few seconds, about 0.2 mL of marrow is aspirated into the syringe.
- After aspiration, trocar is replaced and the needle withdrawn.
- The puncture site is pressed with a finger for 3–5 minutes.

- A sterile dressing is applied over the site.
- The aspirate is smeared in equal amounts on 8–10 glass slides, which are waved in the air to accomplish fast drying.

Postprocedure Care

- Apply a small pressure bandage over the puncture site.
- No activity restriction is necessary after the bone marrow test, although the site is usually sore and the child may prefer to remain quiet.
- Send the specimens to the laboratory with the request form for diagnosis.
- Document the procedure on nursing chart with date and time, approach used, and site selection.

Highlights ●●●●

- ✦ Bone marrow aspiration is an invasive procedure by which a marrow is obtained through a fine bore needle for diagnosis of malignant cells and aplastic anemia and bone marrow suppression.
- ✦ Sternum is usually avoided in children because the bone is more fragile and adjacent to vital organs.
- ✦ The sites for the aspiration are a point on the anterior-medial aspect of tibia about 2.5 cm below the tibial tubercle in young children and posterior or anterior iliac spine in older children.
- ✦ Bone marrow aspiration is one of the most painful procedures. Hence, adequate explanation should be given to parents and child as appropriate.
- ✦ Apply a small pressure bandage over the puncture site upon the completion of procedure.
- ✦ No activity restriction is necessary after the bone marrow test, although the site is usually sore and the child may prefer to remain quiet.

CARDIAC CATHETERIZATION

Definition

Cardiac catheterization is an invasive procedure in which a radio-opaque catheter is inserted through the peripheral blood vessel into the heart. It usually combined with angiography (angiocardiography) in which a radio-opaque contrast material is injected through the catheter and into the circulation.

Purposes

Cardiac catheterization provides information regarding the following:

- Oxygen saturation of blood within the chamber and great vessels
- Pressure changes within these structures
- Cardiac output or stroke volume
- Anatomical abnormalitie, such as septal defects or obstruction to flow

Indications

- For diagnostic purposes
- For interventional purposes
- For electrophysiologic purposes

Types of Diagnostic Cardiac Catheterization

1. *Right-sided or venous catheterization*: In which the catheter is introduced from a vein into the right atrium.
2. *Left-sided or arterial catheterization*: In which the catheter is threaded by a way of a systemic artery retrograde in the aorta and left ventricle or from a right-sided approach across the left atrium by means of a septal puncture or through an existing abnormal septal opening.

Types of Interventional Cardiac Catheterization Procedure in Children

- Balloon arterioseptostomy—transposition of great arteries (TGA)
- Balloon dilation—valvular pulmonic stenosis (PS), aortic stenosis, recurrent coarctation of aorta, etc.
- Coil occlusion—patent ductus arteriosus [PDA (<4 mm)]
- Transcatheter device closure—atrial septal defect (ASD)
- Amplatzer septal occluder (ASO)
- Stent placement—PS, coarctation of aorta
- Radiofrequency ablation—some tachydysrhythmias

Equipment Needed

A sterile trolley contains:
- Sterile gowns
- Disposable sheets with center hole
- Sterile gloves of different sizes
- A sterile basin with two bowls for heparin solution to flush the catheters and needles and to pour betadine solution
- Catheters of different types and size
- Sponge holder
- Contrast material
- Sterile gauze pieces
- Plasters to seal the catheterized site after the procedure
- Xylocaine injection 1 or 2%
- Syringe and needle
- Heparin solution—injectable heparin and sterile NS
- Intravenous (IV) set—IV cannula (different sizes)
- Scissors
- Head roll to support the head
- IV stand
- Oxygen supply
- Pulse oximeter
- Electrocardiogram (ECG) monitor
- Dustbin to collect the waste to be kept at the foot end of the table

Preprocedural Care

Psychological Preparation

- Explain the procedure to the parents and child emphasizing what they will see, feel, and hear.
- Preparation materials, such as picture books or video tapes or tours of the cath laboratory may be helpful.
- Preparation should be geared to the developmental level of the child. Additional information, such as the expected length of catheterization procedure, description of the child's appearance after catheterization, and usual postprocedure care, should be outlined.
- Obtain a written consent.

Physical Preparation

- A complete nursing assessment is necessary to ensure the safety of the procedure and minimize complications.
  It includes the following:
  - Accurate measurement of height and weight.
  - Obtain history of allergic reaction because some contrast agents used are iodine based.
  - Give specific attention to signs of infection.
  - Assess and mark the dorsalis pedis and posterior tibial pulse before the child goes to the cath laboratory.
  - The presence and quality of pulse in both feet are clearly documented.
  - Baseline oxygen saturation with cyanosis should be recorded.
- Methods of sedation vary among institutions and may include oral or IV medications.
- Typically the child is allowed nil by mouth (NBM) before catheterization; although

polycythemic infants and children may require IV fluids to prevent dehydration and neonates may need dextrose solution for up to 2 hours before the procedure to prevent hypoglycemia.
- Usually the morning dose of all oral medication is withheld, although this is clarified beforehand with the practitioner.

Procedure

- Perform surgical scrub.
- Paint the peripheral site with antiseptic swabs.
- Create a sterile field.
- The catheter is usually introduced through a percutaneous puncture into the femoral vein (the catheter is threaded over a guide wire inserted through a large bore needle) (**Fig. 3.11**).
- Rarely a cutdown procedure is needed to gain access to the vein.
- Once the vessel is entered, the catheter is guided through the heart with the aid of fluoroscopy.
- As the tubing is advanced, the child may feel pressure at the insertion site and vasospasm (fluttering) of the small vessels.
- Once the catheter is within the heart, blood samples and pressure readings are taken for analysis.
- Then contrast material may be injected and films taken of the dilution and circulation of the material.

Note: As the contrast medium is administered, the child may experience warmth, nausea, vomiting, restlessness, or headache.

Postprocedure Care

- Patients may recover from the catheterization procedure in recovery unit or in their hospital rooms. Some may require care in the intensive care unit (ICU).
- If bleeding occurs, direct pressure is applied 2.5 cm above the percutaneous site to localize pressure over the vessel punctured.
- Children are usually placed on a cardiac monitor and a pulse oximeter for the first few hours following catheterization.
- The most important nursing responsibility is observation of the following for signs of complications:
    - Pulse, especially below the catheterization site, for equality and symmetry (pulse distal to the site may be weaker for the first few hours after catheterization but should gradually increase in strength).
    - Temperature and color of the affected extremity, because coolness or blanching may indicate arterial obstruction.
    - Vital signs, which may be taken as frequently as every 15 minutes, with special emphasis on the heart rate, which is counted for 1 full minute for evidence of dysrhythmias or bradycardia.

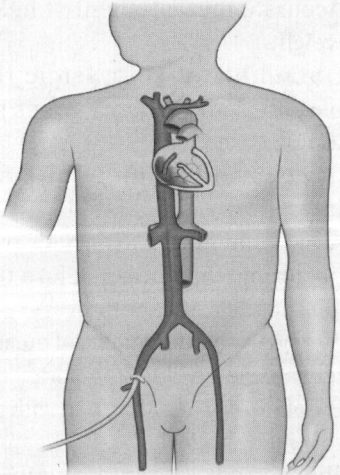

Fig. 3.11: Cardiac catheterization.

Chapter 3: Assisting in Diagnostic Procedures

- BP, especially for hypotension, which may indicate hemorrhage from cardiac perforation or bleeding at the site of initial catheterization.
- Dressing for evidence of bleeding or hematoma formation in the femoral or antecubital area.
- Fluid intake, both IV and oral to ensure adequate hydration (blood loss in the cath laboratory, the child's preprocedure status of NBM, and diuretic actions of contrast material used during the procedure put the child at risk for hypovolemia and dehydration).

- Infants are particularly at risk for hypoglycemia. They should receive dextrose containing IV fluids and blood glucose levels should be checked.
- Depending on hospital policy, the child may be kept in bed with the affected extremity maintained straight for 4–6 hours after venous catheterization and 6–8 hours for arterial catheterization to facilitate healing of the cannulated vessel.
- If younger children have difficulty complying, they can be held in parent's lap with the leg maintained in the correct position.
- The child's usual diet can be resumed as tolerated beginning with sips of clear fluids and advancing as the condition allows it.
- Generally, there is only slight discomfort at the percutaneous site.
- Acetaminophen, with or without codeine or ibuprofen can be given for pain.
- The catheterization site is covered with an occlusive waterproof pressure dressing (usually a foam tape dressing tightly applied) to prevent bleeding and contamination that could cause infection.
- The dressing is left on until the next day.

Home Care Management (Health Education)

- Remove the pressure dressing the day after catheterization.
- Cover site with an adhesive bandage strip for several days.
- Keep site clean and dry.
- Avoid tub bath for several days, may shower.
- Observe site for redness, swelling, drainage, and bleeding.
- Monitor for fever. Notify practitioner if it occurs.
- Avoid strenuous exercise for several days but can attend school.
- Resume regular diet without restrictions.
- Use acetaminophen or ibuprofen for pain.
- Keep follow-up appointments per practitioner's instruction.

Highlights

- Cardiac catheterization is an invasive procedure in which a radio-opaque catheter is inserted through the peripheral blood vessel into the heart.
- It usually combined with angiography (angiocardiography) in which a radio-opaque contrast material is injected through the catheter and into the circulation.
- It is done to assess oxygen saturation of blood within the chamber and great vessels, pressure changes within these structures, cardiac output or stroke volume and anatomical abnormalities.
- Polycythemic infants and children may require IV fluids to prevent dehydration and neonates may need dextrose solution for up to 2 hours before the procedure to prevent hypoglycemia.
- As the contrast medium is administered, the child may experience warmth, nausea, vomiting, restlessness, or headache.
- If bleeding occurs, direct pressure is applied 2.5 cm above the percutaneous site to localize pressure over the vessel punctured.

Contd...

Contd...

- Children are usually placed on a cardiac monitor and a pulse oximeter for the first few hours following catheterization.
- The catheterization site is covered with an occlusive waterproof pressure dressing (usually a foam tape dressing tightly applied) to prevent bleeding and contamination that could cause infection.
- Observe site for redness, swelling, drainage, and bleeding.

ELECTROCARDIOGRAM

Definition

Electrocardiogram (ECG or EKG from Greek: *Kardia*, meaning heart) is the recording of the electrical activity of the heart. Traditionally, this is in the form of a transthoracic (across the thorax or chest) interpretation of the electrical activity of the heart over a period of time, as detected by electrodes attached or displayed by a device external to the body. The recording produced by this noninvasive procedure is termed an ECG.

Function

An ECG produces a pattern reflecting the electrical activity of the heart, which can give information regarding the rhythm of the heart (whether or not the electrical impulse consistently arises from the part of the heart where it should and at what rate), whether that impulses are conducted normally throughout the heart, or whether any part of the heart is contributing more or less than expected to the electrolyte activity of the heart. It can give information regarding the balance of electrolytes in the blood (e.g., hyperkalemia) or even reveal problems with sodium channels within the heart muscle.

Drawbacks of Electrocardiogram

The ECG cannot reliably measure the pumping ability of the heart, for which echocardiography is used. It is possible for a human to be in cardiac arrest, but still have a normal ECG signal (a condition known as pulseless electrical activity).

Working Principles of Electrocardiogram

The ECG device detects and amplifies the tiny electrical changes on the skin that are caused when the heart muscle depolarizes during each heartbeat. At rest, each heart muscle cell has a negative change, called the membrane potential, across its cell membrane. Decreasing this negative charge toward zero, via the influx of the positive cations, Na^+ and CA^{++}, is called depolarization, which activates the mechanisms in the cell that cause it to contract. During each heartbeat, a healthy heart will have an orderly progression of a wave of depolarization that is triggered by the cells in the sinoatrial node, spreads out through the atrium, and passes through the atrioventricular node and then spreads all over the ventricles. This is detected as tiny rises and falls in the voltage between two electrodes placed either side of the heart, which is displayed as wavy line either on a screen or on paper. This display indicates the overall rhythm of the heart and weakness in different parts of the heart muscles.

Usually, more than two electrodes are used, and they can be combined into a number of pairs [e.g., left arm (LA), right arm (RA), and left leg (LL) electrodes from the each pairs LA + RA, LA + LL, and RA + LL]. The output from each pairs is known as a lead. Each lead looks at the heart from a different angle. Different type of ECG can be referred by the number of leads that are recorded, for example, 3-lead, 5-lead, or 12-lead. A 12-lead ECG is one in which 12 different electrical signals are recorded at approximately the same time and will often be used as one-off recording of an ECG, traditionally printed out as a paper copy. Three- and five-lead ECGs tend to be monitored continuously and viewed only on the screen of an appropriate monitoring device, for example, during an operation or while being transported in an ambulance. There may or may not be any permanent record of a 3- or 5-lead ECG, depending on the equipment used.

Preparation of Child and Parents for Electrocardiogram

- Explain the procedure to the parents and child appropriately.
- Make the child to be calm to get proper reading.
- Use therapeutic play: Allow the child to touch the leads and provide play materials.
- Assure the child that this procedure will not cause any pain or discomfort.
- Maintain privacy of the older children.
- Remove the shirt for connecting the leads.

Placement of Electrocardiogram Leads in Pediatric Clients

In young children, the right ventricle normally extends to the right side of the sternum. To appropriately display right ventricular potentials, ECGs for children in the under 5-year age-group must include an extra lead (V4R) on the right side of the chest at a point analogous to the left-sided V4.

Periodical Leads

- R4V: 5th intercostal space, right midclavicular line.
- V1: 4th intercostal space, right sternal border.
- V2: 4th intercostal space, left sternal border.
- V3: Use this lead for V4R, must label as much on ECG.
- V4: 5th intercostal space, right midclavicular line.

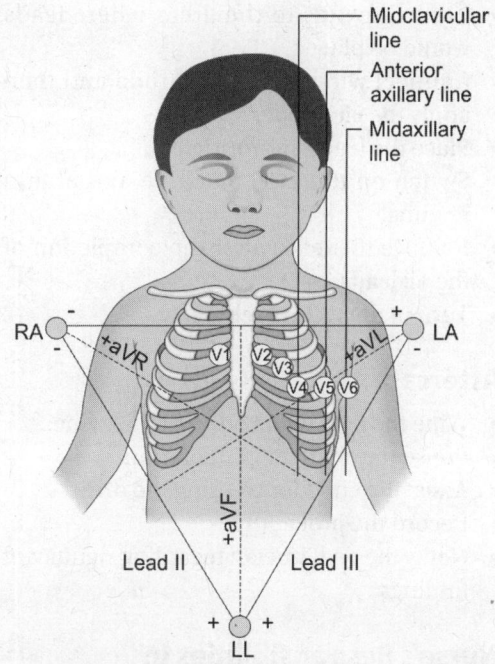

Fig. 3.12: Landmarks for the placement of ECG leads in children. (ECG: electrocardiogram)

- V5: Anterior axillary line, same horizontal plane as V4
- V6: Midaxillary line, same horizontal line as V4

Limb leads: Place on the top part of arm or leg (less muscle interference) (**Fig. 3.12**).

Procedure

- Gather necessary supplies. Check the working conditions of leads and cables.
- Perform hand hygiene and wear gloves.
- Lay the child in supine position. Have the parents to be present at the bed side.
- Clean the area, that is, right and left side of the chest; left upper quadrant of the abdomen with soap and water.
- Remove the gloves and dispose it in kidney tray.
- Apply the gel to the areas where leads would be placed.

- Connect wires to the areas where leads would be placed.
- Connect wires to the electrode and then apply the electrode.
- Place the leads appropriately.
- Switch on the ECG machine and obtain reading.
- Remove the leads after the completion of the all leads.
- Turn of the ECG machine.

Aftercare

- Wipe the area with cotton/tissue wipe.
- Praise the child for cooperation.
- Assist the child for wearing the dress.
- Record the procedure.
- Notify the pediatrician regarding significant findings.

Nurse's Responsibilities in Monitoring Electrocardiogram Using Cardiac Monitor

- Check the monitor screen for correlating heart rate and respiratory rate.
- Adjust the monitor for complex sensitivities as necessary. Leads I, II, and III are most commonly used in children.
- Check the manufacture's guidelines for operational instructions.
- Ensure that electrodes are correctly placed. Change the electrodes as needed for infants and every 72 hours for older children.
- Assess the skin condition. Rotate the site when applying new electrodes.
- Notify the pediatrician when the heart and respiratory rates out of normal limits.

The stepwise assessment of the ECG is as follows:

1. **Rhythm**
   - *Sinus*: Atrial depolarization starts from the sinoatrial node. This requires:
     » P wave preceding each QRS complex, with a constant PR interval
     » Normal P-wave axis (0 to +90°), that is, P wave is upright in leads I and atrioventricular fibrillation (aVF).
   - *Nonsinus*: Some atrial rhythms may have P waves in front of every QRS but with an abnormal P axis (inverted in lead II).
2. **Rate:** Usual paper speed is 25 mm/s so 1 mm (small square) = 0.04 second, and 5 mm (big square) = 0.2 second. Calculate atrial and ventricular rates separately if different (**Fig. 3.13**). Many methods to estimate the rate, for example:
   - *For regular rhythms:* 300/number of large square in between each consecutive R wave
   - *For very fast rates:* 1,500/number of small square in between each consecutive R wave
   - *For irregular rhythms:* Number of complexes on the rhythm strip × 6.

   Note: Refer vital signs for resting heart of various age-groups.
3. **QRS axis:** It is calculated using the hexaxial reference system that shows the frontal view of the electrical activity of the heart via the six limb leads.
   - In lead I, the R wave represents the leftward force, the S wave the rightward force.
   - In aVF, the R wave represents the downward force, the S wave the upward force.
   - Normal QRS axis varies with age:
     » 1 week–1 month: +110° (range +30° to +180°)
     » 1 month–3 months: +70° (range +10° to +125°)
     » 3 months–3 years: +60° (range +10° to +110°).
4. **ECG intervals:** The intervals of the ECG are illustrated below:
   - PR interval
     » The normal PR interval varies with age and heart rate.

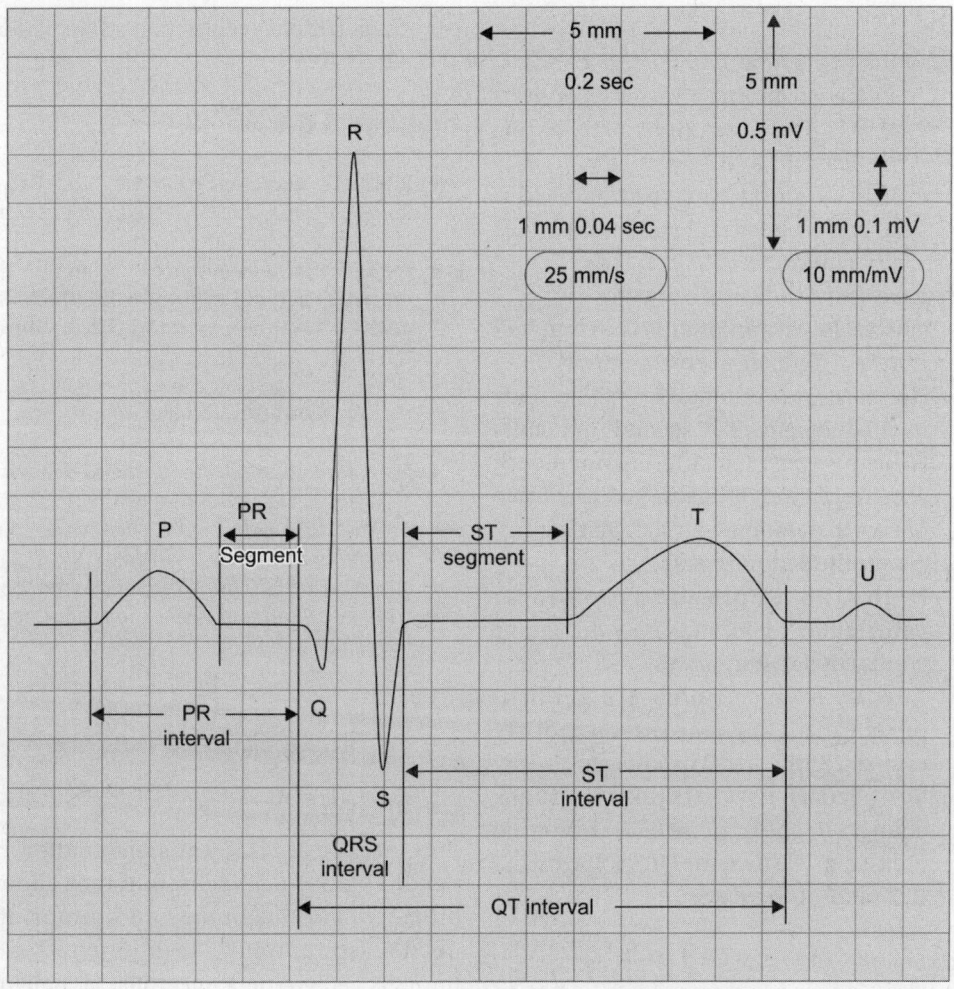

Fig. 3.13: Normal ECG. (ECG: electrocardiogram)

- » Prolonged PR intervals (first-degree heart block) may be normal or be seen in:
  Viral or rheumatic myocarditis and other myocardial dysfunctions
  Certain congenital heart disease (ASD)
  Digitalis toxicity
  Hyperkalemia
- » Short PR interval occurs in:
  - Preexcitation (e.g., Wolff-Parkinson-White)
  - Glycogen storage disease

- QRS duration:
  » QRS duration varies with age.
  » Prolonged QRS is characteristic of ventricular conduction disturbances such as bundle branch blocks: intraventricular block or ventricular arrhythmias.
- QT interval
  » QT interval varies with heart rate.
  » Bazett's formula is used to correct the QT for heart rate (HR):
  $QTc = QT\ measured/(\sqrt{R\text{-}R\ interval})$

» Normal QTc
Infant < 6 months = <0.49 seconds
Infant > 6 months = <0.44 seconds
» QTc is prolonged in hypocalcemia, myocarditis and head injury.
» QTc is short in hypercalcemia: digitalis effect and congenital short QT syndrome.
5. **P-wave amplitude and duration**
   - Normal P-wave amplitude is <3 mm (tall P wave = right atrial enlargement).
   - Normal P-wave duration is > 0.09 seconds in children and <0.07 seconds in infants (wide P waves = left atrial enlargement).
   - A combination of tall and wide P wave occurs in combined atrial hypertrophy.
6. **QRS amplitude (voltages)**
   - High QRS amplitude is found in ventricular hypertrophy: ventricular conduction disturbances.
   - Low QRS amplitudes are seen in pericarditis, myocarditis, hypothyroidism, and normal newborns.
   - Ventricular hypertrophy produces changes in one or more of the following areas: the QRS axis, the QRS voltages, the R/S ratio, or the *T* axis.
7. **Q waves**
   Characteristics of normal Q waves:
   - Narrow (average 0.02 seconds and < 0.03 seconds)
   - Usually < 5-mm deep in left pericardial leads and aVF
   - May be as deep as 8 mm in lead III in children younger than 3 years.
8. **ST segment**
   - The normal ST is isoelectric. Elevation or depression is judged in a relation to the TP segment.
   - Pathological ST segment changes are commonly associated with T waves.
   - Changes occur in pericarditis, myocardial ischemia, or infarction: severe ventricular hypertrophy (ventricular strain pattern); digitalis effect.

Highlights

✦ Electrocardiogram (ECG or EKG from Greek: *Kardia*, meaning heart) is the recording of the electrical activity of the heart.
✦ An ECG produces a pattern reflecting the electrical activity of the heart, which can give information regarding the rhythm of the heart.
✦ Use therapeutic play: allow the child to touch the leads and provide play materials to get cooperation.
✦ ECGs for children in the under 5-year age-group must include an extra lead ("V4R") on the right side of the chest at a point analogous to the left-sided V4.
✦ When taking ECG using cardiac monitor note that leads I, II, and III are most commonly used in children.

FINE NEEDLE ASPIRATION

Definition

Fine needle aspiration is also called fine needle biopsy is a technique that allows a biopsy of various bumps and lumps. Fine needle aspiration is a test done to see if a tumor is benign (noncancerous) or malignant (cancerous).

Indications

- For cytological and bacteriological examination of a mass or a lymph node.
- It aids in tissue diagnosis and in determining what the course of management should be.

Equipment Needed

A sterile tray containing:
- 2.4- to 4-cm (20- to 25-ga) needle (a small bore needle causes less shearing force on tissues but obtains a very prompt sample)

- 10- to 20-mL plastic disposable syringe
- Clean glass slides
- 70–90% ethanol for routine wet fixation
- Containers with specific culture media (if necessary)
- Antiseptic cotton wipes in a bowl
- Pair of gloves
- Kidney tray

Preparation

- Explain the procedure to the child and parents.
- Demonstrate on stuffed toys if age appropriate.
- Use distraction techniques.

Procedure

- Perform hand hygiene and don gloves.
- Sterilize the site with antiseptic wipes.
- Local anesthesia, though usually not required, may be employed in anxious children.
- Immobilize the lump or the skin over the area to be biopsied between your thumb and finger with one hand.
- Hold the syringe in the other hand and insert the needle into assigned area, perpendicular to skin surface and position the needle within target tissues.
- Pull the syringe plunger to apply negative pressure.
- As pressure is maintained, make several punctures through the lump.
- Release the negative pressure.
- While the needle remains in target tissue, withdraw the needle.
- Detach the needle, clear some air, 2–3 mL into the syringe.
- Reattach the needle and blow aspirate on to the slide.

Postprocedure Care

- Apply a plaster over the site.
- Send the specimen for laboratory test.
- Document the procedure with date and time.

Precautions to be Taken

The following factors may contribute to an unsatisfactory yield during fine needle aspiration cytology (FNAC):
- When the needle misses the lesion tangentially
- When the central area is cystic/necrotic/hemorrhagic and devoid of diagnostic material
- When there is a small malignant lesion close to a dominant benign mass
- When the target tissue is fibrosclerotic and poor in cells

General Instructions

- As the sample tissue is very small, it gets stuck into the syringe lumen and is hard to remove. So, there is need to repeat the procedure.
- Deep biopsies can be obtained with the assistance of radiological and imaging techniques, such as ultrasonography.

Highlights ●●●●

- ✦ Fine needle aspiration is also called fine needle biopsy is a technique that allows a biopsy of various bumps and lumps.
- ✦ Fine needle aspiration is a test done to see if a tumor is benign (noncancerous) or malignant (cancerous).
- ✦ As the sample tissue is very small, it gets stuck into the syringe lumen and is hard to remove. So, there is need to repeat the procedure.
- ✦ Deep biopsies can be obtained with the assistance of radiological and imaging techniques, such as ultrasonography.
- ✦ Some factors may contribute to an unsatisfactory yield during fine needle aspiration cytology (FNAC).

MEMORY EXERCISE

1. Bone marrow aspiration is planned for a 3-year old child at 10 AM. What is an appropriate time to apply EMLA cream to achieve the intended purpose?
   a. 7 AM
   b. 8 AM
   c. 9 AM
   d. 9.30 AM

2. Which of the following methods give accurate information regarding urine protein excretion?
   a. Dipstick testing
   b. Frothy urine
   c. Spot urine for protein/creatinine ratio
   d. 24-hour urine for protein and creatinine excretion

3. A 10-year-old child had undergone lumbar puncture procedure. The best postprocedure position to be given to the child is:
   a. Prone for 2 hours to prevent aspiration, if vomits
   b. Semi-Fowler's position for 5 hours so that the child can watch television
   c. Supine for several hours, to prevent headache
   d. Right lateral position to encourage return of CSF

4. ECG lead R4V is placed in:
   a. 3rd intercostal space, right midclavicular line
   b. 4th intercostal space, right midclavicular line
   c. 5th intercostal space, right midclavicular line
   d. Right sterna border

5. The pulse that must be assessed and noted before the child goes for cardiac catheterization:
   a. Radial pulse
   b. Apical pulse
   c. Dorsalis pedis pulse
   d. Femoral pulse

CHAPTER 4

Meeting Nutritional Needs

LEARNING OBJECTIVES

Upon the completion of this chapter, the learners will be able to:
- List the needs for nutritional support.
- Counsel the mothers regarding exclusive breastfeeding.
- Demonstrate sterilization of feeding articles.
- Collect the equipment needed for feeding.
- Explain the children and parents need for nutritional support.
- Perform various feeding procedures.

Keywords: breast milk, Ryle's tube, gastrostomy, jejunostomy, total parenteral nutrition, peripheral venous access, complications, nutrition

ASSISTING IN BREASTFEEDING

Introduction

Lactation is the physiological process that leads to the secretion of milk in alveoli of the female breast, its passage along the ducts due to the "let-down" reflex, and its ejection into the mouth of the baby by suckling.

Breastfeeding comprises more than lactation. It adds to the interaction between the mother and baby, her response to his signals and his response to hers, the tactile contact between the nursing couple and the ingestion of milk by the baby.

Advantages of Breastfeeding

- The breastfeeding provides close physical contact between the neonate and the mother, which provides satisfaction. It provides an opportunity for bonding.
- Breast milk is available at the required temperature in required strength and is fresh and free of contamination.
- It contains more lactalbumin, which can be easily digested because of soft curds.
- Presence of extra lactose helps in synthesis of some vitamins. It also contains cystine, an amino acid that may be essential during the neonatal period.
- Early breastfeeding helps the mother in rapid involution of the uterus.
- Confers passive immunity
- Is protective against measles and other communicable diseases.
- Provides optimal growth and neurological development.

- Protects against cold weather
- Reduces the incidence of childhood cancer
- Enhances visual development
- Provides natural way of spacing pregnancy
- Decreases the incidence of breast and ovarian cancer among women
- Removes the economic burden on families due to the high cost of artificial feeding

Indications for Assisting in Breastfeeding

- Primi mothers
- With cesarean section
- Those who delivered a premature baby
- Those who delivered a low-birth-weight baby
- Those who delivered twins/triplets
- Those who delivered baby with cleft lip/palate

Nurse's Responsibility in Breastfeeding

Antenatal Preparation

- During antenatal checkup, the nurse needs to help the mother if she has any specific problems relating to breastfeeding, such as the size of the breasts, nipples, etc. Provide strong emotional support after delivery when they are going through a lot of mood swings due to hormonal changes.
- Examine the nipples to see whether they are normal and protractile.
- The care of nipples is necessary to prevent mechanical problems of feeding. If nipples are retracted, they should be pulled out at least once a day.
- Advice the mother to wear appropriate-size brassiere during pregnancy.
  - Calculating brassiere size during pregnancy:
  Measure the rib cage of expectant mother under the breast in inches and add 4–5 inches for an even number. This is the brassiere size (S1)—32, 34, etc. Measure the top of the mother's breast without a bra on (S2). S2 - S1 = cup size (AA, A, B, C, D, DD, etc.). For example, <1 inch means A.
- Advice the mother to eat well-balanced diet with extra proteins, calcium, and iron.
- Mother should be informed during pregnancy of the following:
  - The advantages of breastfeeding
  - The importance of rooming in policy
  - The importance of unrestricted feeding
  - Correct technique of breastfeeding
  - Importance of colostrum
  - The mother should be told that the adequate milk is secreted from the third day of the postpartum.

Positioning

Any position that is comfortable to the mother is acceptable because she has to feed frequently and for longer durations. There are many ways a mother can hold the baby to breastfeed (**Figs. 4.1A to D**).

The most common methods are:

- *Indian method*: Sitting on the floor cross-legged with one thigh drawn up on which the baby's back is resting; the mother has her baby close to her.
- *Cradle position*: Sitting, the mother cradles the baby in her arm.
- *Modified cradle position*: Sitting, the mother cradles the baby in her arm. Her hand supports the baby's head and neck.
- *Football hold*: Sitting or leaning back, the baby is under the mother's arm with his feet pointing back. His abdomen touches the side of the mother's chest. The baby's body is supported by the mother's arm. This position is good for feeding twins simultaneously.
- *Side lying position*: Lying on her side, with baby facing the mother supports the baby's head and neck with her arm. This position

Chapter 4: Meeting Nutritional Needs

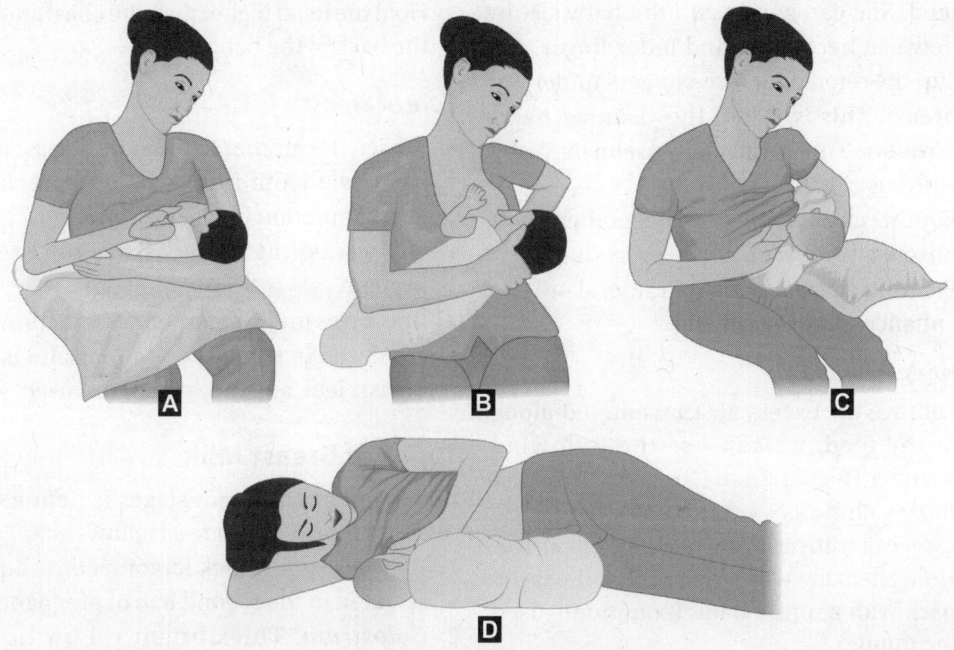

Figs. 4.1A to D: Different positions for breastfeeding. (A) Cradle hold; (B) Cross-cradle hold; (C) Football hold; (D) Lying down.

is comfortable for night feeds and when the mother has a cesarean operation.
- *Supine position*: Lying on her back with baby's face down on her chest, the mother's hand supports the baby's head on her breast. She uses the other hand to hold the breast and helps the baby attach (latch on) well to the nipple and areola. The supine position helps to avoid pain immediately after cesarean section and makes it possible for a drowsy mother to breastfeed.

In all these positions:
- The baby's head and body should be in straight line.
- Baby's face should face the breast, with nose opposite the nipple.
- Mother should hold the baby's body close to hers.
- Mother should support the newborn's bottom also, and not just the head and shoulders.

Attachment

Good attachment at the breast ensures sufficient production, release, and flow of milk.

Help the mother to attach the baby well to the breast as follows:
- Her nipple should touch the baby's upper lip, cheek, or side of the mouth (rooting reflex).
- As soon as the baby opens its mouth wide, mother should bring the baby to the breast by aiming baby's lower lip toward the base of the areola (lower portion).
- She may use one of the hands to support and offer the breast. This support can be provided either with the mother's fingers placed flat against her ribs at the base of her breast or with her hand cupping her breast.
- If the baby has difficulty staying attached to the breast, the mother can support her breast, baby's chin and jaw to stabilize and maintain good attachment throughout the

feed. She can gently cup the baby's chin between her thumb and index finger and cup the remaining three fingers under the breast. This is called the "Dancer hand position." This is especially useful in a baby who has cleft lip.
- Educate and demonstrate the mother about burping in between and after feeding.
- Position the baby in right lateral side to enhance gastric emptying.

Burping technique

To remove the excess air that entered along with the feed, we can use the following techniques (**Figs. 4.2A to C**):
- Baby's chin rests on the shoulder of the caregiver with head and neck are supported. Hold the baby with one hand and pat the back with another hand (commonly used technique).
- Keep the baby in sitting position on the caregiver's lap, supporting the chest with base of hand and cupping the chin with thumb and index fingers. Pat the back of the baby with another hand.
- Lay the baby across the lap in prone position with abdomen rest on the thigh of caregiver. Hold the head higher than the chest and pat the back of the baby.

Care of Breast
- Advice the mother to clean the breast with clean wet cloth from nipple to areola in circular motion before feeding.
- Daily washing is necessary for breast hygiene.
- Brassieres may be worn in order to provide comfortable support and are useful if the breasts leak and breast pads are used.

Types of Breast Milk

Breast milk at different stages is defined by different terms. They are as follows:
1. *Precolostrum*: Thick lemon yellow liquid secreted in the second half of pregnancy.
2. *Colostrum*: Thick bright yellow liquid secreted during the first 3–6 days after the delivery of the baby. It contains more protein than mature milk.
3. *Transition milk*: During the second week that follows the colostrum stage, the milk increases in quantity and changes in appearance and composition. The

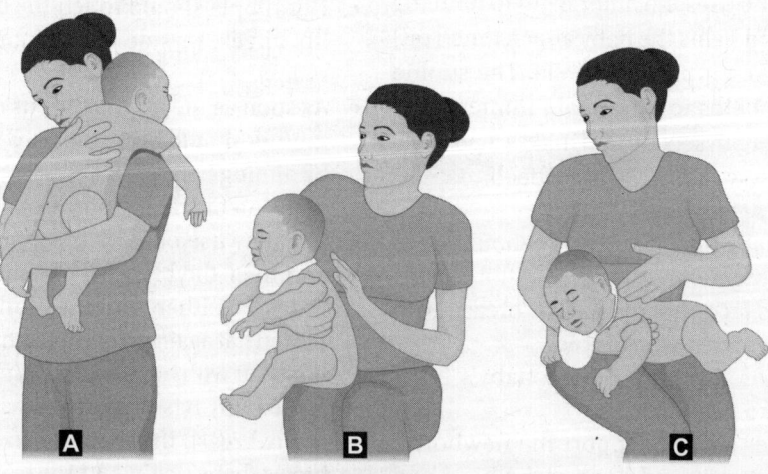

Figs. 4.2A to C: Burping technique.

immunoglobulin and protein content decreases, while the fat and sugar content increases. The breasts feel full, hard, and heavy. Some people call this phase as the breast milk "coming in."

4. *Preterm milk*: Milk produced by a woman who has delivered prematurely. This milk has more protein, minerals, immunoglobulin, and lactoferrin than mature milk, making it more suited for the needs of a premature baby. Preterm milk is essential and best suited for the survival and growth of a premature baby.

5. *Mature milk*: Mature milk increases in quantity and contains all the nutrients needed for healthy physical and mental development of the baby, though it appears more watery than cow's milk. Mature milk changes even during the length of a single feed exactly suit the needs of a particular baby.

6. *Foremilk*: The milk that comes at the start of a feed is called foremilk. This milk is watery and pearl blue in color; has low level of fat; and is high in lactose, protein, vitamins, and minerals. It satisfies the baby's thirst and is produced in large quantity than hind milk.

7. *Hind milk*: The milk that comes later in the feed is four times rich in fat, which makes it appear white than foremilk. It satisfies the baby's hunger and supplies much energy of a breastfeed.

Signs of Adequate Feeding

- *Adequate urine output:* An exclusively breastfed baby usually passes dilute urine at least six to eight times in 24 hours except the first 3 days of birth, when the baby is on colostrum.
- *Weight gain:* For the first 6 months of life, a baby should gain at least 500 g of weight each month or 125 g each week.
- Abundant milk flow in 2–4 days of delivery.
- Correct latch on and rhythmical sucking.
- At least 8–12 feeds/day.
- Baby should appear satisfied after nursing and probably will fall asleep at the second breast.

Contraindications to Breastfeeding

- *Drugs:* When the mother is on certain drugs, breastfeeding may be suspended temporarily.
- *Cancer:* If the mother has cancer, the treatment she receives will make it impossible to breastfeed without harming the baby.
- Breast surgery
- Breast injury
- Human immunodeficiency virus (HIV) infection

Problems with Breastfeeding

Difficulties Due to Mother

- Breast engorgement
- Deep breast pain
- Mastitis
- Breast abscess
- Blocked ducts
- *Breast problems:* Sore and damaged nipples, dermatitis, anatomical variations (long nipples, short nipples, abnormally large nipples, and inverted and flat nipples)

Difficulties Due to Baby

- Cleft lip and cleft palate
- Tongue-tie
- Blocked nose
- Down syndrome babies
- Prematurity
- Illness or surgery

Expressing Breast Milk

Indications

- Where there is concern about the interval between feeds in the early newborn period

Chapter 4: Meeting Nutritional Needs

Table 4.1: Breast milk storage.

Type of breast milk	Storage location and temperatures		
	Countertop 77°F (25°C) or colder (room temperature)	*Refrigerator 40°F (4°C)*	*Freezer 0°F (−18°C) or colder*
Freshly expressed or pumped	Up to 4 hours	Up to 4 days	▪ Within 6 months is best ▪ Up to 12 months is acceptable
Thawed, previously frozen	1–2 hours	Up to 1 day (24 hours)	Never refreeze human milk after it has been thawed
Leftover feeding (expressed milk is fed through bottle)	Use within 2 hours after the baby is finished feeding		

- Where there are problems in attaching the baby to the breast.
- Where the baby is separated from the mother, owing to prematurity or illness.
- Where there is concern about the baby's rate of growth, or the mother's milk supply (expressing to top up with the mother's own milk may be necessary in the short-term while the cause of the problem is resolved).
- Later in lactation, when the mother may need to be separated from her baby for periods (occasionally or regularly).

Methods of Expressing Breast Milk

- Manual expression of milk
- Expressing with a breast pump
- Hand pumps
  - Manually controlled
  - Electrically controlled

General Guidelines for Storage of Breast Milk

- The lactating mothers and the family members can be educated about storage of breast milk in home setting.
- Various factors, such as amount of milk, temperature of the atmosphere during milk expression, temperature fluctuations if any in refrigerator and freezer, and hygiene have influence on duration of breast milk storage (**Table 4.1**).

Highlights ●●●●

✦ Lactation is the physiological process that leads to the secretion of milk in alveoli of the female breast, its passage along the ducts due to the "let-down" reflex, and its ejection into the mouth of the baby by suckling.

✦ Breastfeeding is the interaction between the mother and baby, her response to his signals and his response to hers, the tactile contact between the nursing couple and the ingestion of milk by the baby.

✦ Breast milk at different stages is defined by different terms: precolostrum, colostrum, transition milk, preterm milk, mature milk, foremilk, and hind milk.

✦ The care of nipples is necessary to prevent mechanical problems of feeding. If nipples are retracted, they should be pulled out at least once a day.

✦ Any position that is comfortable to the mother is acceptable because she has to feed frequently and for longer durations.

✦ Good attachment at the breast ensures sufficient production, release, and flow of milk.

✦ To remove the excess air that entered along with the feed, we need to burp the baby.

Contd...

Contd...

> ✦ Advice the mother to clean the breast before feeding with clean wet cloth from nipple to areola in circular motion.
> ✦ Signs of adequate feeding are adequate urine output, weight gain, abundant milk flow in 2–4 days of delivery, correct latch on and rhythmical sucking, at least 8–12 feeds/day, and baby will fall asleep at the second breast.

CLEANING AND STERILIZATION OF FEEDING ARTICLES

Equipment
- Bottle with cap, rim, and teat
- Strainer
- Spoon
- Saucepan with lid or any stainless steel vessel with lid
- Cups with lid
- Measuring glass
- Paladai
- Soap solution with scrubber
- Bottle brush
- Water source
- Sterilizer or big pan with lid

Procedure
- Rinse the feeding bottle with running water, then using soap solution clean the bottle with bottle brush.
- Mouth of the bottle should be washed first using rotatory movement, then wash the inside and outside of the bottle using the same motion.
- Clean the teat by inverting it.
- Wash all other equipment using the scrubber.
- Put all the articles, including feeding bottle, in sterilizer or big vessel containing water.
- Boil for 7–10 minutes after it reaches boiling point.
- Then put all the plastic articles and boil for 3–5 minutes.
- Remove all the sterile equipment from the vessel or sterilizer and place it in sterile container.

Highlights ● ● ● ●

> ✦ Mouth of the bottle should be washed first using rotatory movement, then wash the inside and outside of the bottle using the same motion.
> ✦ Wash all other equipment using the scrubber.
> ✦ Put all the articles, including feeding bottle, in sterilizer or big vessel containing water and boil.
> ✦ The sterile equipment should be placed in a sterile container.

FORMULA FEEDING

Definition
Artificial feeding is a form of supplementary or substituted feeding given instead of breastfeeding.

Indications (May be Absolute or Relative)
- Insufficient breast milk
- Death of the mother
- Working mother
- Pregnancy
- Diseases of the breasts, for example, mastitis
- Mother who is on any medications incompatible to breastfeeding, for example, sulfonamides
- Infectious disease of the mother, for example, tuberculosis (TB) and HIV
- Chronic diseases, for example, heart and kidney diseases, communicable diseases, and major injuries
- Mental illness
- A child with poor sucking reflex, for example, prematurity and birth trauma

Equipment Needed

- *A sterile vessel contains:* Bottle, teat, cap, rim, cups with lid, paladai (**Fig. 4.3**), strainer, ounce glass, and spoon
- *A clean tray contains:*
  - Duster
  - Transferring forceps
  - Boiled cooled water in a kettle
  - Sugar
  - A jug with milk, or prescribed formula tin
  - Saucepan with lid to boil milk
  - Big bowl with water to cool the milk
  - Bib
  - Draw sheet and mackintosh
  - Gown

Procedure

Formula Preparation

- Check the doctor's order and do the calculation accordingly.
- Collect the necessary equipment.
- Wash hands with soap and water.
- Measure the required amount of water and milk and pour in saucepan.
- Add 1 teaspoon of sugar to 90 mL of liquid.
- Boil the milk until it reaches boiling point.
- Cool the milk in the bowl of water till it is warm enough for the child to drink.
- Strain the milk into a cup.
- Pour into the feeding bottle.
- Place teat, cover the bottle, and take it to bedside.

Feeding

- Wash hands and wear gown.
- Make sure that the baby is dry and clean.
- Place a mackintosh and a draw sheet under the infant buttocks to prevent soiling of cloth as a result of gastrocolic reflex that is stimulated by feeding.
- Mummify the infant if needed.
- Put towel or bib under the chin to prevent the soiling of infant's dress.
- The nurse or the mother should sit comfortably on a chair with legs crossed.
- The infant should be held in semi-Fowler's position with head on the crook of the arm.
- Test the temperature of the milk and rate of flow. Drop a few drops on the inner aspect of the palm.
- The size of the teat hole must be according to the formula (rice porridge—big hole, newborn—small hole).
- Place the entire nipple tip in the infant's mouth.
- Bottle should be held in upright throughout the feeding to prevent air entering.
- The nipple should be always filled with milk otherwise the infant will suck in air.
- In between and after feeding, the baby should be burped and cuddled.
- Place the baby in bed in right lateral position to facilitate gastric emptying.
- Wash and replace the articles.
- Record accurately the amount offered, amount taken, any vomiting, etc.

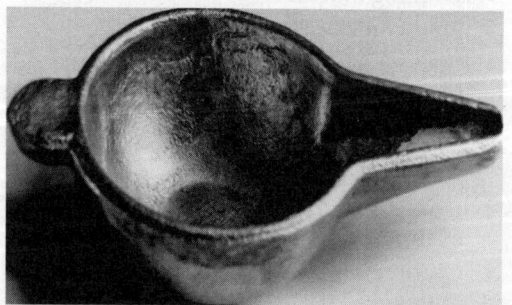

Fig. 4.3: Paladai.

Highlights ● ● ● ●

- ✦ Artificial feeding is a form of supplementary or substituted feeding given instead of breastfeeding.
- ✦ The indications may be absolute or relative, such as death of mother and insufficient milk production.
- ✦ To test the temperature of the milk and rate of flow, put a few drops on the inner aspect of the palm.
- ✦ The infant should be held in semi-Fowler's position with head on the crook of the arm for feeding.
- ✦ The size of the teat hole must be according to the formula. Bottle should be held in upright throughout the feeding to prevent air entering.
- ✦ The nipple should be always filled with milk otherwise the infant will suck in air.
- ✦ Place the baby in bed in right lateral position to facilitate gastric emptying.

GAVAGE FEEDING

Definition
Commonly called tube feeding involves insertion of tube via nose or mouth with the tube ending in the stomach. It is otherwise called nasogastric (NG) or orogastric feedings.

Indications

Short-term Enteral Feeding

It is indicated for the children who have a functioning gastrointestinal (GI) tract but cannot ingest enough nutrients orally.
- The child may be unconscious or have a severely debilitating condition that interferes with his/her ability to consume adequate food and fluids.

Other Conditions Include
- Failure to thrive
- Inability to suck or tiring easily during sucking
- Abnormalities of throat or esophagus
- Swallowing difficulties or risk for aspiration
- Respiratory distress
- Metabolic conditions
- Surgery
- Severe trauma

Equipment Needed
A tray containing:
- Ryle's tube (6–8 Fr) for insertion
- Sterile water in a bowl to lubricate the tube and check placement of the tube
- 5-mL syringe for aspirating gastric contents and feeding
- Feeding cup with water for flushing the tube
- Prescribed formula for feeding
- Adhesive tape and scissors to fix the tube in position
- Cotton tip applicators to clean the nostrils

General Instructions
- Position the baby on the back with folded towel placed under the shoulders to elevate the head slightly.
- In the case of older children, head end of the bed to be elevated during feeding.
- Application of mummy restraint may be necessary to control the child's movement during tube insertion.
- Infant's hands may be restrained using a soft restraint to prevent grasp of gavage tube and its removal.
- For gavage feeding of infants, sterile equipment should be used.
- Feeding amount should be calculated.
- Use sterile water or saline to lubricate the tube. Do not use oil because of the dangers of aspiration into the lungs.
- For small infants, pass the tube through mouth because infants are nasal breathers.
- The flow of feeding should be slow. Do not apply pressure.
- Elevate the reservoir of feed 15–20 cm above the child's head.

- Feeding should be given about 5 mL/5–10 minutes or 15–20 minutes total time.
- Weigh the child daily.
- The feeding formula should be at room temperature.

Preparation
- Verify the order for the gavage feeding.
- Explain the procedure to the child and parents using appropriate language geared to the child's developmental level.
- Gather necessary equipment.

Procedure
- Wash hands and put on gloves.
- Inspect the child's nose and mouth for any deformities that may interfere with the passage of the tube.
- Position the infant supine with the head slightly elevated and with the neck hyperextended so that nose is pointed upward.
- Assist the older child to sitting position if appropriate.
- Alternatively have the parents or another person to hold the child to promote comfort and reassurance.
- Determine the tubing length for insertion measure from the tip of the nose to the earlobe to the middle of the area between the xiphoid process and umbilicus. Mark this measurement on the tube with indelible pen or with a piece of tape (**Fig. 4.4**).
- Lubricate the tube with generous amount of sterile water or water-soluble lubricant to promote the passage of the tube and minimize trauma to the child's mucosa.
- Insert the tube into one of the nares or the mouth. Direct nasally insert tube straight back toward the occiput; direct an orally inserted tube toward the back of the throat.
- Advance the tube slowly to the designated length. Encourage the child if capable of swallowing frequently to assist with advancing the tube.
- Watch for signs of distress, such as gasping, coughing, or cyanosis indicating that tube is in airway.
- If these signs develop withdraw the tube and allow the child to rest before attempting reinsertion.
- Check for proper placement of the tube by attaching a syringe to the end of tube and aspirate stomach content.
- Return any aspirated contents to the stomach.
- Secure the tube in cheek.

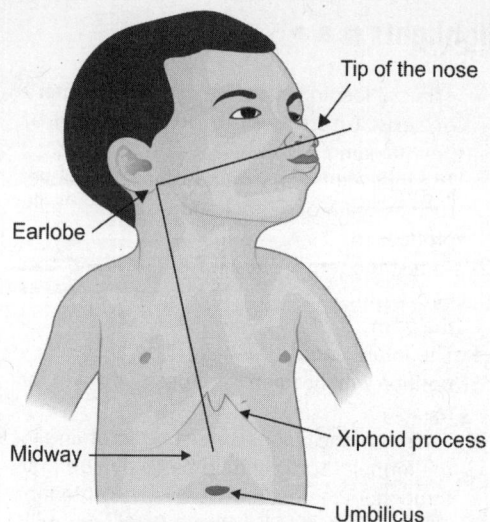

Fig. 4.4: Measuring the length of nasogastric tube in children.

Postprocedure Care
Document the type of tube inserted, length of tubing inserted, measurement of external tubing length after insertion, and conformation of placement.

Administering Tube Feeding
Tube feeding can be given continuously or intermittently (bolus feeding).

Bolus feedings: A specified amount of feeding solution is given at specific intervals, usually over a short period of time, such as 15–30 minutes. It can be given via syringe, feeding bag, or infusion pump.

Continuous feeding: Given at a slower rate over long period of time and enteral feeding pump is used to administer the solution at a prescribed rate.

Steps

1. Check for the tube placement.
2. Measure the gastric residual (the amount remaining in the stomach indicates gastric emptying time) by aspirating gastric contents.
3. Place the child in supine position with the head and shoulders elevated approximately 30°.
4. Flush the tube with small amount of water to clear it.
5. Place the feed in barrel of syringe or into a feeding bag attached to the feeding tube and allow it to flow by gravity.
6. Monitor the child's tolerance to the feeding.
7. Once the feeding is complete but before the formula completely empty from the container, flush the tube with water.
8. As the water leaves the syringe, clamp the tube to prevent air from entering the stomach.
9. Disconnect the syringe or tube feeding bag from the tube.
10. Burp the infant during and after tube feeding.
11. Position the baby on his or her right side with head slightly elevated (30°) for about 1 hour after the feeding to facilitate gastric emptying and reduce the risk of aspiration and regurgitation.

Points to Remember

- Instilling air into the stomach and then auscultating for the sound is no longer considered a viable method for checking tube placement.
- Air instilled into the tube that is positioned above the gastroesophageal sphincter can still be auscultated as air in the stomach there by giving a false positive result.
- Small diameter feeding tubes, though more comfortable, may easily become dislodged if the child coughs vigorously.
- Tube should be changed every 72 hours or as per institutional policy.
- If the child vomits during feeding, stop feeding immediately and turn him on to his side or sit him up.

Highlights ●●●●

- Tube feeding involves insertion of tube via nose or mouth with the tube ending in the stomach. It is otherwise called NG or orogastric feedings.
- It is indicated for the children who have a functioning GI tract but cannot ingest enough nutrients orally.
- Use Ryle's tube (6–8 Fr) for insertion.
- For small infants, pass the tube through mouth because infants are nasal breathers.
- Feeding should be given about 5 mL/5–10 minutes or 15–20 minutes total time.
- Determine the tubing length for insertion measure from the tip of the nose to the earlobe to the middle of the area between the xiphoid process and umbilicus.
- Check for proper placement of the tube by attaching a syringe to the end of tube and aspirate stomach content. Instilling air into the stomach and then auscultating for the sound is no longer considered a viable method for checking tube placement.
- Tube feeding can be given continuously or intermittently (bolus feeding).
- Once the feeding is complete but before the formula completely empty from the container, flush the tube with water.
- If the child vomits during feeding, stop feeding immediately and turn him on to his side or sit him up.

GASTROSTOMY FEEDING

Definition
Gastrostomy feeding is a method of administration of fluids through the surgical opening into the stomach via the opening at abdominal wall.

Indications
- Congenital abnormalities, such as esophageal/choanal atresia or tracheo-esophageal fistula
- Conditions that require long-term enteral feeding
- Esophageal injury
- Esophageal dysmotility
- Child has a functioning GI tract but is unable to meet his/her total nutritional requirements orally.

Contraindications
- Gross ascites/severe obesity
- Clotting abnormalities
- Gastroparesis
- Esophageal/gastric varices and ulceration
- Complete intestinal obstruction
- Uncontrolled gastroesophageal reflux with a risk of pulmonary aspiration

Methods of Gastrostomy Feeding
- *Continuous*: Over an extended time period feeding is given by a pump at a slow rate, for example, 30 mL/24 h (**Fig. 4.5**).
- *Bolus*: A large amount of feeding is given 3–6 times/day, sometimes given by a pump over a certain amount of time (1 hour), or simply allowed to run into the stomach by gravity using a roller clamp to slow down flow as necessary.
- *Direct*: Direct feeds are given with the feeding set hooked directly into the gastrostomy tube.
- *Chimney*: Chimney feeds are given by dripping the feeding into a vent that is attached to the gastrostomy tube.

Equipment Needed
- Feeding syringe (about 60–100 mL)
- Disposable gavage bag with tubing
- IV stand, measuring cup, formula, glass of water

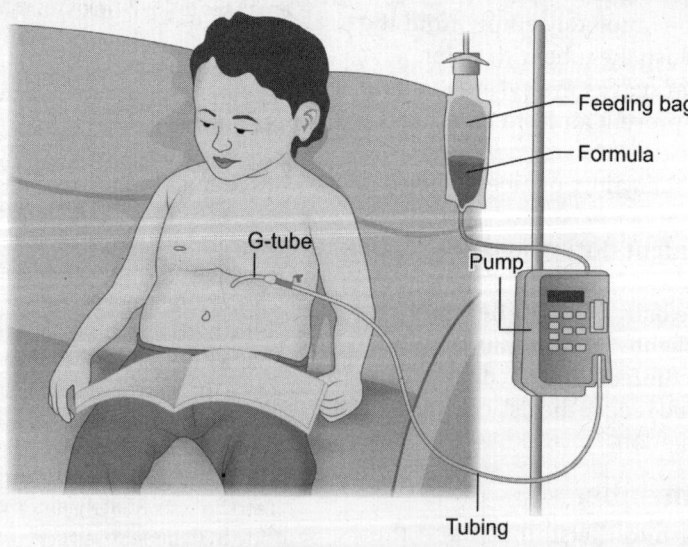

Fig. 4.5: Pump method.

- Administration set
- Pair of gloves
- Stethoscope to auscultate the bowel sounds

Preparation
- Confirm the patient, instructions, and order.
- Explain the procedure to the child and parents as appropriate.
- Auscultate for bowel sounds.
- Check the condition of gastrostomy site.
- Check if your formula is warm or at room temperature by putting a few drops on your wrist.

Procedure (Syringe Method)
- Perform hand hygiene.
- Pour correct amount of formula into a clean measuring cup or clean baby bottle.
- Place the child in a comfortable position. If possible place the child in a high chair or at the table during mealtime.
- Insert the syringe tip into the feeding tube or bolus extension set for the MIC-KEY or Bard Button (**Fig. 4.6**).
- Flush tubing with 3–5 mL of water before starting the formula feeding.
- Slowly pour the formula into the syringe.
- Unclamp the feeding tube. The feeding rate can be controlled by raising or lowering the syringe.
- The feeding should take about the same amount of time as it would take a child drink the formula, about 15–20 minutes.
- When all the formula has been given, flush the tubing with water.
- Burp the child after each feeding if appropriate.
- Rinse the feeding supplies with warm water after each feeding and allow to air-dry.

Procedure (Drip Method)
- Connect the bag with tubing and fill the bag with feed.

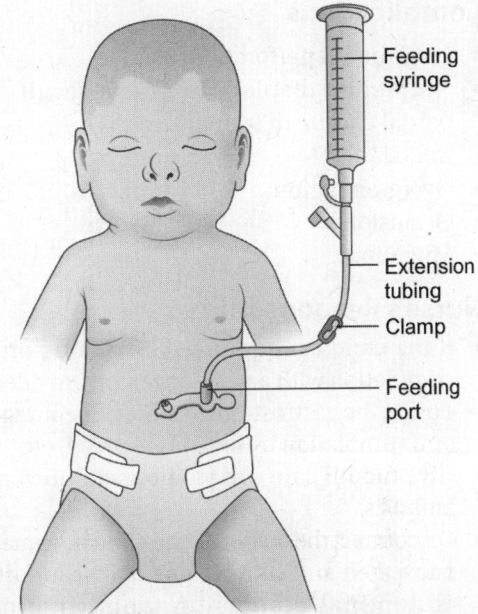

Fig. 4.6: Syringe method.

- Hang it on the IV stand and expel air.
- Open the clamp so that the food fills with no air.
- Close the clamp.
- Insert the catheter tip into the G-tube
- On finishing, flush the tube with water.
- Clamp the G-tube
- Remove the feeding system

Switching to a Skin Level Device or Button

Once the child's gastrostomy site is well healed and the tract is developed, it is possible to switch to a skin level feeding device. These devices are commonly called "buttons."

There are several types of buttons. The most common are the Bard and the MIC-KEY. The change to the button can be done once the tube has been in place for a minimum of 8 weeks.

Complications
- Large bowel perforation/fistula
- Accidental displacement can result in partial closure of stoma
- Infection
- Overgranulation
- Occlusion
- Migration

Nurse's Responsibility
- If the child cannot be fed by mouth, oral stimulation with a pacifier can be provided during the gastrostomy feeding. Encourage oral stimulation by blowing, kissing, etc.
- Give mouth care every 4 hours to prevent halitosis.
- Disconnect the feeding if the child becomes nauseated and shows signs of discomfort, abdominal distension, vomiting, or difficulty in breathing.
- Remember to flush the feeding tube with water between all feeding and medications.
- *Care of the tube:* In the first 2–3 days, the gastrostomy site should be cleaned 2–3 times/day with half-strength hydrogen peroxide. After 2–3 days, the site should be cleaned with mild soap and water.
- Take measure to prevent contamination of feed.
- *Bathing:* Sponging can be given for first 2–3 days to keep the child's new gastrostomy site dry.
- Showering can be given after 2 days. Clean the site and pat dry after showering.
- Swimming is restricted until the stitch is removed.
- *Venting the tube:* Place a 60-cc syringe with the plunger removed into the end of the gastrostomy tube. If the tube is clamped, open the clamp.
- Hold the syringe above the child's stomach for a few minutes. If gas is present, you can hear the gas bubbles up through the tube or sometimes even see stomach contents back up into the tube and syringe.
- Once the gas is removed, allow the formula to flow slowly back into the stomach.
- Make early referral to speech therapist for children requiring long-term feeding.

Accidental Tube Expulsion
- If tube comes out, cover the site with a clean, dry gauze pad or cloth.
- Once the tube is out, hole will begin to close and may close completely in 4–6 hours.
- So the child should be replaced with new gastrostomy tube immediately and should be checked under X-ray for proper placement.
- Balloon devices should be deflated and reinforced weekly to ensure that correct amount of fluid remains in the balloon.

Activity Restrictions
- Child should not lift anything heavier than 5 lb (4.4 kg) and should not participate in vigorous activity for 2 weeks after surgery.
- The school nurse/teacher needs instruction filled by the hospital and signed by doctor.

Highlights ●●●

✦ Gastrostomy feeding is a method of administration of fluids through the surgical opening into the stomach via the opening at abdominal wall.
✦ It can be given as continuous, bolus, direct, or chimney method.
✦ Once the child's gastrostomy site is well healed and the tract is developed, it is possible to switch to a skin level feeding device. These devices are commonly called "buttons."
✦ Oral stimulation with a pacifier can be provided during the gastrostomy feeding. Encourage oral stimulation by blowing, kissing, etc.
✦ Gastrostomy site should be cleaned 2–3 times/day with half-strength hydrogen peroxide for first 2–3 days. After 2–3 days, the site should be cleaned with mild soap and water.
✦ Make early referral to speech therapist for children requiring long-term feeding.

JEJUNOSTOMY FEEDING (POSTPYLORIC OR TRANSPYLORIC FEEDING)

Definition
Jejunostomy feeding is the method of feeding directly into the small intestine. In this procedure, the feeding tube is passed into the stomach, through the pylorus and into the jejunum.

Purposes
To provide full enteral nutrition via catheter directly into the jejunum.

Indications
- Children who have absent gag reflex with normal GI function
- Persistent vomiting resulting in failure to thrive
- Gastric dysmotility
- Gastric outlet obstruction
- Gastroparesis
- Pancreatitis
- Gastroesophageal reflux with high risk for aspiration
- *In case of newborns:* Low birth weight and respiratory distress to reduce effort.

Disadvantages
- Difficulty in placing tube
- High risk for GI infection due bypassing of natural microbiological defenses (acidic medium of stomach)
- Frequent tube blockage
- Need frequent flushing
- Decreased ambulation of the child because of long duration of feeding
- Need for frequent follow-up to check the placement, which may lead to repeated radiological exposure of the child

Equipment Needed
- 50–60 mL Asepto syringe (**Fig. 4.7**)
- Ounce glass
- Sterile water
- Prepared formula brought to room temperature
- Clamp
- Protective bed covering
- Enteral feeding bag and tubing/enteral feeding pump (optional)
- Gloves

Preparation of Child and Parents
- Explain the procedure to parents and child as appropriate.
- Elevate the child's bed to semi-Fowler's position to prevent aspiration and to facilitate digestion. In case of infants, they can be held in mother's lap as like regular feeding with head of baby in crook of mother's arm.
- Pacifier can be kept in mouth of infant for nonnutritive sucking unless contraindicated.

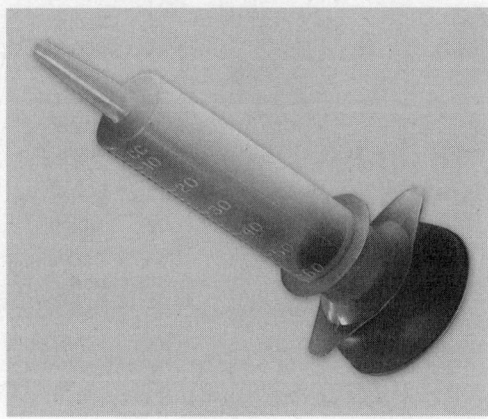

Fig. 4.7: Asepto syringe.

Procedure

- Wash hands and wear gloves.
- Prepare the measured amount of formula in appropriate container.
- Place the protective bed covering under tubing to protect bedding and clothes.
- Remove clamp or plug from the feeding tube.
- Check the placement by aspirating the contents with syringe.
- Connect syringe or enteral bag or pump tubing to Jejunostomy tube.
- Flush the tubing with at least 3 mL of sterile water to clear the lumen (**Fig. 4.8**).
- Fill the syringe with formula and release the feeding tube to allow formula to flow through (in the case of enteral tube or pump, open the regulator clamp and adjust flow rate).
- When syringe is three-quarters empty, add more solution.
- Instill the required amount of water to flush the tubing once the feeding is about to finish.
- Pinch the tubing and remove the syringe/enteral bag and clamp (or cap) the feeding tube.
- Burp the infant and position the child to right side with head end elevated.

Aftercare

- Discard the soiled supplies according to hospital policy.
- Clean all reusable articles dry and keep ready for next feeding.
- Document the procedure in nurses' record:
  - Amount, color, and consistency of contents aspirated before feeding
  - Type and amount of feeding formula
  - Child's response to the procedure
  - Findings of jejunostomy tube site assessment
  - If any medication is administered, details of name, dose, frequency, etc.

Complications

- Diarrhea
- Malabsorption
- Abdominal pain
- Dumping syndrome
- Abdominal cramps
- Abdominal distension

Nursing Considerations

- The formula should have low osmolality and at room temperature.
- The prepared formulas should not be kept for more than 24 hours.
- Formula can be administered intermittently or continuously as needed.
- In case of continuous feeding, assess the child frequently for abdominal distension.

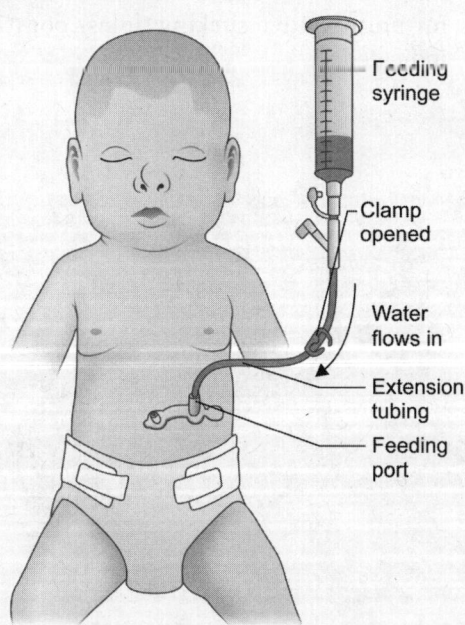

Fig. 4.8: Jejunostomy feeding in child.

- The formula should be liquid for easy feeding and preventing lumen block.
- Flushing of tube should be as per hospital policy.

Guidelines for Flushing the Jejunal Feeding Tubes

- Jejunal feeding tubes should be flushed regularly to maintain patency. Since there is a repeated blockage of tube due to narrow lumen, flushing can be done at least every 6 hours. Common flushing should be done:
  - Before feeding
  - After completion of feeding
  - Before and after administering medications through tube
  - Every fourth hourly if the tube is not used
  - Before changing each bottle in the case of continuous feeding
- Sterile water must be used to flush tubing to prevent infection.
- The amount of water for flushing should be based on child's fluid balance and size:
  - Older children: 3–5 mL
  - Newborn: 1–3 mL

Highlights ● ● ● ●

> - Jejunostomy feeding is the method of feeding directly into the small intestine. In this procedure, the feeding tube is passed into the stomach, through the pylorus and into the jejunum.
> - Jejunal feeding tubes should be flushed regularly to maintain patency.
> - Need for frequent follow-up to check the placement, which may lead to repeated radiological exposure of the child.
> - Formula can be administered intermittently or continuously as needed.
> - In case of continuous feeding, assess the child frequently for abdominal distension.

TOTAL PARENTERAL NUTRITION

Definition

Nutritional support can be administered through a central venous access is termed total parenteral nutrition (TNP). It is also called IV alimentation.

Indications

- Child with a prolonged starvation with a nonfunctioning GI tract, for example, intestinal obstruction, extensive bowel resection, and gastroschisis
- Severe failure to thrive
- Multisystem trauma or organ involvement
- Preterm newborns
- Bowel fistula, inadequate intestinal length with subsequent malabsorption
- Chronic nonremitting severe diarrhea
- Extensive body burns
- Abdominal tumors treated by surgery, irradiation, or chemotherapy

Purposes

- To provide all nutrients to meet child's needs
- To supply enough calories to maintain a positive nitrogen balance
- To maintain water and electrolyte homeostasis

Types/Components of Total Parenteral Nutrition Solution

1. Highly concentrated solution of carbohydrates (CHO)
2. Lipid emulsion to supply need for essential fatty acids
3. Total nutrient admixture (TNA) with components of total parenteral nutrition (TPN) plus lipids and other additives

TNA refers to a PN formula with CHO, lipids, amino acids, vitamins, minerals, water, trace elements, and other additives in a single container. It is also known as three-in-one admixture, trimix, or all-in-one parenteral admixture.

Methods of Total Parenteral Nutrition Administration

1. Continuous administration (over a 24-hour period)
2. Cyclic basis (over a 12-hour period during night)

Sites for Inserting Central Venous Catheter

- Superior vena cava or intrathoracic subclavian veins approached by way of external or internal jugular veins (**Fig. 4.9**)
- Inferior vena cava from a femoral vein (sometimes)

Note: The solutions require infusion into a vessel with sufficient volume to allow for rapid dilution to minimize phlebitis or irritation.

Venous Access Devices

There are various types of venous access devices available. The selection of the device is based on the factors, such as age of child, purpose, and duration of TPN (**Table 4.2**).

Complications

- Air embolism from inadvertent of air into the system during cap changes or accidental disconnections.
- Cardiac tamponade due to catheter advancement with movement of the arm, neck, or shoulder.
- Catheter occlusion from the development of a fibrin sheath or thrombus, kinking, malpositioning, deposition of precipitate, or blood clot.
- Venous thrombosis from injury to the vessel wall or administration of medications.
- Hyperglycemia (too rapid infusion)
- Hypoglycemia (rapid cessation)
- Dehydration due to increased renal excretions of excess glucose
- Electrolyte imbalance
- Infection at the insertion site, pathway, or in the bloodstream

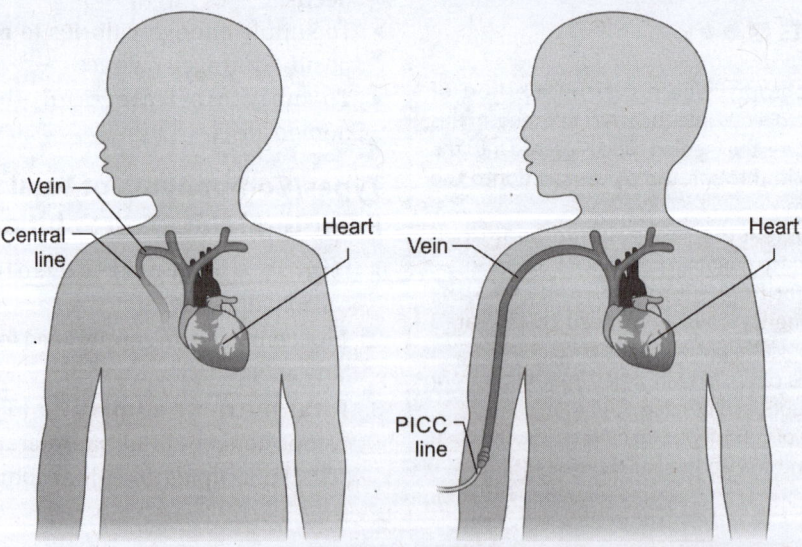

Fig. 4.9: Intravenous catheterization sites for total parenteral nutrition. (PICC: peripherally inserted central catheter)

Table 4.2: Types of venous access devices.

Types of catheter	Benefits	Care considerations
1. Tunneled catheter made of silicon, flexible radio-opaque with open ends - May have >1 lumen, for example, Hickman or Broviac	■ Reduced risk of bacterial migration ■ Easy to use for self-administered infusion	■ Daily heparin flushes ■ Must be clamped ■ Restriction of activities ■ Risk for infection ■ Susceptible to damage ■ May affect the body image ■ Patient and family must learn catheter care
2. Groshong catheter clean, flexible, radio-opaque with closed tip and two-way valve at proximal end may have >1 lumen	■ Less expensive ■ Decreased risk of damage ■ Increased patient safety ■ Easy to use self-administered intravenous (IV) infusions	■ Requires weekly irrigation with normal saline (NS) ■ Heavy activity restricted ■ Must keep exit site dry ■ Water sports must be restricted ■ Susceptible to damage ■ Patient and family must learn catheter care
3. Implanted ports totally implantable metal or plastic device that consist of self-sealing injection port with top or side access with preconnected or attachable silicon catheter that is placed in large blood vessel	■ Reduced risk of infection ■ Less prone to damage ■ Less expensive ■ Heparinized monthly and after each infusion to maintain patency ■ No limitations on physical activity ■ No or slight changes in body image	■ Must pierce skin for access, pain with insertion of needle (EMLA can be used) ■ Special noncoring needle (HUBER) with straight or angled design used to inject into ports ■ Skin preparation needed ■ Catheter may dislodge from the port

Nurse's Responsibility

- When administered cycled TPN, the solution is infused at half the prescribed rate for the first and last hour to prevent hyper- and hypoglycemia.
- Initiation of infusion should be slow and then gradually increase the rate of flow.
- Monitor the blood glucose level frequently such as every 4–6 hours at early stage, and every 12th hourly thereafter.
- If blood glucose levels are elevated, subcutaneous administration of insulin may be needed.
- Perform catheter site care, tubing and filter changes, and dressing changes according to institutional policy.
- Inspect the insertion site closely for signs of infection.
- Monitor the child's daily weight, vital signs, and intake/output.
- Review laboratory test results, which can aid in early detection of problems, such as infection or electrolyte deficits/excess.
- Adhere to strict aseptic technique.
- Adhere to institutional policy for flushing of the catheter and maintaining catheter patency (**Table 4.3**).
- Ensure that the system remains closed at all times. Secure all the connections, use occlusive dressing, and clamp the catheter or have a child perform the Valsalva maneuver during tubing and cap changes.

Table 4.3: Heparin flush guidelines.

Type of catheter	Newborn and infant	≤2 years	>2 years
Tunneled (intermittent)		10 U/mL, 3 mL after medications	
Tunneled (dormant)		10 U/mL, 3-mL heparin everyday	100 U/mL, 3 mL everyday
Surgically placed CVC with <5 Fr (dormant)	2 U/mL, 2 mL every eighth hourly		
Surgically placed CVC with 5 Fr (intermittent)	2 U/mL, 2 mL between TPN or medications		
Surgically placed CVC with 5 Fr (dormant)	10 U/mL, every 12 hours		

(TPN: total parenteral nutrition, CVC: central venous catheters)

Points to Remember

- If any reason the TPN infusion is interrupted or stops, begin an infusion of a 10% dextrose solution at the same infusion rate as of TPN. This helps to prevent rebound hypoglycemia that may occur due to increased insulin secretion by the child's body in response to the use of highly concentrated TPN solution.
- Never administer any medication, blood, or other solution through the TPN lumen. Doing so will increase the risk for contamination of the system and infection.

Health Education of the Child and Family

Children who require long-term TPN therapy may receive TPN in home.

- Provide written and verbal instructions about the care involved.
- Demonstrate the care to parents and child (if appropriate).
- Develop plans for troubleshooting problem with devices and equipment and give instructions to how to recognize and treat complications.
- Also teach them about danger signs and symptoms that require immediate notification.
- Significant others, for example, teacher should be informed about venous access devices.

Promoting Growth and Development

- Vigorous sports should be avoided.
- Provide love, comfort, support, and socialization to the child during TPN as like enteral feeding.
- Provide opportunities for holding and cuddling the child.
- Allow the older child to participate in activities that can help to occupy the time associated with meals.
- Child's dental care should not be neglected.
- Encourage the child and parents to participate in the care to promote a sense of independence as well as a sense of control over the situation.
- Infants and toddlers should be allowed to crawl and pull up to standing position to promote optimum development.
- Running the tubing under one-piece clothing outfit and out the back often encourages ambulation.

Highlights ●●●●

- Nutritional support can be administered through a central venous access is termed total parenteral nutrition (TNP). It is also called IV alimentation.
- TPN can be administered through continuous administration (over a 24-hour period) or cyclic basis (over a 12-hour period during night).
- The selection of the venous access device is based on the factors such as age of child, purpose, and duration of TPN.
- Monitor the blood glucose level frequently such as every 4–6 hours at early stage, and every 12th hourly thereafter.
- Ensure that the system remains closed at all times. Secure all the connections, use occlusive dressing, and clamp the catheter or have a child perform the Valsalva maneuver during tubing and cap changes.
- Never administer any medication, blood, or other solution through the TPN lumen.

MEMORY EXERCISE

1. **Breast milk at room temperature can be stored for:**
   a. 4 hours
   b. 8 hours
   c. 12 hours
   d. 24 hours

2. **Which of the following stamen is true about breastfeeding?**
   a. Has no effect on mother
   b. Likely to affect mother's appearance
   c. May cause breast cancer
   d. Good for mother

3. **Inadvertent of air into the IV alimentation system during cap changes or accidental disconnections results in:**
   a. Venous thrombosis
   b. Cardiac tamponade
   c. Air embolism
   d. Thrombophlebitis

4. **The method by which feeds are given by dripping the feeding into a vent that is attached to the gastrostomy tube is called:**
   a. Chimney feeds
   b. Bolus feeds
   c. Direct feeds
   d. Continuous feeds

5. **After nasogastric tube feeding, the child must be positioned in:**
   a. Left side with head slightly elevated
   b. Right side with head slightly elevated
   c. Supine position
   d. Upright position

CHAPTER 5

Respiratory Care

LEARNING OBJECTIVES

After reading this chapter, the readers should be able to:
- Explain the different methods of oxygen administration.
- Perform postural drainage.
- Demonstrate respiratory care procedures.

Keywords: respiratory tract, oxygen, inhalation, pulmonary function, air

STEAM INHALATION

Definition
Breathing warm and moist air into the mucous membrane of respiratory tract is called steam inhalation.

Indications
Children with:
- Bronchitis
- Asthma
- Acute bronchiolitis
- Cystic fibrosis
- Croup
- Postoperative period

Purposes
- To relieve the inflammation and congestion of the mucous membrane of the respiratory tract and paranasal sinuses
- To soften thick tenacious mucous and help it expel from the respiratory tract
- To provide moisture and heat and to prevent dryness of mucus membrane of the lungs
- To aid in the absorption of the oxygen
- To relieve the spastic condition of the larynx and bronchi
- To provide aseptic action on the respiratory tract

Equipment Needed
- Boiled water in a vessel with lid
- Blanket
- Kidney basin
- Any solution if prescribed, for example, menthol and tincture benzoin

Preparation
- Explain the procedure to the mother and child as appropriate.
- Ensure safety measures to prevent burns and scalds.
- Assemble all the necessary equipment.

Procedure

- Take boiling water with lid covered.
- Make the child to sit on the mother's lap.
- Cover the mother and the child with the blanket.
- Slowly remove the lid and give it for 10–15 minutes.
- Instruct the mother to hold the child carefully.

Postprocedure Care

- Remove the vessel.
- Wipe the child.
- Give chest physiotherapy and postural drainage if needed.
- Record the procedure.

Highlights ●●●●

- ✦ Breathing warm and moist air into the mucous membrane of respiratory tract is called steam inhalation.
- ✦ The most important use of steam inhalation is to relieve the inflammation and congestion of the mucous membrane of the respiratory tract and paranasal sinuses.
- ✦ Give proper instruction to the mother to hold the child carefully during the procedure.
- ✦ Chest physiotherapy and postural drainage can help to remove secretions after steam inhalation.

NEBULIZATION

Definition

A method of administering a drug in which the drug is dissolved in a solution, vaporized, and the vapor is inhaled.

A nebulizer is an electrically powered machine that turns a liquid medication into a mist so that it can be breathed directly into the lungs through a face mask or mouthpiece.

Purposes

- To dilute the secretion
- To induce a productive cough
- To deposit pharmacologic agents in upper and lower respiratory tract
- To decrease bronchial edema

Indications

- Children with acute respiratory tract infection, for example, asthma and pneumonia
- As a part of bronchial drainage to increase the effectiveness of the procedure

Contraindication

Hypersensitivity

Complications

- Infections due to contaminated equipment
- Adverse reactions

Drugs Used for Nebulization Therapy

- Bronchodilators
- Mucolytic drugs
- Decongestant drugs
- Anti-inflammatory drugs (e.g., salbutamol, terbutaline, salmeterol, beclomethasone, budesonide, and ipratropium)

Dosage and Frequency

Usually depends on doctor's prescription. For the salbutamol the dosage is:

- Up to 3 years: 0.1 mL Asthalin + normal saline 2 mL } 6 or 8 hourly
- 3–12 years: 0.5 + 2 mL

Equipment Needed

A clean tray containing:

- Nebulizer machine with accessories
- Sputum cup with disinfectant solution to collect if coughed out

Chapter 5: Respiratory Care

- Kidney tray to collect the waste
- Stethoscope to auscultate the breath sounds
- Face towel for wiping the face
- Hand towel to dry the hands
- Medicine as prescribed
- Bowl with sterile swabs to clean the accessories before and after the procedure
- Spirit for disinfection of accessories
- Dropper or disposable syringe to measure and to pour the medicine
- Additional set of face mask, tube, and accessories to meet the emergency
- Watch to note the timing

Parts of Nebulizer

- Compressor (**Fig. 5.1**)
  - Lid
  - Air outlet connector
  - Power switch
  - Handle

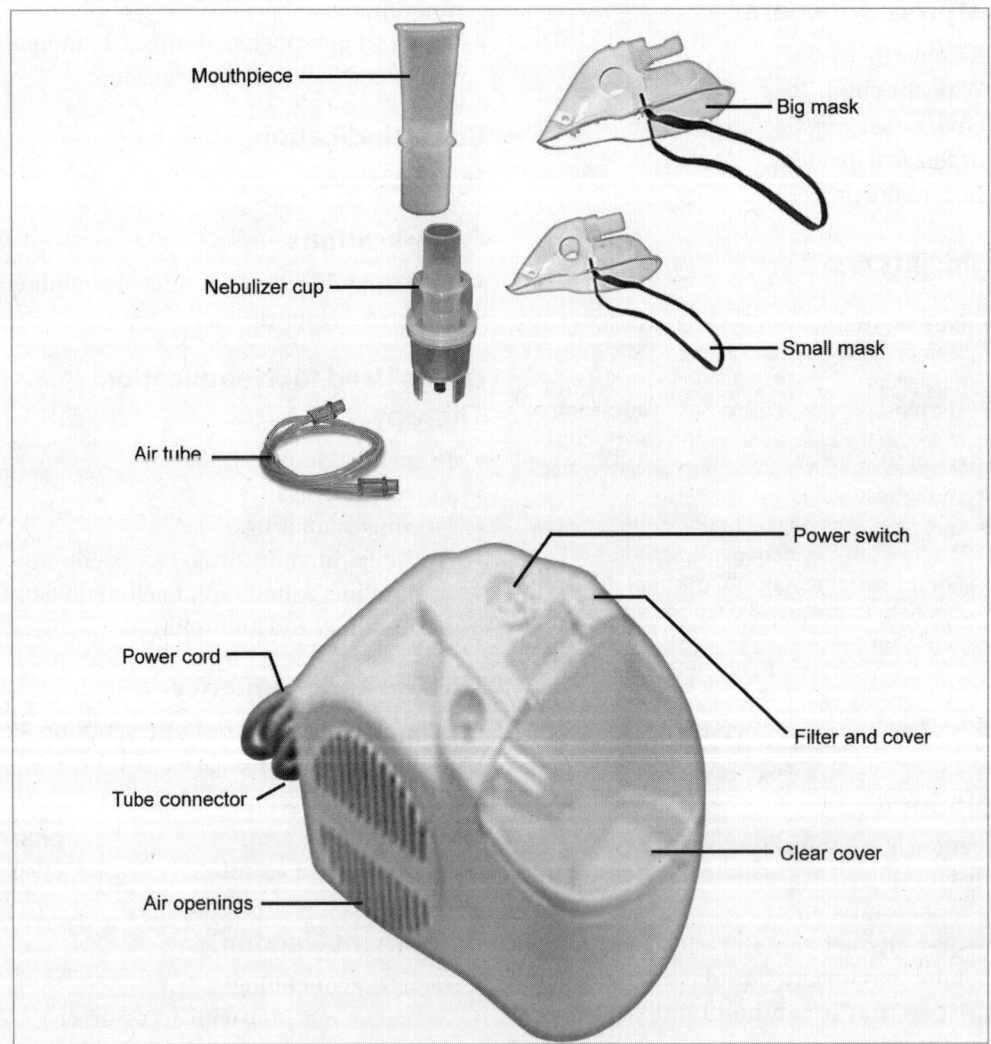

Fig. 5.1: Parts of nebulizer.

- Air filter
- Power cord
- Power cord storage access
- Air inlet connector
- Medication cup
- Cap or dome
- Baffle
- Mouthpiece
- Face mask
- Tubing
- Accessories storage recess

Instructions

- Always keep an extra nebulizer or its accessories in hand. Prior to using the machine, check for its working condition.
- If the treatment is longer than 10–15 minutes, check if the mist output nebulization may be clogged or dirt can obstruct the airflow from the compressor.
- If the treatment is shorter than the normal, check to see if the medicine is leaking out of the nebulizer.
- The nebulizer must not be touched with wet or soaked hands.
- No smoking, no fire around the equipment when in use.
- Do not pour medication solution >10 mL into the medication cup.
- Filter should be changed when it turns completely gray in color.

Nebulization Therapy

Methods

- Mouthpiece treatments for children ages 8 years and older. The child places the mouthpiece between the teeth, using the lips to form a tight seal.
  Disadvantages:
  – May not be effective when the child is sleeping.
- Mask treatment (children <8 years): An aerosol mask is placed on the nebulizer and then secured over the nose and mouth of the child. The mist breathed in through the child's mouth and nose. Placing the mask on a young child can be scary.
- Blow by treatment (very small infants or children who cannot tolerate mask treatment).

This method directs the mists at the patient's nose or mouth through a flex tube. It sends very little medication to the infant's lungs.

Preparation

- Explain the procedure to the parents and child.
- Select the quite area for the treatment to avoid disturbance and enhance comfort.
- Clean the nebulizer and its accessories with spirit swab.
- Prior to using, check the nebulizer parts for cracks or damage of material inside.

Procedure

- Assemble the articles near to the procedure area.
- Pour prescribed medicine in correct dilution in nebulizer and cover it with dome tightly.
- Wash hands.
- Place the child in an upright position and auscultate for breath sounds.
- Place the face mask/mouthpiece correctly in place and instruct the child to take a deep breath through the mouth.
- Switch on the nebulizer and keep it upright.
- Depending on the amount of medication to be used, the treatment will usually last 10–15 minutes.
- When the nebulizer splutters, shake or tap it once or twice. If it continues to splutter, the treatment is done.

Postprocedure Care

- Provide the child a comfortable position and encourage the child to effectively cough.

- Check the breath sounds and corelate with the preprocedural auscultation for changes.
- Check vital signs.
- If perspiration is present wipe the child's face with the face towel.
- Wash hands and replace the articles.
- Record the procedure and the vital signs in nurse's record.

Care of Nebulizer

- After each use the nebulizer must be cleaned.
- Dismantle the mouthpiece, nose piece, or face mask from cap, open nebulizer cup and remove baffle.
- Wash it with soap and rinse under hot tap water.
- Allow to air-dry.
- Keep the outer surface of the tubing dust free by wiping regularly with the clean and dry cotton swab daily.
- Use dry clean cloth to clean the outer part of the nebulizer.

Highlights

> - Nebulization is a method of administering a drug in which the drug is dissolved in a solution, vaporized, and the vapor is inhaled.
> - It is commonly indicated in children with acute respiratory tract infection.
> - If the treatment is longer than 10–15 minutes, check if the mist output nebulization may be clogged or dirt can obstruct the airflow from the compressor.
> - If the treatment is shorter than the normal, check to see if the medicine is leaking out of the nebulizer.
> - When the nebulizer splutters, shake or tap it once or twice. If it continues to splutter, the treatment is done.
> - Nebulization can be given either through mouthpiece for children ages 8 year and older or mask (children <8 years).
> - In very small infants or children who cannot tolerate mask, blow method can be employed.

OXYGEN THERAPY

Definition

Oxygen therapy is the administration of the oxygen for treatment of the conditions resulting from oxygen deficiency.

Purposes

- To increase the oxygen tension of blood plasma
- To restore the oxyhemoglobin in the red blood cells (RBCs) to the normal proportion
- To manage the condition of the hypoxia
- To maintain the ability of the cells to carry out the normal metabolic function
- To reduce the risk of complications

Indications

The indications for administering the oxygen are to correct:

- Hypoxemia (reduction in the oxygen content of the blood below physiologic levels)
- Hypoxia or anoxia (absence of adequate tissue oxygenation)
  The conditions are as follows:
  – Deficiency of O_2 in atmospheric air
  – Ventilation perfusion abnormalities
  – Impaired diffusion
  – Inadequate tissue oxygenation, for example, abnormal tissue demand
  – Poisoning with chemicals that alter the tissues ability to utilize oxygen, for example, cyanide poisoning
  – Hemorrhage
  – Shock and circulatory failure
  – Children who are under anesthesia
  – Asphyxia, for example, drowning, foreign body aspiration, strangulation, etc.

Principles

- The choice of system will depend upon the clinical status of the patient and desired dose

of oxygen. For example, child with irregular respiration needs bag-mask ventilation with as high dose of O_2 as possible.
- Oxygen should be humidified, whenever possible to prevent dried secretions from obstructing the smaller airways.
- The effectiveness of the oxygen delivery should be monitored with pulse oximeter.
- Young children may become frightened or agitated when O_2 is administered, causing their clinical conditions to deteriorate. Therefore they should remain in a position of comfort whenever possible. A caregiver can often hold the O_2 source in proximity to or over the child's face.
- The O_2 is a drug and as such should be prescribed accordingly.

Methods of Administration

It is important to consider both the nature of respiratory illness and also the age of the child when determining the method of administration.

Methods of oxygen administration are majorly divided into two types:
- Low-flow delivery method: It provides oxygen at flow rates that are lower than patients' inspiratory demand:
  - Simple face mask
  - Non-rebreather face mask (mask with oxygen reservoir bag and one-way valves, which aims to prevent/reduce room air entrainment)
  - Nasal prongs (low flow)
  - Tracheotomy mask
  - Venturi mask
  - Oxyhood
- High-flow delivery method (discussed in later sections)
  - Ventilators
  - continuous positive airway pressure (CPAP)/bilevel positive airway pressure (BiPAP) drivers

LOW-FLOW DELIVERY SYSTEM

Simple Masks

Semirigid and have vents within the mask to enable dilution of O_2 (**Fig. 5.2**).

Indications
- Medium-flow oxygen desired, mild-to-moderate respiratory distress
- When increased oxygen delivery for short period(<12 hours)

Contraindications

Poor respiratory efforts, apnea, severe hypoxia

Advantage

High concentration can be given.

Disadvantages
- In low concentrations (<4 L), it can cause exhaled CO_2 to be rebreathed
- Uncomfortable
- Require tight seal
- Do not deliver high FiO_2
- FiO_2 varies with breathing efforts
- Interfere with eating, drinking, and communication

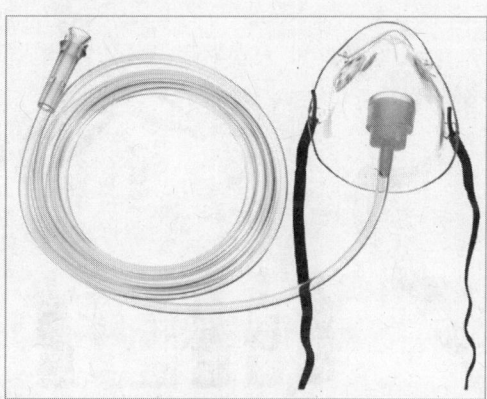

Fig. 5.2: Simple mask.

- Difficult to keep in position for long duration
- Skin breakdown

Venturi Masks or Hudson Masks

On the bottom of the mask is a barrel with holes in the side. The position and size of these holes determine the percentage of O_2 that is administered to the child.

These masks are available in 24, 28, 35, 40, and 60% (**Fig. 5.3**).

Indications

The situations where exact amount of oxygen needs to be delivered.

Contraindications

Poor respiratory efforts, apnea, and severe hypoxia

Advantages

- Provide a fixed concentration of O_2 safely.
- For example, chronic lung condition reduces the risk of rebreathing the exhaled CO_2.

Disadvantages

- Expensive
- Need to be discarded if a higher or lower concentration of O_2 is required

Nonbreathing Masks

These masks are used in emergency situation as they have a large reservoir that enables only O_2 to be breathed by the child, preventing the inhalation of the mixed gases, the percentage administered is approximately 99. The initial amount of O_2 flow through this mask should be set at 15 L but it is important to make sure that the bag attached to the mask is inflated before putting the mask on the child (**Fig. 5.4**).

Indications

High FiO_2 requirement >40%

Contraindications

Poor respiratory efforts, apnea, severe hypoxia

Advantages

- Highest possible FiO_2 without intubation
- Suitable for spontaneously breathing patients with severe hypoxia

Disadvantages

- Expensive
- Require tight seal, uncomfortable, interfere with eating and drinking, not suitable for long-term use
- Malfunction can cause CO_2 buildup, suffocation

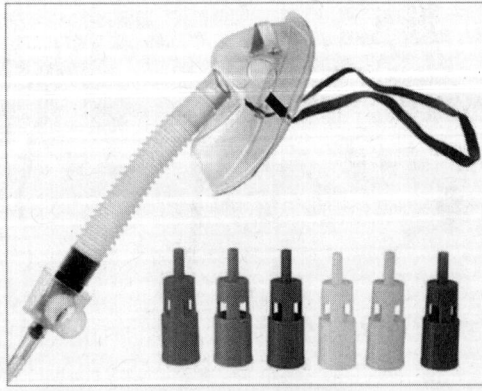

Fig. 5.3: Venturi mask.

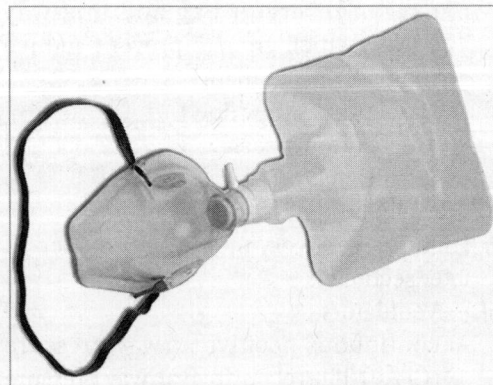

Fig. 5.4: Nonbreathing mask.

Nasal Cannula or Prongs

These are small plastic tubes that are inserted into each nostril. If the child is very young then, the prongs need to be secured with tape on the cheeks (**Fig. 5.5**).

Advantages

- Often tolerated well by children
- They can continue to feed and play without mask coming in the way and can be easily observed.

Disadvantages

It is difficult to give a higher flow rate of O_2 as humidification is said to be inadequate and nasal mucosa became uncomfortable for the patient.

Tracheostomy Mask

A tracheostomy mask, sometimes referred to as a tracheostomy collar, is a small mask that fits over the patient's tracheostomy site. An adjustable elastic strap that fits around the patient's neck holds it in place (**Fig. 5.6**).

The mask has an exhalation port that remains patent at all times and a port that connects to the oxygen source with large-bore tubing. The flow rate is usually set at 10 L/min, with a nebulizer set at the appropriate oxygen concentration.

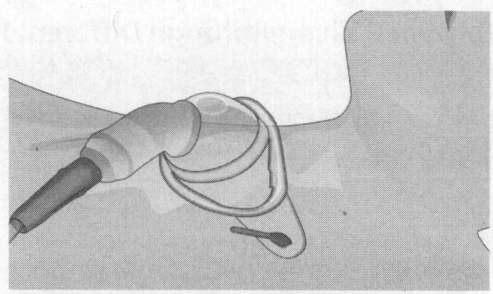

Fig. 5.6: Tracheostomy mask.

Head Boxes (Hood)

The box is placed over the top of the infant's head and also his or her upper body.

Advantages

- It will enable the administration of O_2 to an infant if he or she will not tolerate nasal prongs or masks or a higher percentage of O_2 is required than can be administered through other methods (**Fig. 5.7**).
- It allows the nurse to be able to see the baby.

Disadvantages

- The O_2 going into the head boxes can be variable and the concentration changes if the top of the box is opened often to care the baby.
- O_2 could be blown directly onto the face of the baby. Cold air can cause the diving reflex and can precipitate bradycardia episodes.

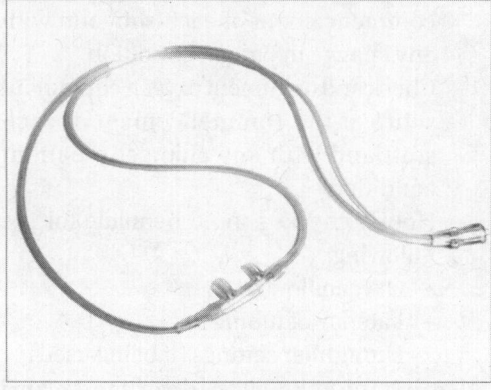

Fig. 5.5: Nasal prongs.

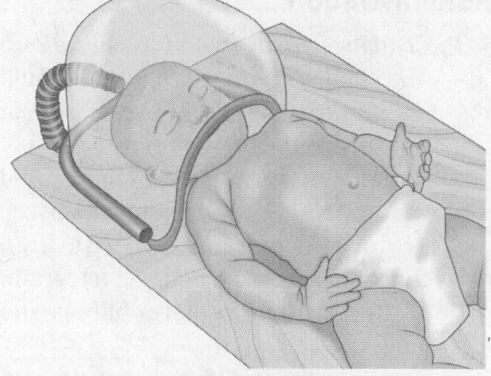

Fig. 5.7: Oxyhood.

Oxygen Delivery through Different Devices

Type of device	Description	Flow rate
Simple mask	Requires a fairly high oxygen flow to prevent rebreathing of carbon dioxide. About 75% of the inspired volume is room air that the patient breathes through the holes in the side of the mask. An accurate FiO_2 is difficult to estimate	8–12 L/min; FiO_2 35–65%
Nonbreather face mask	The reservoir bag allows a higher FiO_2 to be administered. At flow rate slower than 6 L/min, the risk of rebreathing carbon dioxide increases. A valve closes during expiration so that exhaled air does not enter the reservoir bag and prevent rebreathing. The valves on the side ports of the mask open during exhalation but close during inspiration; thus prevent the rebreathing of room air	6–15 L/min; FiO_2 60–100%
Venturi mask	Different size adaptors are used to deliver a fixed or predicted FiO_2. The FiO_2 level depends upon the flow rate and port size	FiO_2 60–100%
Nasal prongs	Can tolerate well and easy to use. FiO_2 varies depending on the flow rate and depth of the patient's breathing	1–2 L/min; FiO_2 24–38% 3–4 L/min; FiO_2: 30–35% 5–6 L/min; FiO_2: 38–44%

Criteria for Selection of Oxygen Delivery Method

Oxygen delivery method selected depends on:
- Age of the patient
- Oxygen requirements/therapeutic goals
- Patient tolerance to selected interface
- Humidification needs

Nurse's Responsibility in O_2 Administration

- *Prevention of accidents and complications:*
  - Any child receiving O_2 therapy should not play friction toys or use a nylon or wool blanket.
  - O_2 concentration must be measured near the child's head with an analyzer. Prolonged exposure to the high concentrations can be toxic to certain tissue (retina in preterm babies and lungs in all children).
  - Observe the child constantly and monitor for any complications.
- *Assessment and documentation:*
  - Proper recording of the procedure includes time of starting, amount of flow, and duration.
  - Assess the airway and position the child accordingly.
  - Clinical assessment and documentation, including, but not limited to, cardiovascular, respiratory, and neurological systems, should be done at the commencement of each shift and with any change in patient condition.
  - Check and document oxygen equipment setup at the commencement of each shift and with any change in patient condition.
  - Hourly checks should be made for the following:
    » Oxygen flow rate
    » Patency of tubing
    » Humidifier settings (if being used).

Hourly checks should be made and recorded on the patient observation chart

for the following (unless otherwise directed by the treating medical team):
- Heart rate
- Respiratory rate
- Signs of respiratory distress, such as nasal flaring
- Oxygen saturation
- *Weaning from oxygen:*
  - Unless clinically contraindicated, an attempt to wean the child from oxygen therapy should be attempted at least once per shift.
  - Criteria for weaning:
    » Child is clinically stable.
    » Vital parameters are within normal limits.
    » No signs of respiratory distress.
    » Taking oral feed.
    » Child is alert and conscious, skin is pink.
  - Monitor the child continuously after cessation of oxygen therapy.

General Guidelines for Commencing/Increasing/Stopping Oxygen Therapy

Commencement or increase of oxygen therapy:
- Oxygen therapy should be commenced if:
  - SpO_2 is <92% (PaO_2 <80 mm Hg) in patients without cyanotic heart disease.
  - SpO_2 is <70% (PaO_2 <37 mm Hg) in patients with cyanotic heart disease who have had cardiac surgery.
  - SpO_2 is <60% (PaO_2 <32 mm Hg) in patients with cyanotic heart disease who are waiting for cardiac surgery.
  - <91% in premature and newborn neonates.
  - Persistently <90% for infants with bronchiolitis.
- Reduction or cessation of oxygen therapy. Oxygen therapy should be reduced or ceased if:
  - SpO_2 is ≥92%.
  - SpO_2 is ≥90% for infants with bronchiolitis.
  - The child with cyanotic heart disease reaches their baseline SpO_2.

Complications

- Retinopathy of prematurity or retrolental fibroplasia
- Bronchopulmonary dysplasia
- Infection
- Fire hazards
- O_2 toxicity causes nausea or vomiting, anxiety and visual disturbance, muscle twitching, and seizures.
- O_2 induced apnea
- Drying of mucus membrane of respiratory tract
- Atelectasis due to increased O_2 concentration and elimination of nitrogen

Highlights ● ● ● ●

✦ Oxygen therapy is the administration of the oxygen for treatment of the conditions resulting from oxygen deficiency.
✦ The indications for administering the oxygen are to correct (1) hypoxemia and (2) hypoxia or anoxia.
✦ The O_2 is a drug and as such should be prescribed accordingly.
✦ It is important to consider both the nature of respiratory illness and also the age of the child when determining the method of administration.
✦ Methods of oxygen administration are majorly divided into two types: low-flow delivery method and high-flow delivery method.
✦ Oxygen therapy should be commenced if:
  - SpO_2 is <92% (PaO_2 <80 mm Hg) in patients without cyanotic heart disease.
  - SpO_2 is <70% (PaO_2 <37 mm Hg) in patients with cyanotic heart disease who have had cardiac surgery.
  - SpO_2 is <60% (PaO_2 <32 mm Hg) in patients with cyanotic heart disease who are waiting for cardiac surgery.

CHEST PHYSIOTHERAPY

Definition

Chest physiotherapy (CPT) is an airway clearance technique that combines manual percussion of the chest wall by the caregiver, strategic positioning of the patients for mucus drainage with cough and breathing techniques.

Indications

- In conditions with copious retention of airway secretions, such as bronchiectasis and cystic fibrosis
- With thick mucus secretion leading on to segmental lesions/collapse
- In children with weak respiratory mechanics, such as cerebral palsy and neuromuscular disorders, for example, spinal muscular atrophy
- In children with weak cough, such as vocal cord palsy and brainstem lesion
- In kyphoscoliosis
- In bedridden children, immobilization may limit or prevent physical exercise, impairing their ability to maintain aerobic capacity and lung volume.
- In acute severe asthma (in the presence of atelectasis)
- In pneumonia (consolidation phase)
- In intensive care unit, CPT is the treatment of choice for only patients with acute lobar atelectasis.
- Prophylactic drainage of contralateral normal lung following the drainage of diseased lung.

Contraindications

Sl. no.	Positioning	Conditions
1.	All positioning	Raised ICP, head and neck injury until stabilized, active hemorrhage with hemodynamic instability, recent spinal surgery or acute spinal injury, active hemoptysis, empyema, bronchopleural fistula, large pleural effusions, pulmonary embolism, pulmonary edema associated with CHF, confused or anxious patients who do not tolerate position change, rib fracture with or without flail chest, surgical wound or healing tissue
2.	Trendelenburg	Raised ICP, patients in whom increased ICP is to be avoided, uncontrolled hypertension, distended abdomen, esophageal surgery, recent gross hemoptysis, uncontrolled airway with risk for aspiration (tube feeding, or recent meal)
3.	Reverse Trendelenburg	Hypotension or vasoactive medication
4.	External manipulation of thorax	Subcutaneous emphysema, pneumatoceles, pneumothorax, recent epidural spinal infusion or spinal anesthesia, recent skin grafts or flaps on the thorax burns, open wounds and skin infection of the thorax, suspected pulmonary TB, lung contusion, bronchospasm, osteomyelitis of the ribs, osteoporosis, coagulopathy, severe thrombocytopenia, complaint of chest wall pain, recently placed transvenous pacemaker or subcutaneous pacemaker

(ICP: intracranial pressure; TB: tuberculosis; CHF: congestive heart failure)

Techniques

- Positioning (postural drainage)
- Chest percussion
- Vibration
- Thoracic squeezing
- Cough stimulation

Positioning (Postural Drainage)

It is mere positioning of the child with assistance of gravity to stabilize the secretions toward the main bronchus (**Fig. 5.8**).

Upper lobe

- *Apical bronchus:* Sitting upright with slight variation according to the position of the lesion, that is, slightly leaning backward, forward, or sideways
- *Anterior bronchus:* Lying supine with the knees slightly flexed
- *Posterior bronchus:*
  - Right—lying on the left side and turn his face 45° resting against a pillow, with another pillow supporting the head
  - Left—lying on the right side turning his/her face 45° with three pillows arranged to lift the shoulders by 12 inches.

Middle lobe (right)

Lateral and medial bronchus—lying supine with the body a quarter turned to the left maintained by a pillow under the left side from shoulder to hip and foot end raised by 14 inches (35 cm).

Lingular (left)

- Superior and inferior bronchus—lying supine with the body a quarter turned to the right maintained by a pillow under the left side from shoulder to hip and foot end raised by 14 inches (35 cm).

Lower lobe

- Apical basal bronchus—lying prone with a pillow under the hips.
- Anterior basal bronchus—lying supine with the buttocks resting on a pillow and the knees flexed. Foot of the bed raised by 18 inches (45 cm).

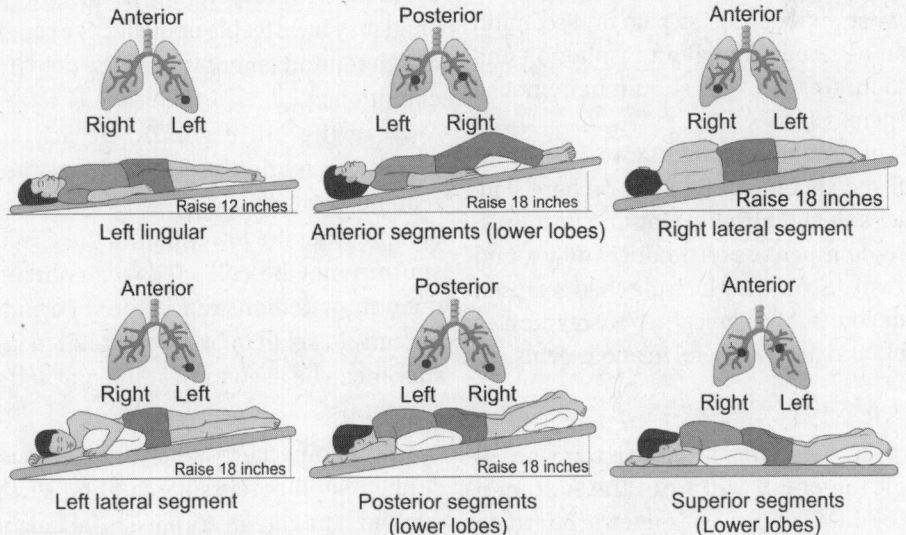

Fig. 5.8: Different positions for postural drainage.

- Posterior basal bronchus—lying prone with a pillow under the hips. Foot of the bed raised by 18 inches (45 cm).
- Lateral basal bronchus—lying on the opposite side with a pillow under the hips. Foot of the bed raised by 18 inches (45 cm).
- Medial basal (cardiac) bronchus—lying on the right side with a pillow under the hips. Foot of the bed raised by 18 inches (45 cm).

Chest Percussion

Depending on the available area, the therapist can use a single or both cupped hands or three fingers with the middle finger tented or a face mask with either the part covered or occluded by a finger and strike repeatedly at a rate of 3/s over that part of the bronchopulmonary segment, which needs to be drained. The cupped hand/mask tends to trap a cushion of air, which softens the blow while striking, and the air column inside the cupped hand causes effective dislodgement of the secretions in the underlying bronchus as the compression wave is presumably transmitted to the underlying bronchus and gravitational aid causes flow of secretions from the bronchus toward the glottis. The movement should be only at the wrist without causing pain or discomfort and can be done throughout inspiration and expiration; rings (if any) should be removed before percussion.

Percussion should be vigorous but not painful and should not be done on bare skin, but over soft comfortable clothing or towels. Properly done percussion produces only sound rather than discomfort which the child gets used to in due course. Mechanical percussors are also available and may be useful in adolescents.

Vibration

In this a rapid vibratory impulse is transmitted through the chest wall from the flattened hands of the therapist by isometric alternate contraction of forearm flexor and extensor muscles, to loosen and dislodge the airway secretions. Vibration is a technical procedure and is usually effectively executed only by a physiotherapist.

Thoracic Squeezing

The expiratory phase is reinforced in this maneuver. The child is asked to take a deep breath and then exhale through the mouth as completely and rapidly as possible, as would be done for a forced expiratory volume determination. The depth of expiration is increased by brief firm pressure from the operator's hand compressing the sides of the thorax (thoracic squeeze). This is usually done by physiotherapist.

Cough Stimulation

Child can be requested to cough. In uncooperative or small children, tracheal stimulation or tickling can be done by placing index finger or thumb on anterior side of the neck against trachea just above sternal notch with gentle but firm inward pressure in circular pattern as the child begins to exhale. In certain diseases with respiratory involvement, the child may have feeble or ineffective cough and cough reinforcement is of much help in such conditions.

Here the child should be advised to cough out while the hand of the operator reinforces anticipated cough by synchronously compressing the lower half of the chest. The sputum may be collected in a container to quantify or demonstrate to the child and their parents. In small infants and children, a bulls sucker can be used to clear the oral and nasal secretions.

Note: For home therapy, postural drainage with cupped hand percussion and oral suction is advised. The caregivers have to be taught and demonstrated about the techniques before discharge.

Timing and Duration of Chest Physiotherapy

Chest physiotherapy should be done one to four times a day, preferably half an hour before meals or 1 and 0.5 hours after meals. The total duration should not exceed 30 minutes with 3–6 minutes in each position. Prior bronchodilator inhalation (preferably salbutamol) may effectively clear the lung secretions in children with associated bronchospasm. Breathing exercise or deep breathing or vigorous activity, such as skipping and jumping can precede postural drainage in order to loosen the secretions, provided such activity is not contraindicated.

A printed sheet with pictures of various drainage positions explaining the procedures should be made available to the parents.

Physiotherapy in Young Infants

Position: Baby lying on the physiotherapist or mother's lap and pillows could be added to achieve the required position.

During physiotherapy, the baby should be positioned in such a way that the facial color and breathing can be checked frequently.

Toys and musical boxes can be shown to hold the attention of the toddlers while doing CPT to overcome their fear and apprehension.

Complications

- Hypoxemia
- Increased intracranial pressure
- Acute hypotension
- Pulmonary hemorrhage
- Pain or injury to muscles, ribs, or spine
- Vomiting and aspiration
- Bronchospasm
- Dysrhythmias

Highlights ● ● ● ●

- ✦ Chest physiotherapy is an airway clearance technique that combines manual percussion of the chest wall by the caregiver, strategic positioning of the patients for mucus drainage with cough and breathing techniques.
- ✦ Chest physiotherapy can be given by the following techniques: (1) positioning (postural drainage), (2) chest percussion, (3) vibration, (4) thoracic squeezing, and (5) cough stimulation.
- ✦ During physiotherapy, the baby should be positioned in such a way that the facial color and breathing can be checked frequently.
- ✦ Toys and musical boxes can be shown to hold the attention of the toddlers while doing CPT to overcome their fear and apprehension.
- ✦ A printed sheet with pictures of various drainage positions explaining the procedures should be made available to the parents.

INCENTIVE SPIROMETRY

Definition

An incentive spirometer is a medical device used to help patients improve the functioning of their lungs.

Purposes

- To increase transpulmonary pressure and inspiratory volume
- To improve inspiratory muscle performance
- To re-establish or stimulate the normal pattern of pulmonary hyperinflation
- To prevent or reverse lung atelectasis

Indications

- Children who undergone any surgery that might jeopardize respiratory function, for example, thoracic surgery or upper abdominal surgery.
- Children recovering from anesthetic effect
- Pulmonary atelectasis

- Presence of a restrictive lung defect associated with quadriplegia and/or dysfunctional diaphragm

Contraindications

- Very young children
- Uncooperative children
- Children unable to breathe effectively, for example, vital capacity <10 mL/kg or inspiratory capacity less than one-third of predicted

Equipment Needed

Incentive spirometer (**Fig. 5.9**)

Preparation

- Explain the procedure to the child and demonstrate it if necessary.
- Take return demonstration during preoperative period. So that he can follow the technique during postoperative period.

Procedure

- With the unit in an upright position, have the child blow the air out of his lungs (exhale). Have him place his lips tightly around the mouthpiece.
- Have the child take a deep breath (inhale) enough air to raise the flow rate guide between the arrows.
- Have the child to hold the deep breath, continue to inhale, and keep the guide as high as he can for as long as he can.
- Have the child exhale and relax. After each deep breath, take a moment to rest, relax, and breathe as normal. Then repeat the steps as directed.
- Cough after 10 deep breaths.

Complications

- Hyperventilation
- Barotrauma (emphysematous lungs)
- Discomfort
- Exacerbation of bronchospasm
- Fatigue

Nurse's Responsibility

- Assess the child's condition, ability to follow instructions.
- Instruct the child and parents about proper technique and an understanding of the importance of preoperative instructions.
- Constantly monitor the child during therapy.
- Encourage the child to perform independently.
- Maintain universal precautions to prevent transmission of infection between children.

Highlights ●●●

- ✦ An incentive spirometer is a medical device used to help patients improve the functioning of their lungs.
- ✦ It is indicated in children who undergone any surgery that might jeopardize respiratory function, for example, thoracic surgery or upper abdominal surgery.
- ✦ Teach and take return demonstration during preoperative period. So that he can follow the technique during postoperative period.

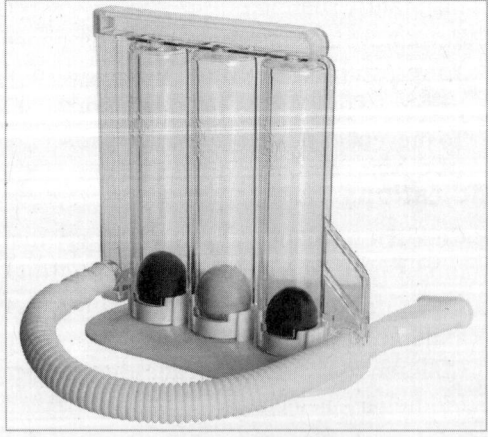

Fig. 5.9: Incentive spirometer.

MEMORY EXERCISE

1. **The most important indication for mechanical ventilation in a child with respiratory acidosis is:**
   a. PCO_2 >75 mm Hg
   b. Concomitant metabolic acidosis
   c. Slowly responsive underlying disease
   d. Hypoxia that responds poorly to oxygen

2. **The percentage of FiO_2 that can be delivered using mask is up to:**
   a. 35
   b. 45
   c. 65
   d. 75

3. **All of the following are controlled mode of mechanical ventilation, *except*:**
   a. Pressure-support ventilation (PSV)
   b. Conventional mechanical ventilation (CMV)
   c. Intermittent mechanical ventilation (IMV)
   d. Synchronized intermittent mechanical ventilation (SIMV)

4. **Amount of oxygen administered to infants by nasal catheter:**
   a. 4 L/min
   b. 5 L/min
   c. 2.5 L/min
   d. 1 L/min

5. **Breathing warm and moist air into the mucous membrane of respiratory tract is called:**
   a. Steam inhalation
   b. Nebulization
   c. Aerosol therapy
   d. Oxygen therapy

CHAPTER 6

Administration of Medications and Vaccines

LEARNING OBJECTIVES

After reading this chapter, the readers should be able to:
- Recall the concepts of medication administration.
- Calculate the correct dosage of given drug.
- Prepare the child for medication administration in age-appropriate manner.
- Administer medications following 10 rights.
- Recognize the side effects of medications.
- Document the medication administration procedure as per the institutional policy.

Keywords: medications, routes, calculation, responsibility, pediatric, application, administration, rights, vaccination, adverse drug reaction

INTRODUCTION TO ADMINISTRATION OF MEDICATIONS IN CHILDREN

General Principles in Medication Administration

- Be confident.
- Approach the child with positive attitude.
- Be honest and understanding.
- Allow the child to have control where appropriate.
- Use appropriate language that the child understands.
- Discuss with the child what they might taste/smell/see/hear/feel.
- Listen to all involved.
- Explain the benefits of compliance with the medicine taking.

Rights in Administration of Medications

- Right child
- Right medication
- Right dose
- Right time
- Right route
- Right of parents and child to know about medicine
- Right to refuse
- Right documentation
- Right assessment
- Right evaluation

Drug Calculations

Pediatric calculation is usually based on either body surface area (BSA) (mg/m²) or body weight (mg/kg) of the child. Body weight is more frequently used for ease of calculations.

Formula

Dose required/present standard quantity of drug × present quantity of liquid in which standard quantity of drug is dissolved.

In other words: What you want/what you have × what is in (dilution)

For example, a child is prescribed 90 mg of paracetamol and the medication supplied is 120 mg of paracetamol in 5 mL: 90/120 × 5 = 3.75 mL.

Dose Determination by Body Surface Area

To determine the dose using BSA, nomogram is needed. A nomogram is a graph divided into three columns: height (left column), surface area (middle column), and weight (right column).

1. Measure the child's height.
2. Determine the child's weight.
3. Using nomogram, draw a line to connect the height measurement in the left column and the weight measurement in the right column. Determine the point where this line intersects the line in the surface area column (**Fig. 6.1**). This is the BSA, expressed in meter square (m^2).

Dose Determination by Body Weight

- Weigh the child.
- Check a drug reference for the safe range (e.g., 5–10 mg/kg).
- Calculate the low safe dose.
- Calculate the high safe dose.
- Determine if the dose is ordered within this range.

Note: The pediatric dose should not exceed the minimum recommended dose of an adult.

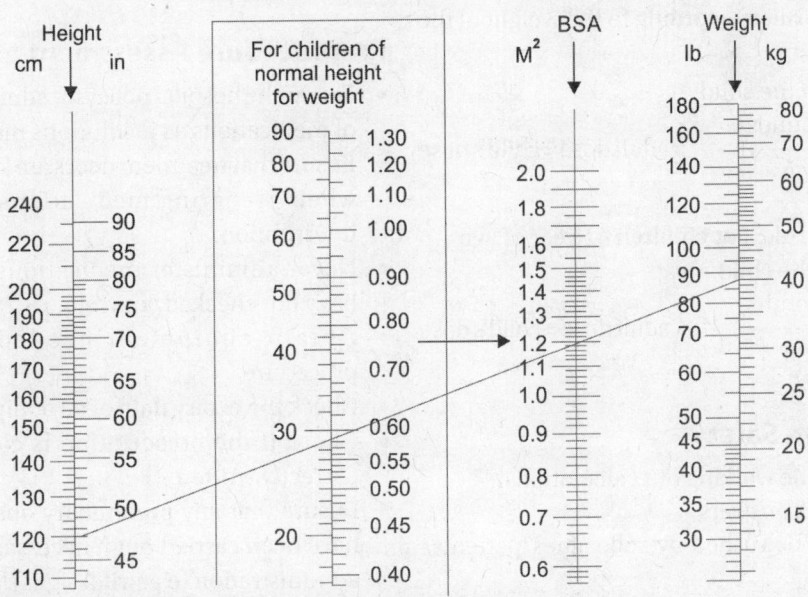

Fig. 6.1: Nomogram.

Calculation of low safe dose:
For example: 5 mg/1 kg = x mg/30 kg
Solve for x by cross-multiplying:
$1 \times x = 5 \times 30$
$x = 150$ mg.

Calculation of high safe dose:
For example: 10 mg/1 kg = x mg/kg

Solve for x by cross-multiplying:
$1 \times x = 10 \times 30$
$x = 300$ mg.
Compare the safe dose range (e.g., 150–300 mg) with the ordered dose. If the dose falls within the range, the dose is safe. If the dose falls outside the range, notify the prescriber.

Other formulas commonly used in calculation of pediatric dosage:

1. Young's rule: For children >1–12 years

$$\frac{\text{Age of the child (in years)}}{\text{Age of the child (in years)} + 12} \times \text{adult dose} = \text{child's dose}$$

2. Clark's rule: According to the weight of the child

$$\frac{\text{Weight of the child (in pounds)}}{150} \times \text{adult dose} = \text{child's dose}$$

3. Fried's rule: For children <1 year of age

$$\frac{\text{Age of the child (in months)}}{150} \times \text{adult dose} = \text{child's dose}$$

To Ensure Safety

- Take time working out calculations.
- Recheck answers.
- Do not be rushed by colleagues/patients/parents.

ORAL MEDICATIONS

Medications to be given via oral route are supplied in many forms, such as liquids (elixirs, syrups, or suspensions), powders, tablets, and capsules.

Equipment Needed

- Medication chart
- Medication drug formulary to ensure correct dosage
- Manufacturer's drug information (if required)
- Medication tray containing:
  - Prescribed medication
  - Medicine cup (with measured volume)
  - Tablet splitter/mortar and pestle
  - Sterile water (for dissolving medicine)
  - Kidney tray
  - Scissors
  - Medication card
  - Face towel
  - Gauze pieces in a small bowl (for wiping the syrup bottle)

Preprocedure Assessment

- Follow the hospital policy for administration of medications as institutions may vary.
- Ensure that treatment doors are kept closed when preparing medications to avoid interruption.
- Never administer medications that you have not checked yourself.
- Obtain equipment needed for the procedure.
- Check the expiry date of all equipment.
- Check if the prescription is clearly and correctly written.
- Ensure that any preliminary observations have been carried out if necessary prior to administration (e.g., vital signs).

Chapter 6: Administration of Medications and Vaccines

- Check if the child does not have any known allergy or contraindication to the prescribed medication.
- Inform the prescribing practitioner if the child does have allergy and do not give medicine.
- Check if a recent and correct weight has been recorded and dated on the prescription chart.
- Check in an approved drug formulary that the dose, route, and frequency of prescribed medication are accurate.
- Check if the medication supplied is suitable for oral administration.
- If more than one medicine is prescribed, check for compatibilities and drug interactions.
- Check if it is necessary for the medication to be given before or after food/fluid.
- If administering more than one medication, ensure that the medications can be given together.
- Liaise with pharmacist or refer to manufacturer's guidelines regarding mixing oral medications with food and fluid.

Procedure

- Follow the protocol for checking and preparing medications:
  - Systematic check of chart, allergies, weight, age, five rights, sign of prescriber, drug commence date, expiry, double checking.
  - Check if the child is available to take medications.
  - Ensure that room door is closed.
- Wash hands.
- Remove the medication from the box and check the name, dose, and expiry date of the medication's original container (e.g., bottle label, tablet strip).
- If using an unopened bottle of medicine, ensure that the date and time of opening are documented on the bottle.
- Dispense medication into the appropriate vessel without directly touching the medication with the hands.
- Take the medication with the prescription chart directly to the child for administration.
- Assist the child in repositioning for administration of medicines.
- Unless contraindicated, the child should be in upright position. A baby can be positioned in a semireclined position with the head elevated on the parent's lap.
- Allow time for the child to take the medicine.
- Oral syringe/spoon can be inserted into the side of the mouth between the cheek and the gum or can be placed on the tip of the tongue.
- Encourage older children to use a medicine cup or spoon to take medications.
- Ensure that the medication is given slowly and use spoon to retrieve any medicine that split or spat out; stroke baby's cheek or under the chin.
- Unless contraindicated, offer the child a flavored drink/ice cube between and after the medicines.
- Provide positive reinforcement as appropriate during and after the procedure.
- Assist the child in repositioning if required after the procedure.

Don'ts

- Don't leave the medication in a room for the parent to administer later.
- Don't take medication that requires administration via different route into the room at the same time [i.e., oral, intravenous (IV) medication].
- Don't attempt to administer oral medicine while the child is asleep/crying.
- Don't force the vessel/medicine into the child's mouth.

Postprocedure Care

- If the child refuses or is unable to take the prescribed medicine, inform the responsible prescriber. Document the incident in the appropriate section of the prescription chart and nurse's notes.
- Discard any unused medicine according to the institutional policy.
- Dispose the equipment.
- Wash and replace the articles.
- Wash hands.
- Sign for the administration of the medication on the child's prescription chart once the administration is complete.
- If the process required "double checking," ensure both signatures are on the prescription chart.
- Monitor the effects of the medicine administered and document in the nursing records.
- Observe for and report immediately to the nurse in charge and responsible prescriber any adverse effects of the medication.
- Stabilize child's condition.

Nurse's Responsibility in Administration of Oral Medications

- Refer to the responsible practitioner if a child is nil by mouth.
- Ensure the child's gag reflex is present.
- Postoperatively, ensure the child is sufficiently awake to take the medicine safely. If the volume of the suspension is large, consider using an alternative preparation.
- The pediatric nurse should understand whether the tablets are suitable for crushing or not. For example, soluble tablets/capsules should not be crushed but dissolved in water.
- Tablets should not be broken in half unless they are scored and an appropriate tablet cutter should be used.
- Consider the constant change of physical, metabolic, and physiological state of infants and children as this has an impact on the pharmacokinetics.
- Liquid medications, primarily suspensions, may be less concentrated at the top of the bottle than at the bottom. Always shake the liquid to ensure even drug distribution.
- Never mix the crushed tablets or the contents of a capsule with formula or other essential foods. Otherwise, the child may associate the bitter taste with the food and later refuse to eat.
- Always use calibrated equipment, such as a medicine cup, spoon, plastic oral syringe, or dropper for administering liquid forms.
- If a dropper is packaged with a certain medication, never use it to administer another medication, since the drop size may vary from one dropper to another.
- When using an oral syringe or dropper for infants and young children, direct the liquid toward the posterior side of the mouth.
- Give the drug slowly in small amounts (0.2–0.5 mL) and allow the child to swallow before more medication is placed in the mouth.
- As the children adapt to swallowing tablets or capsules, administration is similar to that of adults.
- When helping the younger child learn how to swallow medication, the tablet or capsule can be placed at the back of the tongue or in a small amount of food such as ice cream or applesauce. Always tell the children if there is medicine in the food; otherwise they may not trust you.
- Never force an oral medication into a child's mouth or pinch the child's nose. Doing so increases the risk for aspiration and interferes with the development of a trusting relationship.

Chapter 6: Administration of Medications and Vaccines

- When the child has nasogastric, gastrostomy, or nasojejunal tubes, oral medications may be given via these devices. The tube allows for the medication to be placed directly into the stomach or jejunal area.
- Medication for administration via a tube may be supplied in a liquid form, or a crushed tablet or opened capsule can be mixed with a liquid.
- Always check the tube placement before administering the medication.
- After administration, flush the tube to maintain patency.

Role of Nurse in Medication Management

- Administering medication safely and efficiently
- Assessing and monitoring the effects of medication
- Establishing interdisciplinary collaboration
- Evaluating desired and undesired effects of medication

Contraindications

- Unconscious child
- Absence of gag reflex
- Inability to swallow
- Vomiting

Precautions for Oral Administration

- Digestive tract trauma/illness
- Post gastrointestinal surgery
- Nil by mouth
- Nausea
- Diarrhea

Guidelines for Administering Medication via Gastrostomy or Jejunostomy Tubes

- Give liquid medication directly into the tube.
- Draw appropriate amount into syringe and clear air.
- Mix powdered medication well with warm water first.
- If medication is in pill form, verify if it is ok to crush.
- Then, crush tablets and mix in warm water to prevent tube occlusion.
- Open capsules and mix the contents in warm water to dissolve the contents and prevent tube occlusion.
- Label each syringe appropriately.
- Flush the tube with water after administering medications to ensure that the entire amount of medication has been given and to prevent tube occlusion.

Highlights ●●●

+ Medications to be given via oral route are supplied in many forms, such as liquids (elixirs, syrups, or suspensions), powders, tablets, and capsules.
+ If using an unopened bottle of medicine, ensure that the date and time of opening are documented on the bottle.
+ Ensure that the medication is given slowly and use spoon to retrieve any medicine that split or spat out; stroke baby's cheek or under the chin.
+ Always use calibrated equipment, such as a medicine cup, spoon, plastic oral syringe, or dropper for administering liquid forms.
+ If a dropper is packaged with a certain medication, never use it to administer another medication, since the drop size may vary from one dropper to another.
+ When using an oral syringe or dropper for infants and young children, direct the liquid toward the posterior side of the mouth.
+ Give the drug slowly in small amounts (0.2–0.5 mL) and allow the child to swallow before more medication is placed in the mouth.
+ Medication for administration via a tube may be supplied in a liquid form, or a crushed tablet or opened capsule can be mixed with a liquid.

INTRAMUSCULAR INJECTION

Definition
Introducing the medications/drugs directly into the muscles.

Advantages
- Absorption of medication is faster than subcutaneous injection.
- Large injections (up to 1–2 mL in child) can be given this way because muscles can absorb more fluid than fatty tissues.

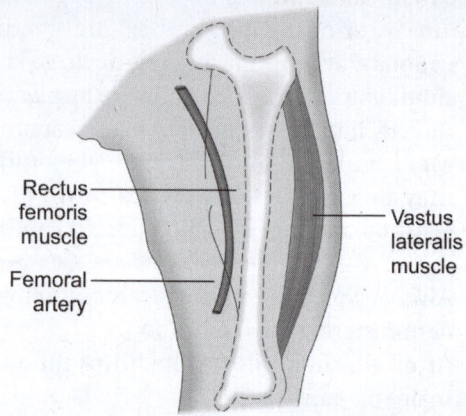

Fig. 6.2: Site for intramuscular (IM) injection in infants and children.

Preferred Sites
- *For infants and young children:* Rectus femoris muscle or vastus lateralis in the middle third of the thigh (**Fig. 6.2**)
  Clinical alert: Never use the dorsogluteal site in the posterior hip for infants or children who are not yet begin to walk.
- *For older children and adolescents:*
  - Ventrogluteal site in the gluteus medius muscle in the posterior hip
  - The deltoid muscles (upper and outer part of arm) (**Fig. 6.3**)

  Clinical alert: Do not inject > 1 mL into the arm of the child.

A clean tray containing:
- Prescribed medicine in ampoules/vial
- Ampoule cutter
- Medication card
- Disposable syringe with needle
- Spirit-soaked cotton swab
- Paper bag or kidney tray

Equipment Needed

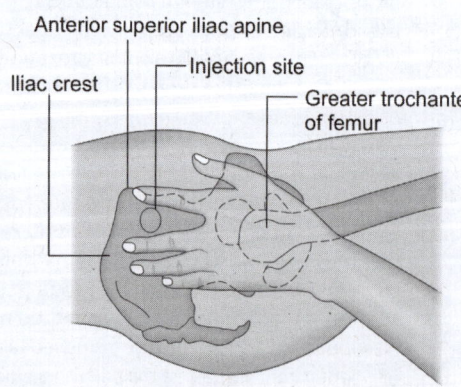

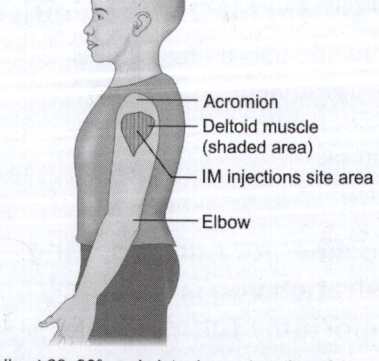

Insert needle at 80–90° angle into densest portion of deltoid muscle above armpit and below acromion.

Fig. 6.3: Ventrogluteal and deltoid sites for IM injection in older toddlers, children and adults. (IM: intramuscular)

Preparation

- Explain the procedure to the parents and child (appropriate to child's development).
- *Provide privacy:* Protect the child's privacy by putting a sheet over the body parts that do not need to be exposed.
- Show the mother how to hold the child.

Procedure

- Perform hand hygiene.
- Choose a site for the injection that has no broken skin, swelling, tenderness, redness, or warmth.
- Locate the exact site and clean it with antiseptic swab using circular motion and extending outward.
- Using your hand, stretch the skin at the site. This makes it firmer so that it is easier to insert the needle.
- Insert the needle quickly at a 90° angle through the skin and into the muscle. If the child is a very small infant or has a small muscle mass, use a 45° angle.
- Aspirate by pulling back on the plunger to inject the medication.
- Quickly remove the needle and apply firm pressure to the site using an antiseptic swab.
- Massage site to hasten absorption unless contraindicated as with irritating drugs.
- Place a small adhesive bandage on puncture site.

Postprocedure Care

- Hold and cuddle the young child and encourage parents to comfort child; praise older child for successful cooperation.
- Allow expression of feelings.
- Discard syringe uncapped; uncut needle in puncture-resistant container located near the site of use.
- Record time of injection, drug, dose, and injection site.
- Wash hands.

Nurse's Responsibility in Intramuscular Injection

- Use safety precautions in administering medication, for example, child's identification.
- Apply EMLA cream topically over site if time permits (at least 60 minutes, preferably 2 hours before injection).
- Select the syringe and needle appropriate to the amount and viscosity of fluid to be administered and amount of tissue to be penetrated.
- Make certain that muscle is large enough to accommodate volume and type of medications.
- Obtain sufficient help in restraining child, children are often uncooperative, and their behavior is unpredictable.
- Place the child in a lying or sitting position; child is not allowed to stand to avoid falling and it is difficult to restrain.
- Use a new, sharp needle with smallest diameter that permits the free flow of the medication.
- Grasp muscle firmly between thumb and fingers to isolate and stabilize muscle for deposition of drug in its deepest part; in obese children spread skin with thumb and index finger to displace subcutaneous tissue and grasp muscle deeply on each side.
- Allow skin preparation to dry completely before skin is penetrated.
- Have medication at room temperature to decrease the intensity of pain.
- Distract child with conversation to decrease the perception of pain.
- Place a cold compress or wrapped ice cube on site about a minute before injection.
- Insert needle quickly, using a dart-like motion in 90° angle unless contraindicated.
- Use separate needle for loading the injection from vial and another new one for administering medication.

- If blood is found, remove syringe from site, change the needle, and reinsert it into new location.
- Place the child on side with upper leg flexed and placed in front of lower leg for ventrogluteal.
- *Vastus lateralis:* Child can be supine, lying on the side, or sitting.
- If medication is given around the clock, the nurse must be careful to wake up the child.

Highlights ●●●

- Large injections (up to 1–2 mL in child) can be given this way because muscles can absorb more fluid than fatty tissues.
- Never use the dorsogluteal site in the posterior hip for infants or children who are not yet begin to walk.
- Apply EMLA cream topically over site if time permits (at least 60 minutes, preferably 2 hours before injection).
- Make certain that muscle is large enough to accommodate volume and type of medications.
- Obtain sufficient help in restraining child, children are often uncooperative, and their behavior is unpredictable.
- Place the child in a lying or sitting position; child is not allowed to stand to avoid falling and it is difficult to restrain.
- Use a new, sharp needle with smallest diameter that permits the free flow of the medication.
- Use separate needle for loading the injection from vial and another new one for administering medication.

INTRADERMAL INJECTION

Definition

An intradermal injection is given in the dermal layer of the skin.

Indications

Intradermal injections are used for:
- Allergy test
- Tuberculin test
- Immunization of BCG vaccine

Preferred Sites

- The most common site for this type of injection is the forearm.
- Other sites include the upper chest and the back beneath the shoulder blade, upper arm, buttock, or upper thigh.

Equipment Needed

A tray containing:
- Disposable syringe with needle
- Prescribed medication
- Alcohol wipes
- Medication card
- Paper bag
- Pen to mark the site

Preparation

- Check the name of the patient.
- Tell the parents and the child (older enough) that the injection will cause a small lump, such as a bite or small blister, but it will disappear quickly.

Procedure

- Wash your hands.
- Select a site that has no discoloration or rash or broken skin.
- Clean the site with alcohol swab using circular motion.
- Load the medicine from the vial and remove the air.
- Pull the patient's skin flat.
- Hold the syringe at about a 15° angle and insert the needle through the epidermis into the dermis (**Fig. 6.4**).
- Inject the fluid slowly until a lump appears. This indicates that the fluid is in the dermis.
- Take the needle out quickly and lightly wipe the site with cotton ball.

Chapter 6: Administration of Medications and Vaccines

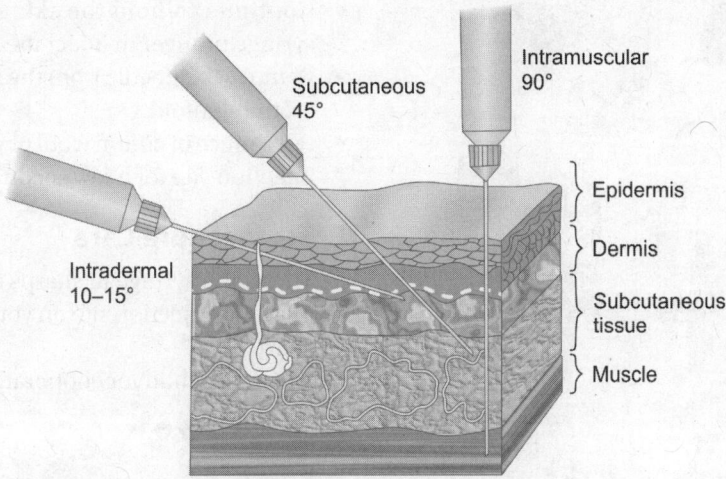

Fig. 6.4: Angle of insertion of needle in giving injection.

- In tuberculin/allergy test, the area should be circled with pen (5-10 cm). Date, time, and name of injection should be written. *Clinical alert:* Do not massage the injection site because that might make the medication absorbed into the tissue or out of the injection site.

Highlights ●●●●

✦ The most common site for intradermal injection is the forearm.
✦ To give ID injection, hold the syringe at about a 15° angle and insert the needle through the epidermis into the dermis.
✦ Do not massage the injection site because that might make the medication go into the tissue or out of the injection site.

SUBCUTANEOUS ADMINISTRATION OF MEDICATIONS

Definition
Medication administered into the subcutaneous fat under the skin.

Indications
The medications that need to be absorbed slowly than others, for example, insulin, growth hormone, and epinephrine.

Preferred Sites
- Thighs
- Buttocks
- Abdomen
- *Older children:* Upper arms (**Fig. 6.5**)

Equipment Needed
A tray containing:
- Syringe package
- Alcohol wipes
- Cotton ball or gauze piece
- Site rotation chart
- Prescribed medicine
- Paper bag

Procedure
- Wash hands
- Wipe the top of the medicine with the alcohol wipe and leave to dry.

Chapter 6: Administration of Medications and Vaccines

- Continue to hold the skin and push the syringe plunger to inject the medicine.
- Remove the needle from the skin and let go off the skinfold.
- Put a piece of cotton wool or gauze over the injection site for a few seconds.

Postprocedure Care

- Throw the syringe in sharps bin.
- Mark the injection site on your site rotation chart.
- Praise the child for cooperation.

Highlights

+ The medications that need to be absorbed slowly than others will be given through subcutaneous route.
+ Holding the needle at 45° angle insert the needle into the skinfold, so that the needle is at an angle of 90°.
+ If you are using a 5- to 6-mm needle, you do not need to lift the skin into a skinfold as described above.

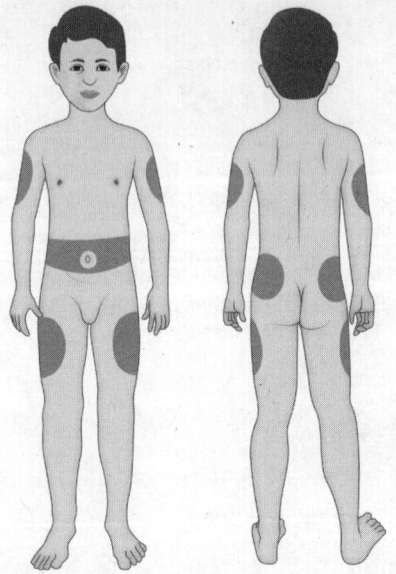

Fig. 6.5: Sites for subcutaneous injection.

- Choose the injection site.
- Open the syringe package and put on a clean surface.
- Insert the needle into the top of the bottle at an angle of 90°.
- Pull back the plunger and draw up slightly more than the prescribed dosage.
- Remove the needle from the bottle.
- By holding the needle upward, tap the syringe gently to move any air bubbles toward the needle.
- Push the plunger gently to remove the air bubbles and squirt a small amount of medicine into the air.
- Lift the skin in the chosen injection site between your thumb and index finger.
- Holding the needle at 45° angle insert the needle into the skinfold, so that the needle is at an angle of 90°. If you are using a 5- to 6-mm needle, you do not need to lift the skin into a skinfold as described above. You can insert the needle at an angle of 90° to the skin surface.

INTRAVENOUS THERAPY

Indications

- To maintain fluid and electrolyte balance
- To administer antibiotic therapy
- To provide nutritional support
- To administer chemotherapy or anticancer drugs
- To administer pain medication

Candidates for Intravenous Therapy

- Children who have poor gastrointestinal absorption caused by diarrhea, vomiting, and dehydration.
- Those in need of high serum concentration of drug.
- Those who have persistent infections that require IV medications.
- Those with emergency problem.
- Those in need of continuous pain relief.

Indications for Intravenous Fluid Maintenance

- *Maintenance replacement:* Children who cannot take food orally, for example, children who underwent surgery, comatose patients, and children with respiratory disorders and inhibited from oral feed.
- *Maintenance+deficit replacement:* Children who have severe dehydration, salt wasting renal disease, pyloric stenosis, and diabetes ketoacidosis.
- *Adjusted maintenance and correction of electrolyte imbalance:* Acute renal failure, nephritic syndrome, and burns.

Preferred Intravenous Sites

Site selection in the pediatric patients varies with the age.

The best choice of site is the one that least restricts the movement of the child.

Common Sites

- Hand, wrist, forearm, foot, and ankle.
- Antecubital fossa should be used if other sites cannot be accessed.
- Scalp vein can be used if no other veins are available (**Fig. 6.6**).

Equipment Needed

A clean tray containing:
- IV tubing
- Solution bottles (**Table 6.1**)
- IV cannula with needles (depending on the child's age) (**Table 6.2**)
- Tourniquet
- Adhesive tape
- Cleansing agent
- Sterile gauze pieces in a bowl
- Syringe with needle
- Arm board
- Infusion pump if (necessary)
- Control chamber
- EMLA cream

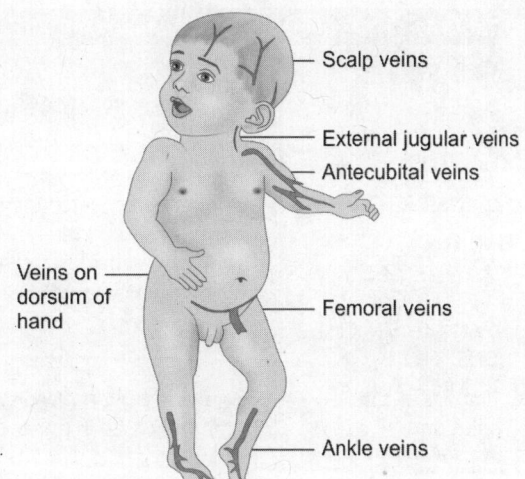

Fig. 6.6: Sites for intravenous cannulation in pediatric clients.

- Rolled towels or small blanket for maintaining position of the head
- IV pole

Preparation of Child and Parents

- Using an age-appropriate developmental approach, explain the procedure to child and parents.
- Furnish information on misconceptions and clarify their doubts.
- Play can be employed during the preparation period to reduce stress and anxiety.
- Allowing child to handle equipment and to start an IV infusion on a toy animal or doll help familiarize them with the frightening aspects of the procedure.
- Introduce a child to another child who is coping well in the same situation.
- Arrange a quiet, private setting for the child during insertion, for example, procedure room, to avoid anxiety and stress concerning loss of control in front of others.
- The child should be provided with some distracting activity.
- Parents are told about the procedure, including the reason for it, how long the

Chapter 6: Administration of Medications and Vaccines

Table 6.1: Types of intravenous (IV) fluids available and their indications.

Type of IV fluid	Indications	Remarks
0.9% NaCl (normal saline) commonly called NS	To provide ECFV replacement	May cause extracellular fluid overload in congestive heart failure and renal failure
0.45% NaCl (1/2 NS)	To provide free water and sodium. Commonly used in treatment of conditions, which causes hypertonic ECFV depleted status	
5%D + 0.45 NaCl (1/2 DNS)	3% NaCl	Severely symptomatic hyponatremia may cause osmotic demyelination
Ringer's lactate solution	To provide ECFV replacement. Commonly used in perioperative period	May cause extracellular fluid overload in congestive heart failure and renal failure
5% dextrose	To give free water and medications	Does not contain sodium; hence there is no chance for ECFV overload
Isolyte P	Used in children with dehydration	
Isolyte M	Used for maintenance fluid therapy	

(ECFV: extracellular fluid volume; NS: normal saline; DNS: dextrose normal saline)

Table 6.2: Size of intravenous (IV) cannula used in children.

Size (G)	Color	Length of cannula (mm)	Flow rate	Uses	Nursing consideration in insertion
26	Violet	19	10–15 mL/min	Newborns	Less painful but difficult to insert
25	Yellow	19	23	■ Infant, toddler, older children ■ Major surgery and trauma among children ■ Can administer fluids and ■ medication	Less painful insertion to though skin is difficult
22	Blue	25	22–50	■ Older children, adolescent ■ IV infusion with moderate flow rates ■ Medication administration	Insertion to though skin is difficult
20	Pink	32	55–80	■ Older children, adolescent ■ Ideal for IV infusion and blood infusion ■ Medication administration ■ Emergency management	■ Easy to insert into small, thin, fragile veins ■ Difficult to insert into though skin
18	Green	45	100–120	■ Adolescent ■ Major surgery and trauma ■ Infusion of large amount of fluids or colloids	Commonly used

Contd...

Contd...

Size (G)	Color	Length of cannula (mm)	Flow rate	Uses	Nursing consideration in insertion
16G	Gray	45	150–240	■ Adolescent ■ Major surgery and trauma ■ Infusion of large amount of fluids or colloids	Painful insertion require large insertion
14G	Orange	45	250–300	■ Adolescent ■ Major surgery and trauma ■ Infusion of large amount of fluids or colloids	Painful insertion require large insertion

catheter must remain in place, and what they can expect during and after the insertion.
- Encourage the parents to participate in procedure.
- One way to control pain during the procedure is by the use of controlled breathing. The child can be taught to inhale slowly and exhale through the mouth through pursed lips.

Position

- Toddlers and young children can be held in parents lap with the child's legs tucked between the parent's legs and the child's arm behind the parents. Ask the parents to hug the child to both restrain the child and provide comfort.
- Do not use any device to restrain the child unless it is necessary.
- Assistant should be prepared to grasp the child gently but firmly during the insertion.

Procedure

- Assemble the equipment.
- Perform hand hygiene. Don the gloves.
- A needle and syringe filled with NS solution is made ready.
- Precut the adhesive tape and keep it ready.
- Connect the IV tubing in the solution bag after checking the clarity and date of expiry and hang it on IV pole.
- Remove the air from the tubing by allowing some amount of fluid to run in.
- Allow the amount of fluid to be infused to run into the microdrip chamber and clamp it again.
- Apply the tourniquet over the extremity proximal to the venipuncture site.
- Locate the vein for needle insertion.

Other methods to visualize the vein include:
- Applying warm compress to the site.
- Running warm water over the extremity.
- Holding the limb in a dependent position below body level will help fill the veins for better visualization.
- Gentle tapping sometimes causes the vein to stand out.
- A commercial vein transilluminator is helpful in locating veins and assessing the depth and patency of vessels.
- A BP cuff can also be used as a tourniquet and can give more control over the pressure needed to make the veins visible.
- If the scalp vein is to be used, the nurse needs to hold the infant or young child or a mummy restraint may be applied. The nurse must hold the head in midline or turned to one side.
- Press the fingers against the bony skull and the prominence of the infant's face.

- The head may then be pressed against the pad on the table or bed. Care must be taken to avoid interference with infant's breathing during restraint.
- A tourniquet in the form of rubber band may be placed over the occiput.
- Clean the site with sterile antiseptic-soaked swabs.
- The IV cannula with the beveled side up is inserted in the skin. When it enters the blood vessels, blood may flow back into the cannula.
- Advance the cannula and remove the stylet (needle) and press the cannula site with the fingers of nondominant hand to prevent bleeding.
- Remove the tourniquet.
- Connect the cannula with the IV set.
- Secure the hub of the cannula with the adhesive tape.
- Transparent dressing is ideal because the insertion site is easily observed.
- Minimum tape should be used at the puncture site and on about 2.5–5 cm of the skin beyond the site to avoid obscuring the insertion site for early detection of infiltration.
- Opaque covering should be avoided. If it is used, the insertion site and extremity distal to the site should be visible to detect an infiltration.
- A protective cover is applied directly over the catheter insertion site to protect the infusion site. A commercial site protector IV house with ventilation holes can be used.
- If not available, padded boards or splints can be used to support the IV site. But its use can be minimized since it poses many disadvantages.
- A colorful and interesting sticker can be applied to the protective device to add a positive note to the procedure.
- Finger or toe areas are left unoccluded by dressings or tape to allow for the assessment of circulation.
- The thumb should not be immobilized because of the danger of contractures with limited movements later on.
- Minimize the use of restraints. If at all it is used frequent removal of the restraints provides the child with the opportunity to move the extremities.
- The flow rate is regulated carefully.
- The child should be positioned comfortably.

Care during Intravenous Therapy

- Calculate both the amount and the rate of flow to avoid fatal cardiac embarrassment.

$$\text{Formula for calculating drops/min} = \frac{\text{Amount of fluid to be infused} \times \text{drop factor}}{\text{Time interval in minutes}}$$

In case of macro drops, the drop factor is 1 mL = 10–15 drops.

In case of microdrops, the drop factor is 1 mL = 60 drops.

- Infusion pump can be used when the rate of flow should be very minimal.
- Monitor the apparatus hourly and keep an accurate record.
- Document the kind and amount of fluid prescribed, the amount given, rate of flow or number of drops/min the amount of fluid remaining, and the condition of the injection site.
- A record of intake–output is maintained.
- Amount of water required to maintain fluid balance is based on the weight of the child **(Table 6.3)**, which can be calculated by using Holliday–Segar's formula.

Table 6.3: Calculation of daily requirements of fluid and electrolytes.

Weight (kg)	Water requirement	Electrolyte (mEq/kg/day)		
		Sodium	Potassium	Chlorine
Infants 3–10	100 mL/kg/day; 4 mL/kg/h	2–3	1–2	2
Children 11–20	1,000 mL + 50 mL/kg/day; 4+2 = 6 mL/kg/h			
Children >20	1,500 mL + 20 mL/kg/day; 4 + 2 + 1 = 7 mL/kg/h			

Nurse's Responsibility in Administration of Intravenous Medication

- Most medications given by the IV route must be given at a specified rate and diluted properly to prevent overdose or toxicity.
- Careful maintenance of the IV site is required to prevent complications.
- Direct IV push medication is typically reserved for emergency situations and when therapeutic blood levels must be reached quickly to achieve the desired effect.
- Direct IV push administration requires that the drug be diluted appropriately and given at a specified rate, such as 2–3 minutes.

Care of Scalp Vein Site

- Family members should be reassured that child's hair will grow back quickly.
- When scalp vein is used, the child's hair is shaved over a small area.
- An inverted medicine cup or a paper cup with the bottom up is often taped over the site to protect it.
- The needle is stabilized with U-shaped taping and a loop of tubing is tapped so that if the child pulls on the tubing, the loop will absorb the pull and the site will remain intact.

Administering Medications via a Syringe Pump

Purpose

To provide accurate and safe administration of IV medication

Procedure

- Verify the medication order.
- Gather the medication and necessary equipment and supplies.
- Wash hands and put on gloves.
- Attach the syringe pump tubing to the medication syringe and purge air from the tubing by gently filling the tubing with the medication from the syringe.
- Insert the syringe into the pump according to the manufacturer's directions.
- Clean the port on the child's IV access device or tubing, flush the device or tubing if appropriate [e.g., an intermittent infusion device (saline lock or heparin lock)], and attach the syringe tubing to the IV tubing or device.
- Set the infusion rate on the pumps as ordered.
- When the medication infusion is completed, flush the syringe pump tubing or deliver any medication remaining on the tubing, according to institution protocol.
- Document the procedure and the child response to it.

Highlights ●●●●

- Most medications by the IV route must be given at a specified rate and diluted properly to prevent overdose or toxicity.
- Careful maintenance of the IV site is required to prevent complications.
- Direct IV push medication typically reserved for emergency situations and when therapeutic blood levels must be reached quickly to achieve the desired effect
- Direct IV push administration requires that the drug be diluted appropriately and given at a specified rate, such as 2–3 minutes.
- Play can be employed during the preparation period to reduce stress and anxiety.
- Allowing child to handle equipment and to start an IV infusion on a toy animal or doll help familiarize them with the frightening aspects of the procedure.
- When scalp vein is used, the child's hair is shaved over a small area.

INSTILLATION

Definition

Instillation means applying medication directly into the eye, ear, or nose.

Eye Medication

Purposes

- To lubricate the eye
- To treat medical conditions
- To treat infection, such as pink eye (conjunctivitis)

Preliminary Assessment

- Check label on medication against medication card.
- Review any special instructions.
- Recheck label and make sure that the medication is marked ophthalmic use only. Also check the expiry date.
- Check solution for color changes or sediment, this mean solution is decomposed. Do not use if it appears abnormal.
- Know which (eyes) gets the medication. (OD = right eye, OS = left eye, OU = both eyes).

Equipment Needed

A tray containing:
- Disposable gloves
- Prescribed medication
- Sterile saline-soaked cotton balls in a bowl
- Paper bag and kidney tray
- Sterile dressing pad (optional)

Preparation

- Explain the procedure to the parents and child (as appropriate)
- Provide comfortable position.
  - Older children—supine position with head should be slightly hyperextended.
  - Infant—supine with mummy restraint or over the mother's lap.

Procedure

- Wash hands and don the gloves.
- If child has discharge or crusting of the eye, make sure the eyelid and lashes are clean before administering the medication.
- Moisten a cotton ball or gauze with warm water.
- Place gauze on closed eye for a minute and gently wipe once from inner to outer canthus and discard after one wipe.
- Continue to moisten gauze and wipe eye until clean.
- Put your thumb directly below the center of the eye and gently pull down, making a pocket (conjunctival sac) (**Fig. 6.7**).
- The medication drops should be instilled on to the outer third of lower conjunctival sac.
- Take care not to touch the eye or eyelid with the dropper (1–2 cm above eye level).

Chapter 6: Administration of Medications and Vaccines

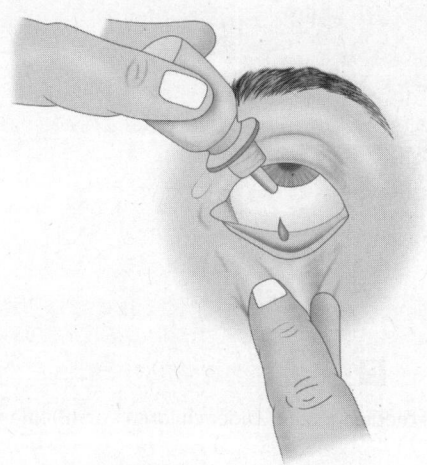

Fig. 6.7: Instillation of eye drops.

In Case of Ointment

- Squeeze a small ribbon (1/4–1/2 inch) of ointment from the inner canthus and move outward.
- With eye closed, gently massage eye with a tissue to distribute over the eyeball.
- Use a clean tissue to remove excess ointment.
- Wash hands.
- If applying two different kinds of ointments, wait at least 10 minutes between ointments.
- Document the procedure immediately.

Ear Drops

Indications

- To treat infection
- To relieve pressure and congestion
- To soften the ear wax
- To relieve pain

Equipment Needed

A clean tray containing:
- Medication bottle with dropper
- Cotton-tipped applicator
- Cotton balls in a bowl
- Kidney tray and paper bag
- Sterile disposable glove

Preparation

- Explain the procedure to the parent and child.
- Provide side lying position with the affected ear upper most.
- Check the label on medication against the medication card.
- Review special instruction.

Procedure

- Wash hands.
- Warm the bottle in the palm of the hand to prevent dizziness and nausea.
- If the medication is a suspension, shake the bottle well.
- Gently pull up and out from center of outer ear. This will straighten the ear canal and ensure the drops will have maximum effect (for infant and young child: pull pinna downward and backward) (**Figs. 6.8A and B**).
- Draw up medication in the dropper and slowly place prescribed number of drops into the ear canal from 1 inch away. Do not touch the dropper to any surface.
- Keep the child in the same position for at least 2 minutes to allow drops to enter ear completely.
- You may loosely tuck a small piece of cotton ball in the ear canal.
- If the drops are orderhed for the other ear, wait 5–10 minutes before turning to the opposite side and then repeat the procedure.
- Wash hands.
- Document administration of the medication immediately.

Nasal Drops

Nasal medications are instilled by means of drops or spray.

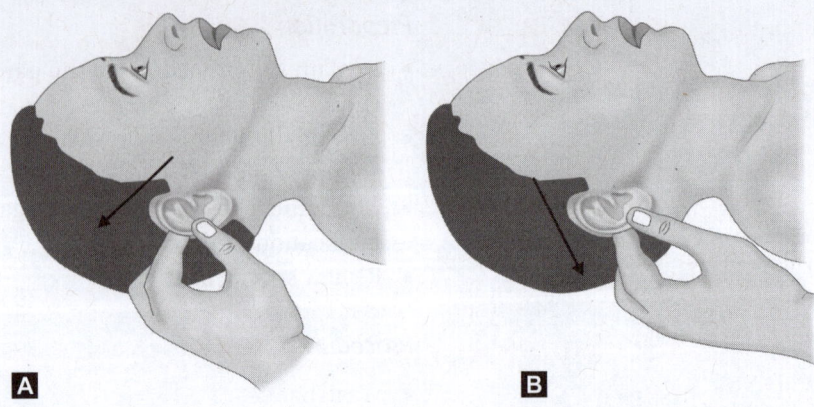

Figs. 6.8A and B: Straightening ear canal for instillation of medication: (A) Older children and (B) Infant.

Indications

- Used for children with allergies to relieve nasal congestion by shrinking swollen membranes
- To soften the mucous secretions
- To treat sinus infection

Equipment Needed

A clean tray containing:

- Pair of gloves
- Medication bottle with a dropper
- Small pillow or rolled linen
- Torch light
- Face towel
- Paper bag and kidney tray

Preparation

- Identify the child's profile.
- Check the physician order.
- Check the label on medication against medication card.
- Explain the procedure to the child and parents.
- Ask the child to gently blow the nose to remove secretions.
- Provide supine position for access to posterior pharynx; tilt the head backward for access to ethmoid or sphenoid sinuses; tilt the head back over the edge of bed or place a small pillow under the shoulder; and tilt the head back.

Procedure

- Wash hands.
- Draw medicine up into the dropper.
- Tilt recipient's head slightly toward you and close the other nostril.
- Ask the child (if older) to breath in and out of the mouth.
- Aim dropper upward toward the eye as you instill the prescribed number of drops (usually 2–3) into each nostril.
- Take care not to touch the sides of the nose with the dropper to prevent contamination of the dropper.
- Keep the child in same position for a few minutes after instillation of the drops.
- Use a face towel or rag piece to wipe off any medication that has escaped from anterior nares.
- Document the procedure immediately.

Instillation of Nasal Spray

- Wash hands.
- Check the label with medication card. Review for special instruction.
- Shake the bottle gently and remove the cover.

Chapter 6: Administration of Medications and Vaccines

- To prime the pump, press downward on the shoulders of the spray bottle. Press down and release several times into the air until a fine spray appears.
- Gently blow the nose and make child to sit down with head tilted slightly forward.
- Close one nostril. Keep bottle upright as you insert nasal applicator into the other nostril.
- Ask the child (older) to breathe in through the nose and while breathing in, press down firmly and quickly once on the applicators.
- Ask the child to breathe out through mouth.
- After spray, lean head backward for a few seconds.
- Repeat the procedure in other nostril (if ordered).
- Avoid blowing nose for 15 minutes after using spray.
- Wipe applicator with a clean tissue and replace cover.
- Wash hands.
- Document the procedure.

Note: If the inhaler contains a cortisone medication, the mouth should be rinsed out with water, without swallowing, after inhaling the dose. This will prevent oral thrush.

Highlights ● ● ● ●

- ✦ In administration of eye drops, if child has discharge or crusting of the eye, make sure that the eye lid and lashes are clean before administering the medication.
- ✦ Instillation means applying medication directly into the eye, ear, or nose.
- ✦ To instill ear drops, gently pull up and out from center of outer ear. This will straighten the ear canal and ensure that the drops will have maximum effect. (For infant and young child: pull pinna downward and backward.)
- ✦ In the case of nasal drops, if the inhaler contains a cortisone medication, the mouth should be rinsed out with water, without swallowing, after inhaling the dose. This will prevent oral thrush.

TOPICAL APPLICATIONS

Definition

A term used to describe medicine that has effects only in a specific area, not throughout the body, particularly medicine that is put directly on the skin.

Indications

- To treat inflammatory conditions
- To protect the intact skin
- To clean the skin of infected weeping lesions
- To prevent and manage pruritus
- To maintain moisture
- To anesthetize the area

Forms of Topical Applications

- Gels
- Ointments
- Pastes
- Lotions
- Creams
- Powder
- Spray
- Adhesive patches

Equipment Needed

A clean tray containing:
- Prescribed medication
- A bowl with warm water
- Washcloth
- A small bowl with gauze pieces
- Tongue blade/spatula/pair of gloves
- Kidney tray

Preparation

- Explain the procedure to the child and parent as appropriate.
- Inspect the skin for cleanliness.
- Assess the skin integrity.

Procedure

- Perform hand hygiene.
- Clean the area with warm water and washcloth. If open wound is present, clean the area with sterile gauze pieces and solution prescribed.
- Dry skin well after washing.
- Apply topical medication to the site.

Nurse's Responsibility in Topical Application

- Administer gels, lotions, pastes, ointments, and creams using cotton swabs, tongue blades, or gloves.
- Gloves help to reduce the transmission of microorganism and protect the nurse from absorbing the medication through her hand.
- If a powder is ordered, sprinkle it over the site; ensure that the child's head is turned away so that none is inhaled.
- If a spray ordered, check with reference source or the manufacturer's recommendations; most sprays must be shaken before administration.
- Spray over the site and ensure that the child's head is turned away to reduce the potential of inhalation.
- Apply a dressing over the site if indicated to prevent the medication from being rubbed off, and to protect the clothing at that site.
- Do not use dressing in case of topical steroids.
- Apply transdermal and topical systemic medication patches to a flat area of the skin; they are self-adhesive.
- Do not cut medication patches to fit area or reduce dose.
- Skin thickness, sensitivity, and condition should be taken into account when applying topical treatments.
- Apply in downward strokes following hair growth to prevent folliculitis.
- Rubbing should be avoided as this creates heat and irritation and can cause damage to delicate skin cells.

Topical Steroids

- Treatment of inflammatory conditions, for example, eczema.
- Apply no more than twice a day.
- Ointments provide better absorption and often less irritation; apply thinly following fingertip units.
- 1% hydrocortisone is safe for infants under 1 year and on face for all ages.
- Occlusive dressing increases the potency up to 10-fold.
- Use the least potent preparation that is effective for severity of condition.
- Avoid prolonged use, especially on the face and around the eyes.

Side Effects

- Skin thinning
- Striae
- Telangiectasia
- Fine hair growth
- Easy bruising
- Perioral dermatitis

Highlights ●●●

+ Topical medication is a term used to describe medicine that has effects only in a specific area, not throughout the body, particularly medicine that is put directly on the skin.
+ Administer gels, lotions, pastes, ointments, and creams using cotton swabs, tongue blades, or gloves.

ADMINISTRATION OF VACCINES

General Principles in Vaccination

- Any number of vaccines can be given on the same day (live/inactivated). However, there should be 5-cm gap between different vaccines site (except BCG and measles/MMR).
- Inactivated vaccines can be given any time in relation to any other live/inactivated vaccines.
- If missed on a single day, gap between any two live vaccines should be at least 4 weeks.

Role of Nurse in Immunization Procedure

- General guidelines for storing vaccines in domestic refrigerator:
  - Maintain the temperature of vaccines; check the log temperature twice a day.
  - Do not keep any other items in the refrigerator other than vaccines.
  - Never leave the vaccine vials outside after use.
  - Stocking of vaccine vials: follow the rule of first in is the first used. Keep the supply for only 1 month as it is a temporary storage.
  - Do not keep vaccines on the door shelves (**Fig. 6.9**).
  - Open the refrigerator only when necessary.
- Administration of vaccines:
  - Be alert about the type of vaccine to be given, its dosage, and route of administration (**Table 6.3**).
  - Ensure that the vaccine is administered immediately or within the prescribed period of use after reconstitution (**Table 6.4**).
  - Educate the parents about possible side effects and home care management (**Table 6.5**).

Common Side Effects of Vaccination

- *BCG:* Axillary lymphadenitis
- *DPT:* Excessive crying, fever, seizures, and encephalopathy
- *OPV:* Diarrhea, vomiting, irritability, and intussusceptions
- *Influenza (inactivated):* Fever, headache, fatigue, Guillain-Barré's syndrome
- *Measles:* Rashes and toxic shock syndrome

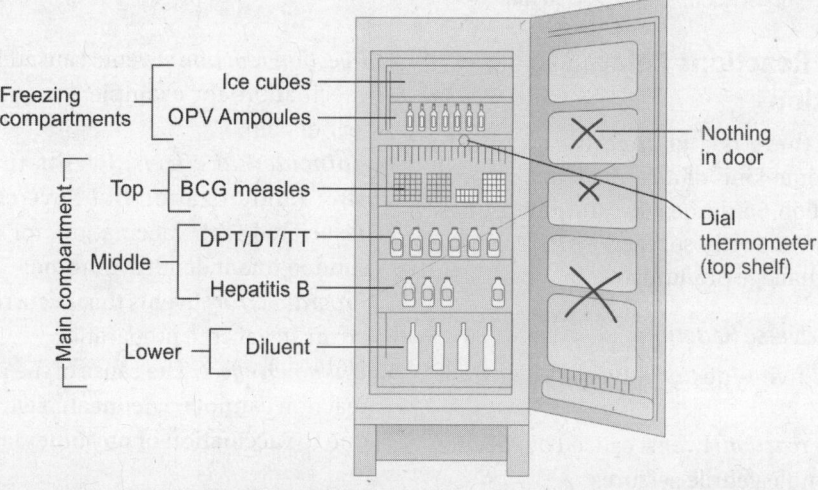

Fig. 6.9: Storing vaccines in refrigerator.

Chapter 6: Administration of Medications and Vaccines

Table 6.4: Route and dosage of vaccines.

Sl. no.	Name of vaccine	Dosage	Route of administration	Common site
1.	TT	0.5 mL	Intramuscular	Deltoid muscle
2.	BCG	0.1 mL	Intradermal	Left upper arm
3.	Hepatitis B	0.5 mL	Intramuscular	Anterolateral side of mid-thigh
4.	OPV	2 drops	Oral	–
5.	Pentavalent vaccine	0.5 mL	Intramuscular	Anterolateral side of mid-thigh
6.	Rotavirus	5 drops	Oral	–
7.	IPV	0.1 mL	Intradermal	Right upper arm
8.	Measles	0.5 mL	Subcutaneous	Right upper arm
9.	JE	0.5 mL	Subcutaneous	Left upper arm
10.	Vitamin A	1–2 mL (1–2 lakhs IU)	Oral	–
11.	DPT	0.5 mL	Intramuscular	Upper arm
12.	MMR	0.5 mL	Subcutaneous	Right upper arm

Table 6.5: Time limits for using vaccines after reconstitution.

Name of vaccine	Time limit
Varicella	30 minutes (should be protected from light)
MMR	30 minutes (should be protected from light)
Yellow fever	1 hour
Measles	4–6 hours
Meningococcal polysaccharide	30 minutes
DTaP/Hib combination	30 minutes

Adverse Reactions Related to Vaccination

At times, there is a chance for a child to develop some kind of adverse reaction after immunization. So, the health-care professionals should be aware of those reactions to recognize early and manage promptly.

Types of Adverse Reaction

There are five types of adverse reactions, including:

1. *Vaccine reaction:* Events caused by vaccine, for example, febrile seizures.
2. *Injection reaction:* Events caused by fear of vaccination, for example, syncope due to fear of pain.
3. *Coincidental effects:* Events that occur after immunization but have chance of associated with vaccination, for example, sudden infant death syndrome.
4. *Program error:* Events that occurred due to errors in vaccine preparation.
5. *Unknown effect:* The cause of the particular reaction cannot be delineated whether it is due to vaccination or any other factors.

Home Management of Common Side Effects

- *Pain:*
  - Keep wet cloth over the injection site.
  - Immobilize the vaccinated limb by keeping soft rolled towels on either side.
  - Give paracetamol if prescribed.
- *Fainting:* Make the child to lie down until he/she is feeling better.
- *Fever:*
  - Administer paracetamol.
  - Ensure adequate fluid intake.
  - Put loose cotton cloth.
  - Monitor the temperature regularly.
- *Seizure:* Child should be immediately brought to the hospital.

Highlights

- Any number of vaccines can be given on the same day (live/inactivated). However, there should be 5-cm gap between different vaccines site (except BCG and measles/MMR).
- Inactivated vaccines can be given any time in relation to any other live/inactivated vaccines.
- Be alert about the type of vaccine to be given, its dosage, and route of administration.
- Ensure that the vaccine is administered immediately or within prescribed period of using after reconstitution.
- At times, there is a chance for a child to develop some kind of adverse reaction after immunization. So, the health-care professionals should be aware of those reactions to recognize early and manage promptly.

MEMORY EXERCISE

1. **Route of administration of Hib vaccine:**
   a. Oral
   b. Intramuscular
   c. Subcutaneous
   d. Intradermal

2. **A preferred site for giving IM injection to a 6-month-old infant is:**
   a. Rectus femoris
   b. Dorsogluteal
   c. Ventrogluteal
   d. Vastus lateralis

3. **Hydrocortisone cream 1% is prescribed for a child with eczema. The correct way of applying the medicine is:**
   a. Apply a thin layer of cream and spread across thoroughly
   b. Avoid cleansing the area before the application
   c. Apply a thick layer of the cream to affected areas only
   d. Apply the cream to other areas to avoid occurrence

4. **When administering IV medication to an adolescent, the most appropriate action of nurse would be:**
   a. Allowing the client to verbalize his concern about the procedure
   b. Covering the insertion site with bandage
   c. Explaining possible adverse reactions
   d. Reassuring the client that only particular part alone will be exposed

5. **When preparing a 7-year-old child for oral medication, which has bitter taste, the correct action of pediatric nurse would be:**
   a. Allowing the child to take their own time in swallowing medications
   b. Getting more staff for assistance
   c. Telling the child that it does not taste bad if it is swallowed
   d. Telling the child that it tastes bad and offering beverages of their choice to drink afterward

CHAPTER 7

Elimination Needs

LEARNING OBJECTIVES

After reading this chapter, the readers should be able to:
- Select appropriate size and type of catheter for urinary catheterization.
- Perform urinary catheterization procedure.
- Assess the stoma condition.
- Demonstrate stoma care.
- Administer suppositories.
- Educate the parents and the child as appropriate regarding care of stoma.

Keywords: catheter, elimination, stoma, suprapubic, suppositories, ostomy, irrigation, bowel, cleansing

URINARY CATHETERIZATION

Definition
Urinary catheterization is the insertion of the catheter through the urethra into the bladder for withdrawal of urine.

Indications
- To obtain a urine specimen
- To relieve urinary retention
- To allow the bladder to restore or heal after a surgery
- To dilate a urethral stricture
- To decompress the bladder
- To measure residual urine
- In management of patients with spinal cord injury, neuromuscular degeneration, or incompetent bladder
- For diagnostic testing such as voiding cystourethrography or urodynamics

Short-term Indwelling Catheterization
- Postsurgery and criticaly-ill patients to monitor urinary output
- Surgical procedures involving pelvic or abdominal surgery
- Repair of bladder urethra and surrounding structures
- Urinary obstructions and acute urinary retention
- Prevention of urethral obstruction from blood clots with continuous or intermittent bladder irrigation
- Instillation of medications into the bladder

Long-term Indwelling Catheterization

- Refractory bladder outlet obstruction and neurogenic bladder with urinary retention
- Prolonged and chronic urinary retention
- To promote healing of perineal ulcer where urine may cause further skin breakdown

Equipment Needed

Catheterization tray consists of:
- Disposable sterile gloves
- Drapes
  - One fenestrated
  - One nonfenestrated
- Lubricant
- Cotton balls with container
- Two artery forceps
- Prefilled 10-cm^3 syringe with sterile water to inflate the balloon
- Sterile specimen container for urine sample collection
- Sterile catheter of appropriate type and size (**Table 7.1**)
- Chlorhexidine 2% aqueous solution
- Sterile water
- Catheter secure device or adhesive tape
- Urinary drainage bag with tubing
- Medicated lubricant

Preparation of the Child and Parents

- A careful explanation of the procedure and its rationale is completed prior to catheterization. The explanation must be tailored to both the developmental level of the child and needs of the parents.
- *For infants:* Reassure the parents that the procedure will not cause pain and neither the bladder nor the urethra will be damaged.
- *Toddlers and older children:* Typically appreciate seeing and manipulating a nonsterile catheter in order to feel its softness and pliability for themselves. The child should be taught to relax the pelvic muscles prior to insertion of the catheter.
- *For infants:* Remain in a supine position and emphasis is placed on leaving the hips flat on the procedure table/bed.
- *For toddlers and young children:* Teach to blow a pinwheel.
- *For preschooler and school aged:* Teach to blow out and gently press the hips against the table. This maneuver is repeated as the catheter is inserted in order to avoid breath-holding and raising hips from the procedure table, which tightens the periurethral muscles and increases discomfort.
- *Adolescents:* Teach to isolate, contract, and relax the pelvic muscle prior to catheterization and to breathe, slowly and deeply as the tube is inserted.

Note: Adolescent girls may prefer to be catheterized by a female staff and adolescent boys may prefer to be catheterized by a male caregiver. The request should be honored whenever feasible.
  - Since catheterization typically provokes anxiety and discomfort, assistance and gentle restraint may be indicated. Parents may be allowed to remain with the child during the procedure to both restrain and distract the child.

Table 7.1: Selecting a catheter for specimen collection.

Age (year)	Size of the catheter
0–1	4–5 Fr feeding tube, 6 Fr in and out catheter
1–12	4–5 Fr feeding tube, 6–10 Fr in and out catheter
12–18	8 Fr feeding tube, 8–12 Fr in and out catheter for adolescent girls; 8–12 Fr straight or tipped catheter for adolescent boys

Chapter 7: Elimination Needs

Table 7.2: Selecting indwelling catheter.	
Age (year)	Size of the catheter*
0–1	5 Fr feeding tube, 6–8 Fr Foley's catheter
1–12	6–8 Fr Foley's catheter with 3 cm^3 retention balloon, hydrophilic material with lubricious coating
12–18	8–14 Fr Foley's catheter with 5 cm^3 retention balloon

*Coude tipped 18–15 Fr Foley's catheter with 5 cm^3 retention balloon may be required for boys.

Catheter Selection

Choosing the appropriate catheter depending on:
- The size of the patient's urethral canal
- Expected duration of catheterization
- Knowledge of any allergy to latex or plastic
- Indication for catheterization (**Tables 7.1 and 7.2**)
- Child's age

Types

- *Straight single-use catheters:* Have a single lumen with a small 11/4-cm opening (**Fig. 7.1**).
- *Two-way Foley's catheters (retention catheter):* Have an inflatable balloon that encircles the tip near the lumen or opening of the catheter (**Fig. 7.2**).
- *Curved or coude catheters:* Have a rounded curved tip (**Fig. 7.3**).

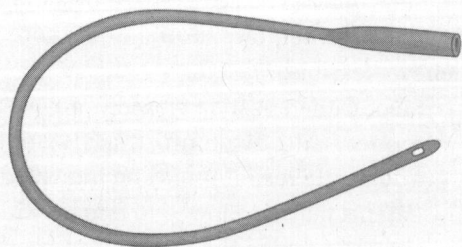
Fig. 7.1: Single-use rubber catheter.

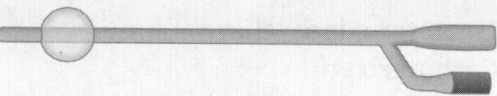
Fig. 7.2: Two-way Foley's catheter.

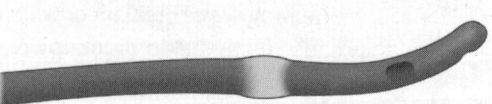
Fig. 7.3: Curved tip catheter.

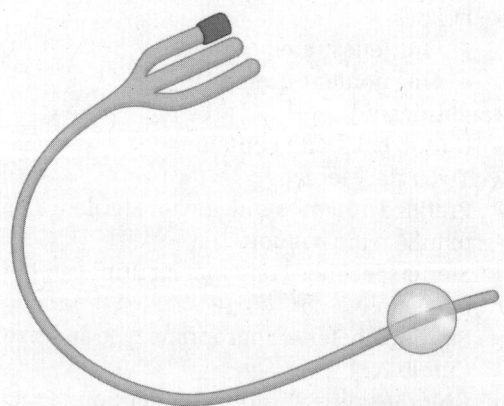
Fig. 7.4: Three-way indwelling catheter.

- *Three-way Foley's catheter:* Often called retention catheter. They have two or more lumens that encircle the body of catheter (**Fig. 7.4**). One lumen drains the urine through the catheter into a collection bag. The second lumen holds the sterile water when the catheter is inflated and is also used to deflate the balloon. The third lumen may be used to instill the medication into the bladder or provide a route for continuous bladder irrigation.

Special Considerations

- Myelodysplastic children may develop hypersensitive reactions, including anaphylaxis when exposed to latex products. So nonlatex catheter (silicon) and

a nonlatex sterile field are routinely used for these patients and careful documentation of latex allergy is recorded in the child's chart.
- *Artificial sphincter:* Meticulous aseptic technique is used. The urethral cuff is deflated immediately prior to catheter insertion.
- *Epispadias or classic exstrophy:* A Young-Dees-Leadbetter procedure is frequently performed to improve the continence. In this, the urethra is angulated with respect to the bladder base to improve continence and this acute angle makes catheterization a challenge.
- In boys with multiple catheterizations, congenital or acquired urethral strictures may be difficult to catheterize. In the above circumstances, a special preparation is needed:
  - Select a smaller coude tipped catheter.
  - Insert 5–10 mL of xylocaine lubricant into the urethra by using the gentle pressure.
  - The urethra is filled until the child perceives pressure and the lubricant is held in place by occluding the meatus. This is to provide the anesthesia of the urethra and encourage slight urethral opening prior to catheter insertion.
  - Insert the catheter without allowing the lubricant to leak from the urethra.
  - In rare instances, systemic sedation may be necessary prior to urethral catheterization.
  - When reasonable efforts are failed, the procedure should be discontinued. Consult the pediatric urologist.
  - Catheterization is completed using endoscopic guidance, urethral dilation, adequate sedation, or local anesthesia.

Risks/Complications
- Urethral trauma
- Bleeding from inappropriate catheter size or use of force
- Urinary tract infection (UTI) related to poor sterile technique or long-term catheterization
- Bladder spasms and pain

Procedure
- Gather appropriate equipment and place into a sterile field.
- Perform hand hygiene and don sterile gloves.

For Female Child
- Place a sterile drape under buttocks.
- Gently separate and pull up the labia minora to visualize the meatus by using nondominant hand and hold the labia open throughout the procedure.
- Swab the meatus from the proximal to distal end using sterile povidone iodine–dipped swabs.
- Lubricate the catheter and insert it into the urethra until urine is obtained.
- Advance the catheter an additional 2.5–5 cm.
- Inflate the balloon with sterile water when using Foley's catheter and gently pull back to test balloon inflation.
- Connect the Foley's catheter to closed drainage system.
- Clean the meatus and labia of povidone iodine and wipe it with wet swab.
- Praise the child for cooperation.

For Male Child
- Grasp the penis with nondominant hand and retract the foreskin and should be remained throughout the procedure.
- Place the sterile drape under the penis.
- Using the sterile cotton swab, clean the glans and meatus with povidone iodine.
- Hold the penile shaft just under the glans to prevent the foreskin from contaminating the area.

- Lubricate and insert the catheter while gently stretching the penis and lifting it to 90° angle to the body.
- Resistance may occur when the catheter meets the urethral sphincter. Ask the child to inhale deeply and advance the catheter at that time.
- Once urine is obtained, advance the catheter to the hub of the catheter (indwelling catheter).
- For intermittent catheter, insert only up to recommended length.
- Inflate the balloon with the sterile water, pull it back gently to test inflation and connect it to the closed drainage system.
- Cleanse the glans and meatus with water to prevent skin irritation.
- Replace the retracted foreskin.

Note: If at any time during the procedure the blood is seen, discontinue the procedure and notify the pediatrician.

- Secure the catheter to either patient's thigh or abdomen. This helps to decrease the risk of bleeding trauma and bladder spasms from pressure and traction.

General Instructions

- If the child says that he/she needs to urinate during catheter insertion, tell the child to go ahead and try to do so. This opens the meatus for passage of the catheter.
- The rule of thumb for catheter length in males is twice the length of the penis plus 4 cm.
- If the child complains of pain or burning, the urinary catheter may not be fully seated in the bladder. Deflate the balloon, advance the catheter further, and reinflate the balloon.
- Daily skin care is essential.
- Adequate fluid intake should be maintained.
- The urine collection bag should be emptied when one-half to two-thirds full or every 3-6 hours. This helps to prevent undue trauma/traction on the urethral related to weight of the bag.
- The frequency of catheter changing should be individually tailored and may be needed every 3-4 weeks.

Instillation of Lidocaine Gel

- Infant ½–1½ mL
- Toddler 1½–2½ mL
- School aged 2½–5 mL
- Adolescent 3–5 mL

Nursing Care of a Child with Indwelling Catheter

- Perform hand hygiene and gather necessary supplies.
- Close the door of the child's room or draw curtains around the child's bed.
- Raise bed to a comfortable working height.
- Don gloves.
- Place a waterproof pad/mackintosh under the child's buttock while positioning the child.
- Girls should be in supine position with their legs spread apart. Boys should be placed in supine with legs straight.
- Place a drape over the child. For girls, place the drape in a diamond configuration with one corner at the child's sternum, one corner over each knee, and one corner over child's perineum. For boys, cover the child's chest and lower extremities with a sheet leaving only the genital area exposed.
- Examine the urethral opening with the help of flashlight.
- Observe for any signs of irritation, trauma, and secretions.
- With the use of syringe, deflate the balloon and assess the amount of water in it and reinflate it.
- Wash the child's genital area with warm water and soap.

- Clean around the urinary meatus and around the catheter itself being careful not to manipulate the catheter. Gently retract the foreskin of boys and clean the area. Return the foreskin to its natural position.
- Rinse and dry the child's perineum.
- Assess the drainage tubing for urine flow and observe that there are no kinks or obstruction in the tubing and make sure that all connections are tightly secured.
- Ensure the collection bag is attached to the frame of the bed below the level of the bladder.
- Ensure the catheter adheres to the thigh or lower abdomen.

Removal of the Indwelling Catheter

- Collaborate with the child's family and health-care personnel regarding the time of removal of indwelling catheter.
- Perform hand hygiene and collect all necessary equipment for removal.
- Provide privacy.
- Raise the bed to a comfortable working height.
- Don gloves.
- Place mackintosh under the child's buttocks while positioning the child. Position the child supine with the legs apart with access to the urinary catheter.
- Place a drape over the child.
- Gently remove the tape holding the urinary catheter in place.
- Attach a syringe to the secondary lumen balloon port of the urinary catheter and deflate the balloon of its entire contents of sterile water.
- Gently remove the urinary catheter by withdrawing slowly and evenly if resistance is felt, do not pull harder, stop, and notify the physician.
- Wash the child's genital area with warm water and soap. Rinse and dry the area.
- Remove the mackintosh and position the child comfortable.
- Lower the height of the bed to an appropriate level.

Highlights ● ● ● ●

✦ Urinary catheterization is the insertion of the catheter through the urethra into the bladder for withdrawal of urine.
✦ Adolescent girls may prefer to be catheterized by a female staff and adolescent boys may prefer to be catheterized by a male caregiver. The request should be honored whenever feasible.
✦ The rule of thumb for catheter length in males is twice the length of the penis plus 4 cm.
✦ If the child complains of pain or burning, the urinary catheter may not be fully seated in the bladder. Deflate the balloon, advance the catheter further, and reinflate the balloon.
✦ The urine collection bag should be emptied when one-half to two-thirds full or every 3–6 hours. This helps to prevent undue trauma/traction on the urethral related to weight of the bag.
✦ The frequency of catheter changing should be individually tailored and may be needed every 3–4 weeks.

SUPRAPUBIC CATHETERIZATION

Definition

A suprapubic catheterization is basically an indwelling catheter that is placed directly through the abdomen. The catheter is inserted above the pubic bone. This catheter must be placed by a urologist.

Indications

- Urine analysis or urine culture in neonates or children younger than 2 years
- Phimosis
- Chronic infection of the urethra or periurethral glands

- Long-term catheterization
- Urethral stricture
- Urethral trauma

Contraindications

Absolute

Empty or unidentifiable bladder (e.g., child's last urination within 1 hour, nonpalpable bladder)

Relative

- Known bladder tumor
- Lower abdominal wounds or scaring
- Overlying cellulitis
- Coagulopathy

Complications

- Bladder stones
- Blood infections
- Hematuria
- Skin breakdown
- Bowel perforation and intra-abdominal visceral injuries
- Urine leakage around the catheter
- UTI
- After many years of catheter use, bladder cancer may also develop.
- *Postobstruction diuresis:* Child should be monitored for 2–3 hours. If it occurs, intravenous (IV) fluid administration and correction of electrolyte is necessary.

Equipment Needed

A sterile tray containing:
- Sterile gloves
- Antiseptic solution
- Gauze pieces
- Sterile drapes
- Anesthetic solutions without epinephrine
- Syringe 10 mL
- Needles 18 and 25 G
- Scalpel blade no. 11
- Syringe 60 mL
- Percutaneous suprapubic catheter set (**Fig. 7.5**)
- Needle obturator
- Connecting tube
- One-way stopcock
- Sterile urine bag
- Drain sponges
- Skin tape or nylon suture (3.0) with a needle driver

Patient Preparation

- Tell the patient or his parents that the doctor will insert a soft plastic tube through the skin of the abdomen and into the bladder, and then connect the tube to an external connection bag.
- Explain that the procedure is done under local anesthesia, that it causes little or no discomfort.
- It takes 15–45 minutes for completion of the procedure.
- Teach the parents about postoperative care of the catheter, collection bag, and surrounding skin.
- If possible, arrange for a visit by an enterostomal therapist for more information.

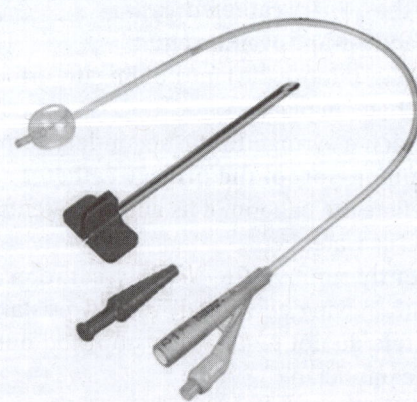

Fig. 7.5: Suprapubic catheter set.

- Ensure that parents or guardian has signed a consent form.
- Place the patient supine on a gurney with his or her legs spread apart.

Procedure

- Perform hand hygiene and don gloves.
- Provide adequate parenteral analgesia with or without sedation.
- Clean the lower abdominal wall.
- Shave the suprapubic area if the patient is hirsute.
- Palpate the distended bladder and mark the insertion site at the midline and 2 inches (4–5 cm) above the symphysis pubis.
- With the use of ultrasonography better to verify the bladder location and to ensure that no loops of bowel are present between the abdominal wall and the bladder.
- Apply an antiseptic solution from the pubis to the umbilicus.
- Repeat the application of the antiseptic solution two more times and allow the area to dry.
- Apply sterile drapes and verify the insertion site by palpating anatomic landmark.
- Fill the 10-mL syringe with the local anesthetic agent and use the 25-gauge needle anesthetize the insertion site.
- Advance the needle through the skin, subcutaneous tissue, rectus sheath, and retropubic space, while alternating injection and aspiration, until urine enters the syringe. Note the direction and depth required to enter the bladder.
- Using the no. 11 blade, make a 4-mm stab incision at the insertion site with the blade facing inferiorly.
- Insert the needle obturator into the malecot catheter and lock it into the part by twisting it so that the needle tip projects 2–5 mm from the distal end of the catheter.
- Connect the 60-mL syringe to the part of the needle obturator.
- Place the tip of the catheter–obturator unit into the skin incision and direct it caudally and at a 20–30° angle from true vertical toward the patient's legs.
- The practitioner's nondominant hand should be placed on the lower abdominal wall, and the unit should be stabilized between the thumb and index finger.
- The dominant hand should be used to advance the unit, while aspirating until urine enters the syringe.
- Once urine enters the syringe, advance the unit 3–4 additional cm into the bladder.
- While securing the unit with the nondominant unscrew the obturator from the catheter.
- Advance the catheter approximately 5 additional cm over the obturator and then completely withdraw the obturator needle.
- Connect the extension tubing to the catheter and connect the tubing to a urinometer or a leg bag.
- Gently withdraw the catheter to lodge the balloon against the bladder wall (**Fig. 7.6**).
- Undrape the patient and apply the skin preparatory solution, for example, Lenzoin to the skin.
- Apply drain dressings around the catheter at the insertion site.
- Stitch the catheter to the skin.

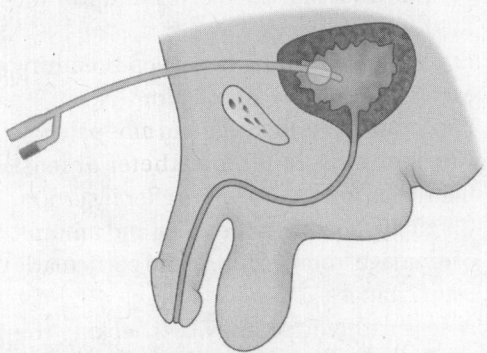

Fig. 7.6: Placement of suprapubic catheter.

Postprocedure Care

- Monitor the child for postobstructive diuresis for 2–3 hours.
- If this complication occurs, patients should be started with IV fluid administration and monitoring and correction of electrolytes.
- The insertion site should be inspected and cleaned with soap and water to prevent cellulitis and abscess formation.
- Simple irrigation with normal saline (NS) should resolve most catheter obstructions.
- If displacement or malpositioning of catheter occurs, the urologist should be notified, cystography can be performed.
- Every effort should be made to ensure the bladder position with palpation and ultrasonography to minimize or prevent the chances of complications.
- Ensure that the child drinks fluids adequately.
- Ensure that drainage bag is below the level of waist.
- Maintain a closed drainage system to minimize the number of times disconnecting the bag.
- Check the catheter for troubleshooting such as kinking of catheter, urine color is cloudy or catheter, balloon not deflated or bleeding. Inform the doctor immediately and take appropriate measures.

Nurse's Responsibility

- Monitor vital signs, intake and output, and fluid status.
- Encourage coughing and deep breathing exercises and early ambulation.
- Ensure adequate drainage and tube patency.
- Check the suprapubic catheter at least hourly for the first 24 hours after insertion.
- Carefully document the color and amount of drainage from the tube, note particularly color changes.
- Assess catheter patency by checking the amount of urine in the drainage bag and by palpation for bladder distention.
- Ensure that collection bag is below waist level to enhance drainage and prevent backflow, which can lead to infection.
- As ordered, perform a voiding trial by closing stopcock (or clamping the tube) for 4 hours asking the child to attempt urination and then reopening the tube and measuring residual urine.
- To prevent kinks in the tube, curve it gently but do not bend it.
- Tape the catheter securely in place on the abdominal skin to reduce tension and prevent dislodgement.
- If it becomes dislodged, immediately notify the doctor.
- Irrigate the suprapubic catheter as ordered.
- Check the catheter frequently for kinks or obstruction. If mucous or a blood clot blocks the tube, try milking it to restore patency.
- If you cannot clean the obstruction promptly, notify the physician.
- Check drainages often and change often at least once per day or as ordered.
- Observe the skin around the insertion site for signs of infection and encrustation.

Home Care Instructions

- Teach the child/his parents how to change the dressing and how to empty and reattach the collection bag.
- Encourage to drink plenty of fluids to reduce the risk of complications.
- Stress the importance of regular follow-up, examination to allow early detection of possible complications.
- Tell the patient/his family to notify the doctor promptly any signs of infection or encrustation such as discolored or foul-smelling discharge, impaired drainage or swelling, redness, and tenderness at the tube insertion site.

Duration of Changing the Catheter

Once a month to decrease infection.

Points to Remember

- When changing a suprapubic catheter, speed is very important. The new catheter should be inserted within 5-10 minutes of removal of the old catheter.
- Never remove a suprapubic catheter unless it is going to be changed immediately.

Highlights ●●●●

> + A suprapubic catheterization is basically an indwelling catheter that is placed directly through the abdomen. The catheter is inserted above the pubic bone.
> + Monitor the child for postobstructive diuresis for 2-3 hours after the procedure.
> + The insertion site should be inspected and cleaned with soap and water to prevent cellulitis and abscess formation.
> + Check the catheter for troubleshooting such as kinking of catheter, urine color is cloudy or catheter balloon not deflated or bleeding. Inform the doctor immediately and take appropriate measures.
> + Never remove a suprapubic catheter unless it is going to be changed immediately.

ENEMA

Definition

Introduction of fluid into the rectum is called enema.

Indications

- To encourage the expulsion of feces and flatus
- To soften stools or soothen the membranes
- To reduce the hyperthermia
- To administer the nutrition and medication

Amount

Amount of fluid to be introduced depends upon the size of the child:
- Infants: 150-250 mL
- Young child: 250-350 mL
- Older child: 300-350 mL
- Adolescent: 500-750 mL

Note: For oil-retention enema, use 10-12 Fr catheter. The catheter should be inserted into the rectum depending on the age of the child as follows:
- Infants: 2.5 cm
- 2-4 years: 5 cm
- 4-10 years: 7.5 cm
- >11 years: 10 cm

Temperature of the solution: 105°F or 45.5°C; for oil-retention enema 100°F (37.7°C)

Equipment Needed

A clean tray containing:
- Enema bag or can and tubing with clamp or syringe with rubber tubing
- Lubricant (liquid paraffin)
- Enema solution
- 10-12 Fr rectal catheter
- Gauze pieces in bowl
- Pair of gloves
- Bedpan padded at the edges
- Kidney tray or paper bag
- Toilet tissue
- Lotion thermometer
- Mackintosh

General Instructions

- The can should not be held >18" above the child's hip. So that solution may run slowly by gravity and pressure into the bowel.
- An isotonic solution or physiologic saline is used. Tap water alone is not used because of the danger of fluid shift and overload.
- Commercially prepared disposable pediatric enemas may be used only when especially prescribed. That can result in rapid harsh action and can be dangerous when used on dehydrated children, children with megacolon or azotemic children.
- A cleansing enema can be given 30-40 minutes after the oil-retention enema.

Position
- Infant and toddler lie on abdomen with knees bent (**Fig. 7.7**).
- Older children and adolescent lie on left side with right leg flexed toward chest (**Fig. 7.8**).

Preparation
- Explain the procedure to the parents and child.
- Allow the child to do it on dummy or toys.
- Provide privacy.

Procedure
- Gather supplies
- Wash hands and don gloves
- Position the child
- Clamp the enema tubing, remove the cap, and apply lubricant to the tip of the catheter.
- Insert the tube into the rectum.
- Unclamp the tubing and administer the prescribed volume of enema solution at a rate of about 100 mL/min.
- Remove the catheter gently and put it in kidney tray.
- Hold the child's buttocks together if needed to encourage retention of enema for 5–10 minutes.
- Offer bedpan.
- In case of ambulatory and older children assist them to go to toilet.

Postprocedure Care
- Praise the child for cooperation.
- Make the child comfortable.
- Record the procedure in nurse's record:
  - Type of solution used
  - Time
  - Any other remarks.
- Clean and replace the supplies.

Use of Other Methods over Enema
- A preoperative bowel preparation solution given orally or through a nasogastric tube.
- The polyethylene glycol electrolyte lavage solution (GoLYTELY) mechanically flushes the bowel without significant absorption, thereby avoiding potential fluid and electrolyte imbalances.
- Another effective oral cathartic is magnesium citrate solution.

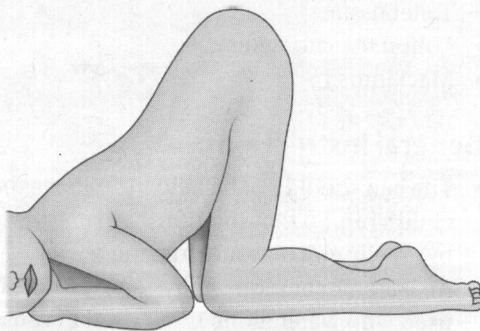

Fig. 7.7: Knee-chest position.

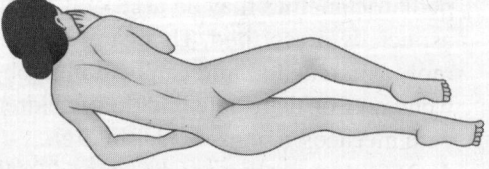

Fig. 7.8: Sims' lateral position.

Highlights
- Introduction of fluid into the rectum is called enema.
- An isotonic solution or physiologic saline is used for enema. Tap water alone is not used because of the danger of fluid shift and overload.
- The polyethylene glycol electrolyte lavage solution (GoLYTELY) mechanically flushes the bowel without significant absorption, thereby avoiding potential fluid and electrolyte imbalances.

COLOSTOMY CARE

Definition
A colostomy consists of an artificial opening created in the large intestine and brought to the surface of the abdomen for the purpose of evacuating the bowels.

Indications
- Anorectal malformations
- Spina bifida
- Ulcerative colitis
- Hirschsprung's disease
- Acquired indications—rectovaginal fistula, perineal injury, and colonic injury

Complications
- Skin excoriations
- Prolapse
- Hemorrhage
- Sepsis/wound infection
- Poor parental acceptance
- Para-colostomy hernia
- Stoma stenosis
- Persistent odor

Purposes of Colostomy Care
- To prevent the excoriation of the skin around the stoma
- To establish regularity of evacuation
- To stop any leakage of feces
- To teach the patient and parents/relatives regarding the care of colostomy

Equipment Needed
A clean tray containing:
- Pair of gloves
- Mackintosh and sheet
- Bowl with cotton swabs and gauze pieces
- Soap and water
- Wash cloth
- Bedpan
- Disposable colostomy bag with clamp
- Zinc oxide ointment
- Towel
- Tissue paper

Preparation
- Explain the procedure to the parents and the child as appropriate.
- Keep all the equipment near the patient site.
- Maintain privacy of the patient.
- Maintain comfortable position, for example, Fowler's, semi-Fowler's, or sitting position.

Procedure
- Assess the location of the ostomy and the type of colostomy performed. Stoma location is an indicator of the section of the bowel in which it is located and a predictor of the type of fecal drainage to expect.
- Wash hands and don gloves.
- Remove the old appliances.
- Empty the appliances in bedpan.
- Remove the excess stool with tissue paper from the stoma.
- Clean the peristomal skin with soap and water or prescribed cleansing agent.
- Dry the area completely with a paper towel.
- Observe the color of stoma: normal stoma looks reddish pink (**Fig. 7.9**).
- Apply zinc oxide ointment and keep it for 1–2 minutes to absorb.
- Apply the skin barrier to the entire area that the appliance will cover.
- Apply the stoma paste around the stoma and the mucus fistula.
- Apply the stoma pouch over the barrier.
- Position a collection bag over the stoma.

Nurse's Responsibility
- Empty a drainable pouch or replace the colostomy bag as needed or when it is not more than one-third full.

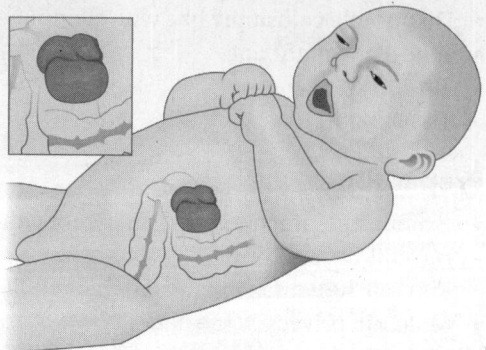

Fig. 7.9: Child with colostomy.

- Assess stoma appearance and surrounding skin condition frequently.
- Use Karaya paste and a skin barrier wafer as needed to maintain a secure ostomy pouch.
- Prior to discharge, provide written, verbal psychomotor instruction on colostomy care, pouch management, skin care, and irrigation for the client.
- Allow ample time for the caregiver and child (older) to practice changing the pouch either on the client or a model.
- Provide dietary teaching regarding the foods that cause stool odor and gas and foods that thicken the stools or cause loose stools.
  - Foods that increase stool odor: asparagus, beans, cabbage, eggs, fish, garlic, onions, and some spices.
  - Foods that increase intestinal gas: broccoli, cabbage, carbonated drinks, cauliflower, corn, cucumber, dairy products, dried beans, peas, radish, and spinach.
  - Foods that thicken Stool: banana, cheese, yogurt, rice, tapioca, pasta, and creamy peanut butter.
  - Foods that loosen the stools: chocolate, fried foods, greasy foods, lightly spiced foods, green leafy vegetables, raw fruits and juices, and raw vegetables.
  - Foods that color stool: beetroot and red gelatin.
- The diet for a child with a colostomy is individualized and may require no alteration from that consumed preoperatively.
- If an abdominoperineal resection has been performed, emphasize the importance of using no rectal suppositories, rectal temperature, or enemas.
- If the child is school-going, he/she should carry medical identification or a medic alert tag or bracelet.

These measures are important to prevent trauma to the tissues when the rectum has been removed.

Highlights ●●●●

- ✦ A colostomy consists of an artificial opening created in the large intestine and brought to the surface of the abdomen for the purpose of evacuating the bowels.
- ✦ Assess stoma appearance and surrounding skin condition frequently.
- ✦ Use Karaya paste and a skin barrier wafer as needed to maintain a secure ostomy pouch.
- ✦ Prior to discharge, provide written, verbal psychomotor instruction on colostomy care, pouch management, skin care, and irrigation for the client.
- ✦ Allow ample time for the caregiver and child (older) to practice changing the pouch either on the client or a model.
- ✦ Provide dietary teaching regarding the foods that cause stool odor and gas and foods that thicken the stools or cause loose stools.
- ✦ The diet for a child with a colostomy is individualized and may require no alteration from that consumed preoperatively.
- ✦ If an abdominoperineal resection has been performed, emphasize the importance of using no rectal suppositories, rectal temperature or enemas.

COLONIC IRRIGATION

Definition
Colonic irrigation refers to a procedure also called colon cleansing, where fluids are pumped through the rectum into the colon in order to clean the bowels.

Indications/Purposes
- To remove toxins and parasites
- Before colonoscopy
- Prior to a surgical procedure
- Enterocolitis
- To prevent stasis of stool in the colon

Complications
- Rectal perforations
- Transmission of communicable diseases if tube is not sterilized properly
- Dehydration and electrolyte imbalance

Equipment Needed
A clean tray containing:
- Silicone catheter: 16 Fr for children <1 year, and 24 Fr for children >1 year
- 60 mL catheter tipped syringe
- Petroleum-based lubricant
- Gauze pieces in a small bowl to apply lubricant
- Plastic apron, pair of gloves
- Mackintosh and towel
- Gown for the patient
- Tissue paper/towels to wipe the anal region after the procedure
- Kidney tray
- Container to discard the return solution
- NS/prescribed solution

Preparation
- Explain the procedure to parents and child as appropriate.
- Review the order for colonic irrigation.
- Assemble the required articles near the working area.
- Provide privacy.
- Remove the clothing below the waist.
- Place the child on the procedure table.
- Provide left lateral position.
- Spread the mackintosh and towel under the waist.

Procedure
- Perform hand hygiene.
- Wear apron and gloves.
- Pour NS solution into the basin or kidney tray.
- Using 60 mL catheter tip syringe, draw 20 mL NS.
- Gently insert the appropriate-size lubricated catheter into the rectum approximately 6 inches.
- Place the catheter tip syringe into the end of the silicone catheter and inject 20 mL NS into the rectum.
- Disconnect syringe from the catheter, allow NS to drip into the container.
- Observe for the return content.
- Continue the procedure till the return fluid is clear or the prescribed amount of solution is completed.

Postprocedure Care
- Remove the catheter gently from the rectum and discard it in the kidney tray.
- Wipe the area. Assist the child in wearing clothes.
- Document the procedure in nurse's record with date, time, type and amount of solution used. Observation made during the procedure.

General Instructions
- The temperature of the solution should be ideal to body temperature (94–100°F).

- Inject 10–20 mL of solution at a time.
- Massage the lower abdomen during the procedure.
- Encourage the child to relax during the procedure.
- Ensure that same amount of fluid is returned, which is injected into the colon.
- Ensure that the size of the catheter should be larger enough to allow passing of stool through the catheter.
- Observe the content of return fluid:
  - Undigested foods indicate improper chewing.
  - Strings indicate tapeworm.
  - Yellow color: toxins.
  - White color: *Candida albicans*.

Highlights ●●●●

> ✦ Colonic irrigation refers to a procedure also called colon cleansing, where fluids are pumped through the rectum into the colon in order to clean the bowels.
> ✦ The temperature of the solution should be ideal to body temperature (94–100°F).
> ✦ Inject 10–20 mL of solution at a time.
> ✦ Massage the lower abdomen during the procedure.
> ✦ Ensure that same amount of fluid is returned, which is injected into the colon.
> ✦ Ensure that the size of the catheter should be larger enough to allow passing of stool through the catheter.

DOUBLE DIAPERING

Definition

Double diapering is a method used to protect the urethra and stent or catheter after surgery where the inner diaper contains stool and the outer diaper contains urine allowing separation between the bowel and bladder output.

Indication

The children underwent surgery for correction of epispadias and hypospadias.

Purposes

- Protection of urethra and stent or catheter after surgery
- To keep the area clean and free from infection

Procedure

- Cut a hole or a cross-shaped slit in the front of the smaller diaper.
- Unfold both diapers and place the smaller diaper (with the hole) inside the larger one.
- Place both diapers under the child.
- Carefully bring the penis (if applicable) and catheter/stent through the hole in the smaller diaper and close the diaper.
- Close the larger diaper, making sure the tip of the catheter/stent is inside the larger diaper.

Nurse's Responsibility

- Change the outside diaper (larger diaper) when the child is wet.
- Change both diapers when the child has a bowel movement.

Highlights ●●●●

> ✦ Double diapering is a method used to protect the urethra and stent or catheter after surgery where the inner diaper contains stool and the outer diaper contains urine allowing separation between the bowel and bladder output.
> ✦ Change the outside diaper (larger diaper) when the child is wet.
> ✦ Change both diapers when the child has a bowel movement.

URETEROSTOMY CARE

Definition
Ureterostomy is a surgical procedure in which the urine bypasses the bladder and exits the body through a surgically created opening (stoma) and collects into a pouch that is worn outside the body (**Fig. 7.10**).

Types
- Loop cutaneous ureterostomy or pyelostomy
- End cutaneous ureterostomy

Based on the number of ureters attached to the stoma and site of diversion, ureterostomy is divided into four types:
- *Single ureterostomy:* Only one ureter is brought to the surface of the abdomen.
- *Bilateral ureterostomy:* Two ureters brought to the surface of the abdomen, one on each side.
- *Double-barrel ureterostomy:* Both ureters are brought to the same side of the abdominal surface.
- *Transureteroureterostomy:* Both ureters are brought to the same side of the abdomen, through the same stoma.

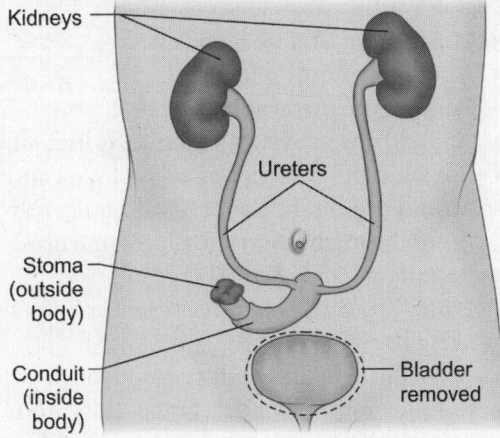

Fig. 7.10: Ureterostomy.

Indications
- Obstructive uropathy unresponsive to lower urinary tract drainage
- Obstruction requiring delayed surgical correction
- High-grade reflux into a solitary kidney obstruction with infection
- Poor bladder function secondary to a variety of congenital anomalies, including prune-belly syndrome, posterior urethral valves, bladder exstrophy, and urogenital sinus defect

Equipment Needed
A tray should contain:
- Clean cloth
- Soap
- Skin wipers
- Pair of gloves

Procedure
- Open the pouches valve and empty the urine.
- Apply soap with cloth
- Rinse thoroughly
- Dry the stoma area well
- Replace the bag

Aftercare
- Place the child in a comfortable position and praise for cooperation
- Clean and replace the articles and dispose the waste
- Document the procedure

Nursing Considerations
- Proper care of the pouch requires regular drainage and changing.
- Drain the pouch when it is between one-third and one-half full. This will be about every 2–4 hours or more often if the child drinks a lot of fluids.

- Change the pouch every 3–7 days or immediately if there is any leakage, remove the old pouch and apply the new pouch putting the sticky side to the skin and passing down to seal all edges.
- The stoma needs regular cleaning to prevent irritation caused by regular contact with urine, which has a high bacterial count.
- Wiping with a wet cloth while changing the bag will usually be enough.
- Soap is safe, but make sure to rinse well afterward.
- Use skin wipes or powder to protect the skin around the stoma, further and under the pouch barrier.

Complications

There is a risk for the child to develop complications during surgery:
- Thrombosis
- Embolism
- Injury to adjacent structures
- Cardiopulmonary complications

Highlights ● ● ● ●

> + Ureterostomy is a surgical procedure in which the urine bypasses the bladder and exits the body through a surgically created opening (stoma) and collects into a pouch that is worn outside the body.
> + Two types of ureterostomy are loop cutaneous ureterostomy or pyelostomy, end cutaneous ureterostomy.
> + Change the pouch every 3–7 days or immediately if there is any leakage, remove the old pouch and apply the new pouch putting the sticky side to the skin and passing down to seal all edges.
> + The stoma needs regular cleaning to prevent irritation caused by regular contact with urine, which has a high bacterial count.

INSERTION OF SUPPOSITORY

Definition

A solid medical preparation in a roughly conical or cylindrical shape, designed to be inserted into the rectum or vagina to dissolve.

Indication

- Constipation

Equipment Needed

- Suppository
- Pair of disposable gloves
- Mackintosh and towel
- Lukewarm water
- Bedpan

Preparation of the Child and Parents

- Explain the parents and the child as appropriate for indication of the procedure and how it will be done.
- Provide privacy.
- Position the child in Sims' position.
- Expose only the anal region.
- Spread the mackintosh and towel under the buttocks.

Procedure

- Wash hands and wear gloves.
- Check the prescription.
- Remove the medication from foil.
- Apply lukewarm water for reducing friction.
- Separate the buttocks by using index and thumb of nondominant hand and gently insert the medication into the rectum using dominant hand (**Fig. 7.11**).
- Hold the buttocks together for fewer seconds.
- Make the child lie in this position for 15–20 minutes to prevent the suppository from coming out.

Chapter 7: Elimination Needs

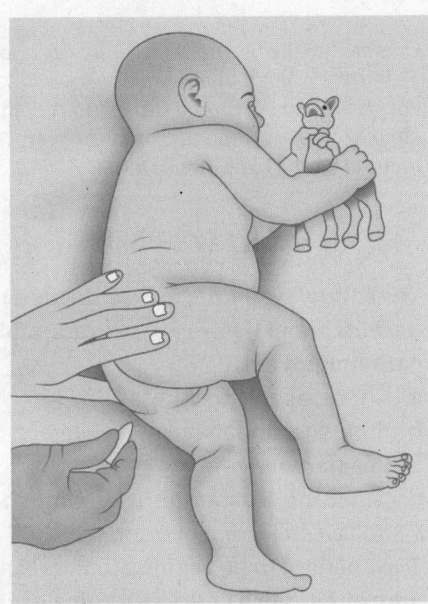

Fig. 7.11: Insertion of suppository.

Aftercare
- Clean and replace the articles
- Remove the gloves
- Offer bedpan as necessary
- Document the procedure in nurse's record

Highlights ●●●●

- ✦ A solid medical preparation in a roughly conical or cylindrical shape, designed to be inserted into the rectum or vagina to dissolve.
- ✦ It is commonly indicated for children with constipation.
- ✦ To insert suppository, position the child in Sims' position.
- ✦ Separate the buttocks by using index and thumb of nondominant hand and gently insert the medication into the rectum using dominant hand.
- ✦ Make the child lie in this position for 15–20 minutes to prevent the suppository from coming out.

ENTEROSTOMY CARE

Definition
An enterostomy is a surgical procedure in which the small intestine is diverted to an artificial opening in the wall.

Indications
- Intestinal gangrene
- Perforated typhoid ileitis
- Anastomotic dehiscence of gastrointestinal (GI) tract
- Intestinal atresias

Equipment Needed
- Drainage pouch
- Adhesive skin barrier
- Ostomy ring
- Skin barrier powder
- Pair of gloves
- Gauze pieces in a bowl
- Receptacle for collecting waste
- A jar with warm water

Procedure
- Wash hands and wear gloves.
- Remove the pouch and skin barrier gently by holding the barrier with one hand and pushing the skin with other hand.
- Keep a gauze piece over the stoma to contain bowel contents during the change of appliance.
- Remove if there is any residue present on the skin with dry gauze piece.
- Wash the skin around the stoma with warm water and dry.
- Apply the adhesive skin barrier firmly to the infant's skin.
- Apply the drainage pouch to the barrier device.

Aftercare

- Clean and replace the articles.
- Wash hands.
- Document the procedure with the date of changing the appliance.
- Mention the observations made.

Nursing Considerations

The condition of stoma should be assessed during each shift. Inspect the stoma for the following:

- *Color:* Should be bright pink to beefy red and moist.
- *Size:* the stoma becomes edematous when exposed while changing the pouch and resolves quickly when it is replaced.
- *Function:* Note the consistency, color, and amount of drainage.
- *Skin:* Note the integrity of skin surrounding the stoma.
- Check the pouch frequently for any leakage.
- Report to the doctor if there is any prolapse of stoma (>1 inch above the skin level) or if there are any abnormal findings such as rashes, skin damage, and bleeding.
- Ostomy usually becomes active for drainage within 48–72 hours after surgery.
- If the pouch is heavily soiled or foul smelling, then need to rinse it thoroughly and reuse.
- Pouch should be changed prior to feeding child so that drainage from stoma can be reduced during appliance changes.

Highlights ●●●●

+ An enterostomy is a surgical procedure in which the small intestine is diverted to an artificial opening in the wall.
+ The condition of stoma should be assessed during each shift.
+ Report the doctor if there is any prolapse of stoma (>1 inch above the skin level) or if there are any abnormal findings such as rashes, skin damage, and bleeding.
+ Ostomy usually becomes active for drainage within 48–72 hours after surgery.
+ Pouch should be changed prior to feeding child so that drainage from stoma can be reduced during appliance changes.

MEMORY EXERCISE

1. The following points to be educated to parents about home care of suprapubic catheter, *except:*
   a. Changing the dressing
   b. Emptying and reattaching bag
   c. Regular follow-up
   d. Drinking less amount of water to avoid fast collection of urine

2. Type of food to be avoided to decrease odorous gas in a child with colostomy:
   a. Onion, cabbage, eggs
   b. Fried foods, rice, nuts
   c. Apple, pear, wheat
   d. Potatoes, carrots, peas

3. Which of the following conditions requires immediate action from the nurse for a child who has undergone colostomy procedure before 8 hours:
   a. The stoma is swollen and large
   b. The stoma is black
   c. The stoma is not draining any stool
   d. The child complains tenderness around the stoma

4. The ideal temperature of solution for colonic irrigation is:
   a. 100°F
   b. 105°F
   c. 110°F
   d. 104°F

5. Which of the following is the most preferred for catheterizing a 6-month-old child?
   a. 6 Fr catheter
   b. 8 Fr catheter
   c. 5 Fr Ryle's tube
   d. 8 Fr Ryle's tube

CHAPTER 8

Emergency Procedures

LEARNING OBJECTIVES

After reading this chapter, the readers should be able to:
- Respond to the needs of a child in emergency situation.
- Assemble the articles needed for various emergency procedures.
- Perform lifesaving procedures.
- Monitor the progress of a child's condition.

Keywords: foreign bodies, Heimlich maneuver, airway, resuscitation, cardiac massage, rescue, tapping, blood, administration

MANUAL REMOVAL OF FOREIGN BODY FROM THE AIRWAY

Common Foreign Bodies
- Offending food items such as nuts, piece of carrot, popcorn, seeds, meat, grapes, and candy.
- Other items include plastic or glass beads, peas, button, and coins.

Signs of Foreign Body Aspiration

Foreign body aspiration should be seriously suspected in the case of spontaneous respiratory distress associated with:
- Coughing
- Gagging
- Stridor
- Hoarseness
- Cyanosis
- Wheezing

Procedure

Removal of Foreign Body in an Infant

Back blow and chest thrust
- Hold the infant face down on your forearm, which in turn should rest on your thigh.
- Support head of your hand between the shoulder blades of the infant.
- Give five forceful blows on the infant's back with heel of your hand (**Fig. 8.1A**).
- Now turn the infant around as a unit to a supine position while firmly supporting the head and neck.
- Administer up to five quick chest thrusts in a similar method and location as used for chest compression (**Fig. 8.1B**).

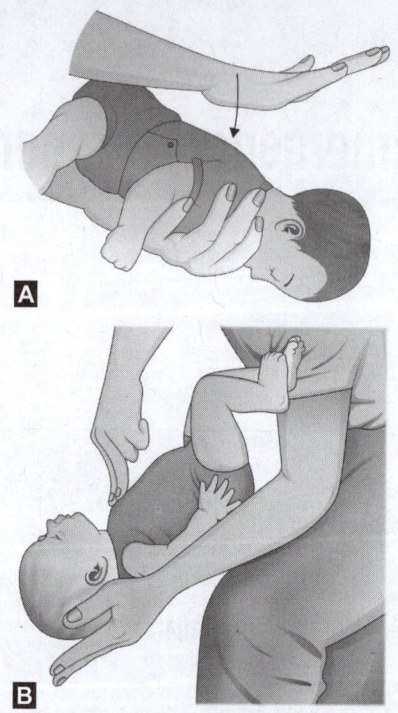

Figs. 8.1A and B: Removal of foreign body in infant: (A) Back blow and (B) Chest thrust.

- The whole process may be repeated until the foreign body is expelled out.

Removal of Foreign Body in a Child Older than 1 Year

Subdiaphragmatic abdominal thrusts (Heimlich maneuver) increase the intrathoracic pressure and create an artificial bout of cough, which forces foreign body out of the airway. This maneuver is not employed in infants because of the risk of liver injury.

Heimlich maneuver in a conscious child

- Stand behind the child and encircle his torso by putting both arms directly under his axillae.
- Place the thumb side of the one fist against the child's abdomen in midline, slightly above naval and well below xiphoid.

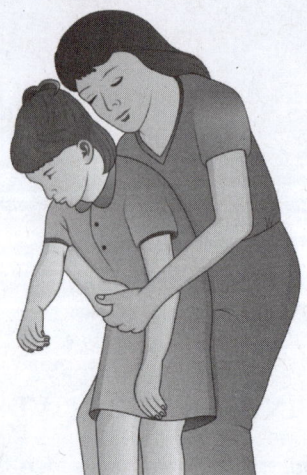

Fig. 8.2: Heimlich maneuver in a conscious child.

- With other hand, grasp the first and exert quick upward thrust taking care not to touch the xiphoid process or lower rib margin (Fig. 8.2).

Each thrust should be forceful enough and intended to relieve obstruction.

Heimlich maneuver in an unconscious child

- Position the child in a supine position and kneel at his feet.
- Place the heel of one hand on child's abdomen in the midline, slightly above the naval and well below the rib cage.
- Place the second hand on top of the first and press into the abdomen with quick upward thrust (Fig. 8.3).

Nurse's Responsibility

- Recognize the signs of foreign body aspiration and implement immediate measures to relieve the obstruction.
- Teach the Heimlich maneuver technique to parents to deal with such situation at home.

Chapter 8: Emergency Procedures

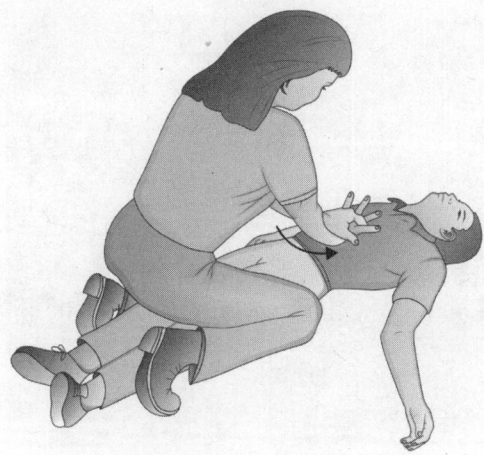

Fig. 8.3: Heimlich maneuver in an unconscious child.

Highlights ● ● ● ●

- Foreign body aspiration should be seriously suspected in case of spontaneous respiratory distress associated with coughing, gagging, stridor, hoarseness, cyanosis, or wheezing.
- To remove foreign body in an infant, give back blow and chest thrust.
- For removal in a child older than 1 year, subdiaphragmatic abdominal thrusts (Heimlich maneuver) increase the intrathoracic pressure and create an artificial bout of cough, which forces foreign body out of the airway.

CARDIOPULMONARY RESUSCITATION

Definition
Manual application of chest compressions and ventilations to patients in cardiac arrest, done in an effort to maintain viability until advance help arrives. This procedure is an essential component of basic life support (BLS), basic cardiac life support (BCLS), and advanced life support (ALS).

Indications
The indications for cardiopulmonary resuscitation (CPR) are majorly divided into two parts:
1. Respiratory failure and arrest
2. Cardiopulmonary failure and arrest

The conditions that lead to either of the above are:
- Drowning
- Suffocation
- Choking
- Injuries—head trauma
- Electric shock
- Excessive bleeding
- Lung disease
- Poisoning
- Suffocation

Procedure
- *Give 2 gentle breaths:* If the baby is not breathing, give 2 small gentle breaths. Cover the baby's mouth and nose with your mouth. Each breath should be 1 second long. You should see the baby's chest rise with each breath.
- *Give 30 compressions:* Give 30 gentle compressions at the rate of 100/min. Use two fingers in the center of the chest below the nipples. Press down approximately one-third depth of the chest.
- Repeat with 2 breathes and 30 compressions until ALS service arrives.

Steps
1. *Determining responsiveness:* The child's state of consciousness and ability to breath and the extent of any injuries should be quickly determined.
2. *Shout and tap:* Shout and gently tap the child on shoulder. If there is no response, position the infant on his or her back.

- Gently shaking the child (assuming there is no risk of cervical spine injury) and speaking in a loud voice are helpful in assessing the level of responsiveness.
- Respiratory effort and effectiveness as well as attempts to speak should be noted. If a head or neck injury is suspected, the cervical spine should be immobilized.
- Look for any deformities, bleeding or environmental clues that indicate trauma.
3. A verbal call for help is made.
4. If there is a lone rescuer and CPR is necessary, it should be performed for five cycles (30 compressions and 2 breaths constitute a cycle for the lone rescuer).
   - Patent airway:
   Airway should be assessed for patency using look, listen, and feel approach.
   - Observe for airway compromise, listen over the patient's nose and mouth for breathing, and/or place a hand or cheek close to the patient's face to feel any air movement.
   - If obstruction is suspected, establish a patent airway.
   - For medical arrest: Head tilt–chin lift maneuver is preferred.
   Note: Any child who suffers a traumatic arrest should have full immobilization of the head and neck, and airway patency is established using the jaw thrust maneuver.
   - Head tilt–chin lift: Place the child in supine position on a firm flat surface. Place one hand on the patient's forehead and one or two fingers of the other hand just lateral to the chin (**Fig. 8.4**). The neck is then extended slightly by gently pushing the forehead while pulling upward on the mandible.

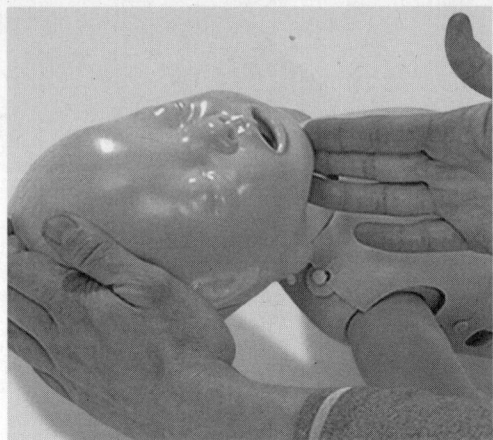

Fig. 8.4: Head tilt–chin lift maneuver.

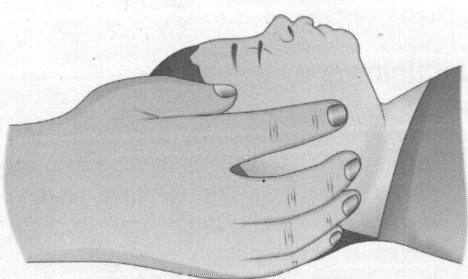

Fig. 8.5: Jaw thrust maneuver.

- Jaw thrust: Three fingers are placed under the angles of jaw, which is lifted upward. The mouth is opened by depressing the chin with thumbs (**Fig. 8.5**).
- Rescue breathing:
  If the child is not breathing:
  » Cover the child's mouth tightly with your mouth.
  » Pinch the nose closed.
  » Keep the chin lifted and head tilted.
  » Give 2 rescue breaths. Each breath should take about a second and make the chest rise (**Fig. 8.6**).
- Perform chest compressions
  » Place the heel of one hand on the breast bone just below the nipples.

Chapter 8: Emergency Procedures | **199**

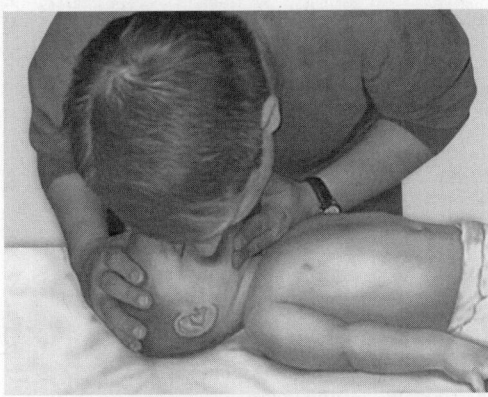

Fig. 8.6: Rescue breathing.

Make sure your heel is not at the very end of the breast bone (**Fig. 8.7**).
» Keep your other hand on the child's forehead, keeping the head tilted back.
» Press down on the child's chest so that it compress about one-third to one-half depth of the chest.
» Give 30 compressions. Each time, let the chest rise completely. These compressions should be fast and hard with no pausing. Count the compressions quickly.
» Give the child 2 more breaths. The chest should rise.

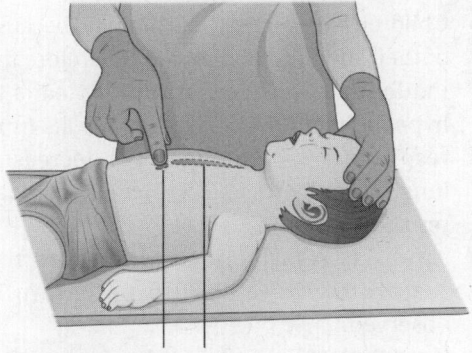

Fig. 8.7: Site for chest compression in pediatric clients.

» Continue CPR (30 chest compressions, followed by 2 breaths then repeat) for about 2 minutes.
» After 2 minutes of CPR if the child still does not have normal breathing, coughing, or any movement, leave the child if you are alone and call for help.
» Repeat rescue breathing and chest compressions until the child recovers or help arrives.
» If the child starts breathing again, place him or her in the recovery position. Periodically recheck for breathing until the help arrives (**Flowchart 8.1**).

Site

- *In infants*: Lower half of the sternum—1 fingerbreadth below the internipple line.
- Two fingers are used to compress the sternum about one-third of the depth.
- *Another technique*: Thumbs are placed on the sternum and the fingers of both hands are placed behind the infant's back (encircling).
- *Small children*: Two fingerbreadth above xiphoid process. The heel of one hand is used to compress the sternum, one-third of the depth of chest.
- *Older children*: Two hands method (as in adult).

General Instructions

Airway
- A cardiopulmonary arrest in children is often caused by respiratory insufficiency. The anatomical and physiological differences in the airway between the child and adult often contribute to this.
- The airway of the child is much narrower than that of the adult. Obstruction from edema or mucus can significantly reduce the airway diameter and increase resistance

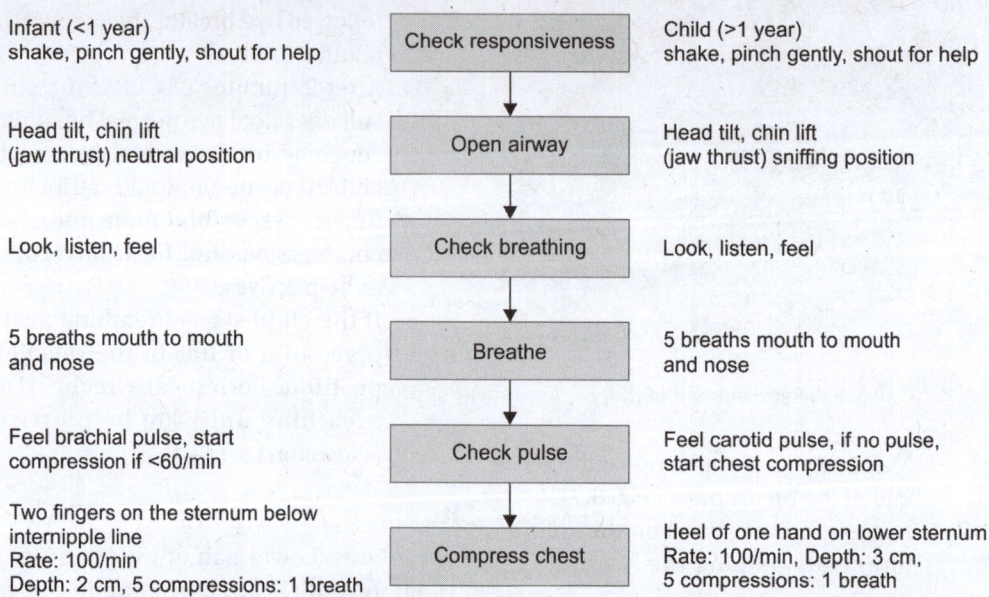

Flowchart 8.1: Primary steps in pediatric CPR.

(ALS: advanced life support; BLS: basic life support; CPR: cardiopulmonary resuscitation; AED: automated external defibrillator)
Source: American Heart Association (2015).

to airflow consequently increasing the work of breathing (WOB).
- Infants under 6 months are obligatory nose breathers, which makes clearing of blocked nostrils essential in this age group. The tongue of the infant is larger in proportion to the oral cavity. Posterior shifting of the tongue can cause severe airway obstruction.
- The epiglottis of young children is short and narrow, angling away from the axis of the trachea. This may cause some difficulties during endotracheal intubation.
- In children under 10 years of age, the narrowest part of the airway is below the vocal cord at the level of the cricoid cartilage.
- In teenagers, the narrowest area is at the glottis inlet.
- Opening the airway is important in the unresponsive children since they may have airway obstruction because of displacement of the tongue.
- Establishing and maintaining airway patent is essential and can be achieved using one of two maneuvers as follows: head tilt and chin lift and jaw thrust.
- Feeling for the expired air movement on the chest.

Breathing
- Children have high oxygen demand because of their high metabolic rate. Therefore the inadequate ventilation rapidly leads to hypoxia in children. Hypoxia results from respiratory failure due to (1) decreased lung's compliance and (2) increased airway resistance.
- Apnea is relatively common and the respiratory rate should be carefully observed.
- If no spontaneous breathing is detected after opening maneuvers, rescue breaths should be administered while maintaining airway patency.

Circulation

- The rescuer should feel for the pulse in a large artery for up to 10 seconds. This should assess rate and volume: palpation of the carotid pulse in older children and brachial pulse in infants. In all age-groups femoral pulse is an alternative.
- Chest compressions are serial, rhythmic compressions of the chest used to circulate the blood to the vital organs until ALS can be provided. To achieve the optimal compressions, the child must be supine on a hard surface **(Flowchart 8.2)**.
- In infants, the area of compression is the lower half of the sternum, which can be located 1 fingerbreadth below the internipple line.

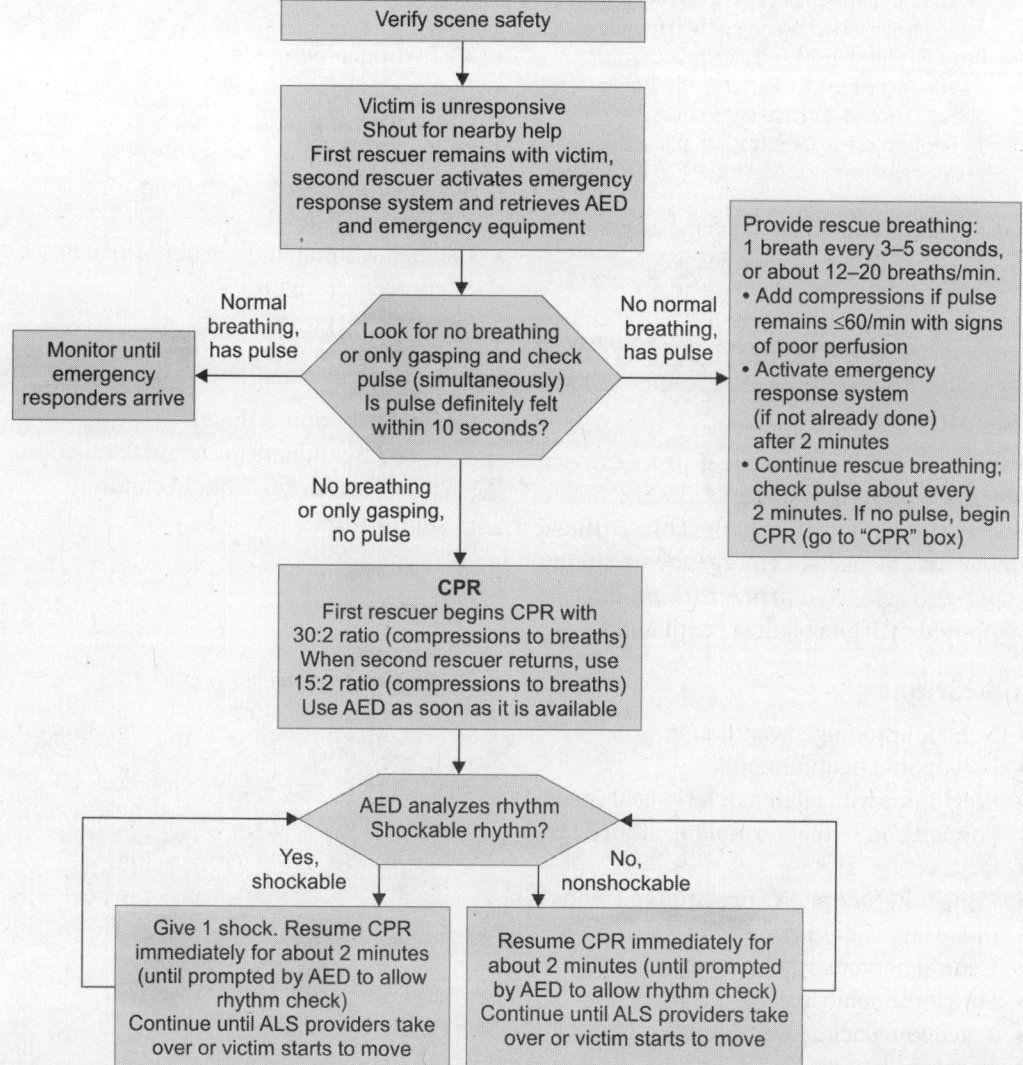

Flowchart 8.2: Pediatric BLS algorithm for two or more rescuers.

(ALS: advanced life support; BLS: basic life support; CPR: cardiopulmonary resuscitation; AED: automated external defibrillator)

Chapter 8: Emergency Procedures

Highlights ●●●●

- Cardiopulmonary resuscitation (CPR) is the manual application of chest compressions and ventilations to patients in cardiac arrest, done in an effort to maintain viability until advance help arrives.
- The indications for CPR are majorly divided into two: (1) respiratory failure and arrest and (2) cardiopulmonary failure and arrest.
- Airway should be assessed for patency using look, listen, and feel approach.
- Establishing and maintaining airway patency can be achieved using one of two maneuvers: head tilt and chin lift and jaw thrust.
- Give 2 rescue breaths. Each breath should take about 1 second and make the chest rise.
- To perform chest compression, place the heel of one hand on the breast bone just below the nipples.
- Make sure your heel is not at the very end of the breast bone.

TRACHEOSTOMY CARE

Definition

A tracheostomy is a surgical procedure in which an opening is made in the trachea to enable the patient to breath. This artificial airway may be used in emergency situations, may be an elective procedure or may be combined with mechanical ventilation.

Indications

- Need for prolonged ventilation
- Laryngotracheobronchitis
- Epiglottitis with edema or laryngeal spasm
- Foreign bodies that cannot be removed via larynx
- Congenital anomalies or acquired stenosis of the larynx or upper trachea
- Central nervous system disorders
- Subglottic stenosis
- Tracheomalacia
- Vocal cord paralysis

Equipment Needed

A sterile tray containing:
- Tracheostomy tube (silastic, polyvinyl chloride, or plastic tubes)
- Extra tracheostomy tube in the case of accidental dislodgement
- Obturator and extra inner cannula (**Fig. 8.8**)
- Tracheostomy ties
- Small curved scissors
- Blunt hemostat
- Cotton-tipped applicators
- Water
- 3% hydrogen peroxide
- Betadine swabs
- Uncut dressing pads
- Oxygen
- Self-inflating resuscitation bag
- Lubricating jelly
- Call bell within child's/parents' reach
- Suction equipment:
  – A pair of sterile gloves
  – Suction apparatus with good negative pressure
  – Sterile suction catheter
  – No 6 Fr catheters for infants and young children, no. 8–10 for old children
  – Sterile saline

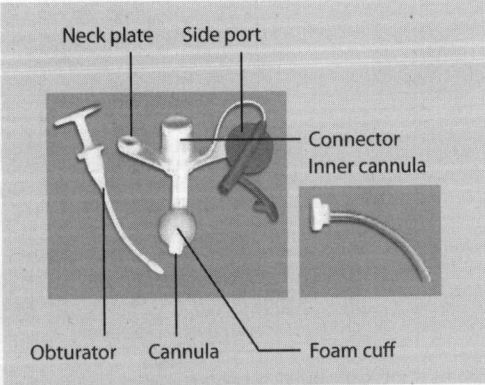

Fig. 8.8: Tracheostomy tube.

Preparation of the Child and Family

- Explain to the parents about surgical procedure.
- Explain the indications.
- Use all the possible means to reduce the anxiety.

Tracheostomy Care Procedure

- Position the infant/child supine with a blanket or towel roll to extend the neck.
- Open all packaging and cut tracheostomy ties to appropriate length if necessary.
- Clean around the tracheostomy site with prescribed solution [half-strength hydrogen peroxide or acetic acid, normal saline (NS), Betadine or soap and water] and cotton-tipped applicators working from just around the tracheostomy tube outward.
- Rinse with sterile water and cotton-tipped applicator in a similar fashion.
- Place the pre-cut sterile gauze under the tracheostomy tube.
- With the assistant holding the tube in place, cut the ties, and remove from the tube.
- Attach the clean ties to the tube and secure in the place.

Nurse's Responsibility

- Nursing care is indispensable to the survival of the patient because blockage of the tube by mucus or other secretions can lead to suffocation.
  - Usually after the procedure, the child is placed in intensive care unit because this is the critical period requiring frequent suctioning and very close observation. When the condition stabilizes, the child is transferred to the regular unit.
  - The child with tracheostomy is placed in an area of high visibility.
  - Infants and children normally communicate their needs by crying but the tracheostomy prohibits vocalization.
  - Whenever possible, one person is assigned to the child and to work with the parents. Reinforce preoperative teaching.
  - Explain what has happened in an age-appropriate manner.
    » For example, "You are having a lot of trouble breathing. The operation called tracheostomy helps you breathe easier. A small opening has been made in your neck. A hallow tube is inserted to keep the area open. It is frightening not able to speak. When you are better, the hole will close by itself and your voice will return."
    » An explanation of suction might be— we have to keep the area in your neck open. This tube goes into the airway and clears it. Demonstrate the use of suction in a glass of water.
    » Prepare the child for unfamiliar sound. You might feel like gagging, but afterward you will feel better. I know this is difficult for you. And I am sorry there is no easier way.
  - Added moisture and humidity are provided using a special tracheostomy collar, or direct attachment to a mechanical ventilator. This is necessary because the nose and the mouth no longer warm and moisten the inspired air.
  - The anatomical difference between a child and adult is the small child's inability to communicate through writing, which increases the need for close observation.
  - Maintaining patency of the tracheostomy tube is of utmost important. Plastic or silastic tubes are generally used because they are flexible and reduce crust formation. They are lightweight and disposable and most do not have

inner cannula. Cuffed tubes are not usually necessary in infants and in small children because their air passages are small and the tracheostomy tube provides a sufficient seal.

Suction Depths

- Shallow suctioning: Suction secretions at the opening of the trach tube that the child has coughed up.
- Premeasured suctioning: Suction the length of the trach tube. Suction depth varies depending on the size of the trach tube. The obturator can be used as a measuring guide.
- Deep suctioning: Insert the catheter until resistance is felt. (Deep suctioning is usually not necessary. Be careful to avoid vigorous suctioning, as this may injure the lining of the airway.)

Signs that a Child Needs Suctioning

- Rattling mucus sounds from the trach.
- Fast breathing.
- Bubbles of mucus in trach opening.
- Dry raspy breathing or a whistling noise from trach.
- Older children may vocalize or signal a need to be suctioned.
- Signs of respiratory distress.

Types of Tracheostomy Care Techniques

1. *Sterile technique:* Sterile catheters and sterile gloves
2. *Modified sterile technique:* Sterile catheters and clean gloves
3. *Clean technique:* Clean catheter and clean hands

Suctioning Procedure

- Explain the procedure in a way appropriate for the child's age and understanding.
- Wash hands
- Set up the equipment and connect suction catheter to machine tubing.
- Pour NS into cup
- Put on gloves (optional)
- Turn on suction machine
- Place tip of catheter into saline cup to moisten and test to see that suction is working.
- Instill sterile NS with plastic squeeze ampoule into the trach tube if needed for thick or dry secretions. Excessive use of saline is not recommended. Use saline only if the mucus is very thick, hard to cough up or difficult to suction. Saline may also be instilled via a syringe or eye dropper, which is less expensive than single-dose units. Recommended amount per instillation is approximately 1 cm^3.
- Gently insert catheter into the trach tube without applying suction. (Suction only length of trach tube—premeasured suctioning. Deeper insertion may be needed if the child has an ineffective cough.)
- Put thumb over opening in catheter to create suction and use a circular motion (twirl catheter between thumb and index finger) while withdrawing the catheter so that the mucus is removed well from all areas. Avoid suctioning longer than 10 seconds because of oxygen loss.
  Note: Research findings had shown that by applying suction both going in and then out of the tube takes less time and therefore results in less hypoxia. Also, there are now holes on all sides of the suction catheters, so twirling is not necessary.
- Draw saline from cup through catheter to clear catheter.
- For trach tubes with cuffs, it may be necessary to deflate the cuff periodically for suctioning to prevent pooling of secretions above trach cuff.
- Let the child rest and breathe, then repeat suction if needed until clear (allow at least 30 seconds between suctioning).

- Oxygenate as ordered (extra oxygen may be given before and after suction to prevent hypoxia).
- Some children need extra breaths with an Ambu bag (approximately 3–5 breaths).
- *Purposes of bagging:* Hyperoxygenation, hyperinflation, and hyperventilation of the lungs. However, this is usually not needed for stable children with no additional respiratory problems.

Nurse's Responsibility

- Withdraw the catheter while rotating and applying suction by covering the part on the catheter with the thumb.
- Hold the suction for no >5 seconds.
- The child should be allowed to rest for about a minute and take 2 or 3 breaths between suctioning.
- Hyperventilate the child with 100% oxygen between suctioning to prevent hypoxia.
- The use of pulse oximeter can provide a measure of the child's oxygenation during and after the procedure.

Additional Measures

- Frequent change of position, the use of arm restraints, oral feeding unless contraindicated.
- Careful bathing to prevent water entering the tube.
- Range of motion exercise is a must for long-term patients and in acute cases, arm restraints are removed one at a time to allow for passive exercises.
- Although the patients, initially may have nothing by mouth, as their condition improves, they progress to a soft or normal diet.
- Fowler's position is preferred during feeding.
- Older children can cooperate by holding their head flexed with chin down. This decreases swallowing difficulties because when the esophagus opens and the airway narrows.
- Monitor feeding of an infant closely so that no food particles aspirated through the tracheostomy.
- Some patients are discharged with the tracheostomy. This should be anticipated, and instruction and demonstration for patients should begin early.
- Parents who are comfortable with the procedure during hospitalization feel more secure when the child returns home.
  - It is advisable for the parents to be "demonstrated" on tracheostomy procedure before discharging and most hospitals now require this.
- Trach ties: Children often may develop rashes or skin breakdown under the trach ties because of leaking secretions, perspiration, and the short length of the child's neck or any skeletal deformities. Treatment of these conditions includes antibiotic or antifungal creams, powders more frequent tie changes, changing the type of ties, using pads to bridge the damaged area. Occasionally, it is necessary to reposition the patient to reduce the pressure on the area. If all these have been failed, ENT specialists may need to suture the trach in the place and thus temporarily eliminate the need for any type of trach ties.

Suction Pressure

Infant: 60–100 mm Hg
Children: 100–110 mm Hg
Adult: 110–150 mm Hg
Chest physiotherapy can be given to remove the secretions.

Complications

Intraoperative: Hemorrhage, tracheoesophageal fistula, pneumothorax, pneumomediastinum, cricoid cartilage injury, cardiopulmonary injury, tube obstruction or displacement, posterior tracheal wall disruption, or death.

Immediate postoperative: Hemorrhage, wound infection, subcutaneous emphysema, pneumothorax, pulmonary edema, dysphagia, pneumonia, sepsis, atelectasis, death.

Late postoperative: Suprasternal collapse, suprasternal/distal tracheal granuloma, tracheoesophageal fistula, tracheocutaneous fistula, laryngotracheal stenosis, tracheal wall erosion, hemorrhage, inability to decannulate, mucus plug, bronchospasm, death.

Highlights

- A tracheostomy is a surgical procedure in which an opening is made in the trachea to enable the patient to breath.
- Before suctioning, instill sterile normal saline with plastic squeeze ampoule into the trach tube if needed for thick or dry secretions.
- Applying suction both going in and then out of the tube takes less time and therefore results in less hypoxia.
- Also, there are now holes on all sides of the suction catheters, so twirling is not necessary.
- Hyperventilate the child with 100% oxygen between suctioning to prevent hypoxia.
- The use of pulse oximeter can provide a measure of the child's oxygenation during and after the procedure.
- Suction should not be done for >5 seconds.

CARE OF A CHILD ON MECHANICAL VENTILATION

Definition

Mechanical ventilation can be defined as the technique through which gas is moved toward and from the lungs through an external device connected directly to the patient.

Indications

- Progressive hypoxia despite oxygen therapy measured by oxygen saturations or blood gas analysis (high $PaCO_2$ and low pH)
- Excessive WOB manifested by retractions, tachypnea, decreasing O_2 saturation, and abnormal respiratory patterns
- Inadequate respiratory effort
- Hyperventilation for treatment of increased intracranial pressure
- Need for mechanical ventilation for any reason.
  The conditions that cause inadequate ventilation are:
  - Apnea
  - Central nervous system injury or infection
  - Alveolar hypoventilation
  - Respiratory muscle weakness
  - Medication toxicity
  - Infectious pathologic condition
  - Foreign body obstruction
- Pulmonary lavage
- Instillation of medication
- Need for short-term ventilation:
  - During surgery
  - Acute lung injury
  - Acute respiratory acidosis
  - CCF

Contraindication

- Unilateral lung disease
- Obstructive lung disease
- Pneumothorax
- Bronchopleural fistula
- Intracardiac shunt
- Increased intracranial pressure

Classifications

Types of Ventilators

1. *Pressure-cycled ventilator*: Terminates the respiratory cycle where a preset inspiratory pressure is reached. Volume differs greatly, depending on the flow rate of the delivery of gas. The lung's compliance affects the tidal volume (VT) even though the pressure remains constant.

2. *Volume-cycled ventilator:* Terminates respiration when a preset volume (VT) is delivered. The lung's compliance and resistance change the pressure needed to deliver the preset volume.
3. *Time-cycled ventilator:* Terminates inspiration when a pressure time is reached.
4. VT is greatly affected by compliance of the ventilator tubing, lung's compliance, and resistance and flow rate of the delivered gas. The duration of the inspiratory pressure is affected by the preset inspiratory time and the flow rate of the delivered gas.
5. *Combined ventilator:* It can be used as either volume- or time-cycled, pressure-limited ventilation.

Some Commonly Used Ventilators

1. *Sechrist (pressure type):* Pressure control/intermittent mandatory ventilation (IMV)/continuous positive airway pressure (CPAP)
2. *Sechrist (volume and pressure type):* PC/VC/Synchronized IMV (SIMV)/SIMV with PS
3. *Servo 300:* Numerous
4. *VIP Bird:* Volume and pressure-numerous
5. *Drager Babylog:* Pressure-numerous
6. *Infant star:* Pressure-SIMV and A/C
7. *LP-10:* V&P-SIMV and A/C

Modes of Ventilation

Control Mechanical Ventilation

Patient receives a preset number of breaths/min, of a preset VT, patient effort, when not trigger a mechanical breath. The ventilator performs all the WOB.

Indications

- Patient with minimal or no respiratory effort, for example, spinal cord lesion
- When negative inspiratory effort is contraindicated, for example, flail chest
- As a backup to assisted ventilation

Disadvantages

- Patient–ventilator asynchrony.
- Prolonged use may result in respiratory muscle weakness and atrophy.

Assist-control Ventilation

Ventilator delivers a preset number of breaths of a preset VT. Between this machines initiated breath, patient may trigger spontaneous breaths. Patient performs negative inspiratory effort.

Indications

Normal respiratory drive but respiratory muscles are too weak to perform WOB.

Advantage

Allows the patient to control the rate of breathing and still it guarantees the delivery of a minimal preset rate and volume.

Disadvantages

- The patient's tendency to hyperventilate because of anxiety, pain, etc. leads to respiratory alkalosis.
- Variation in patient's hemodynamic status.

Synchronized Intermittent Mandatory Ventilation

It is the same as A/C mode. The main difference between the IMV and A/C mode is the volume of the patient-initiated breaths. In A/C, the VT is guaranteed, whereas in IMV it is variable.

Mandatory breaths may be synchronized with a patient's spontaneous effort (SIMV) to avoid mandatory breaths occurring during a spontaneous breath. This effort known as "stacking" may lead to excessive VTs, high airway pressure, incomplete exhalation, and air trapping.

Indications

- Normal respiratory drive but respiratory muscles unable to perform all WOB.
- Need to wean the patient from mechanical ventilation.

Advantages
- Decreased rate of hyperventilation
- Less respiratory muscle atrophy
- Less hemodynamic efforts of positive-pressure ventilation
- Improves patient's comfort and reduces competition between ventilator and patient.

Disadvantages
- Fatigue
- Atelectasis
- Reduction in compliance leads to increased WOB and greater need for ventilator support.

Time-cycled, Pressure-limited Ventilation

The rate and inspiratory time (I:E) are preset. A preset PIP is determined.

Indication

Neonates and infants where VT is small.

Advantages
- Precise control of inspiratory time and a rapid respiratory rate
- Less chance for barotrauma

Disadvantage

Inability to detect airway obstruction or kinking due to preset limited PIP (high pressure alarm may go off).

Pressure-controlled, Inverse Ratio Ventilation (PCIRV)

PCIRV is a new and potentially promising method of ventilation in which the pressure ventilation with an inspiratory/expiratory (I:E) ratio greater than 1:1 is used. this helps to maintain a high mean airway pressure and hold peak alveolar pressure within a safe range. All breaths are pressure limited and time cycled and the inspiration is longer than expiration.

Indication

Child with specific noncompliant lung conditions.

Advantages
- Decrease in both PIP and positive-end expiratory pressure (PEEP) levels.
- Stabilizes the alveoli equilibration of volume.

Disadvantages
- PCIRV can cause hemodynamic instability due to increase intrinsic PEEP and mean airway pressure.
- It can lead to stacking of breaths.
- Can cause ventilator induced lung injuries
- Can result in significant decrease in cardiac output

Pressure Support Ventilation

Patient's spontaneous respiratory activity is augmented by the delivery of a preset amount of inspiratory positive pressure and the VT is variable based on patient's effort.

Indications
- During weaning from mechanical ventilation
- Long-term mechanical ventilation.

Disadvantage
- Tidal volume would decrease if compliance decreases or resistance increases (bronchospasm or significant secretions).

Positive-end Expiratory Pressure

Positive-end expiratory pressure is the application of a constant, positive pressure in the airways so that at end expiration the pressure is never allowed to return to the atmospheric pressure.

Positive-end expiratory pressure, measured in centimeter of water, ranges from 5 to 20 cm of H_2O.

Advantages
- Recruits alveoli, counteracts alveoli and small airway closure during expiration.
- Redistributes lung water so it decreases shunting.
- Increases functional residual capacity.

- Improves compliance and oxygenation.
- It can be added to every type of mechanical ventilation, including spontaneous respiration, where it is known as CPAP.

Ventilation Methods

Artificial ventilation methods are mainly divided into positive-pressure and negative-pressure ventilations. Based on the devices used, further it has been classified as given in **Table 8.1**.

Formula for calculating appropriate size of ET tube:

$$\text{Size of ET tube} = \frac{\text{Age in years} + 16}{4}$$

Equipment for ET Tube Insertion

An emergency trolley containing:
- *Laryngoscope blades:*
  - Straight blades (Miller)—for infants and young children
  - Curved blades (Macintosh)—for older children
- ET tubes (three sizes)
- Oxygen source, bag valve mask
- Suction apparatus, appropriate-size suction catheters
- Pulse oximeter, cardiac monitor
- Gloves, gown, and mask
- Adhesive tapes
- Gauze pads

Table 8.1: Ventilation methods.

Method	Description	Remarks
Anesthesia bag or flow ventilation systems	A small collapsible bag that consists of a reservoir bag, an overflow port, and a fresh gas inflow port	<ul><li>Adjustment of the O_2 flow and outlet control valve is necessary</li><li>Useful in providing PEEP or CPAP</li><li>Adequate training and skill are needed to operate</li><li>Hypercapnia and barotrauma may result with improper use</li><li>Used more commonly in recovery rooms and NICU</li></ul>
Bag valve mask device or manual resuscitator	A self-inflating O_2 delivery bag that does not require an O_2 source for resuscitation and ventilation. The bag can be connected to O_2 to provide higher O_2 levels than room air. When the child exhales, nonbreathing valve closes allowing exhaled deoxygenated air to escape	<ul><li>Effective in providing O_2 to a child who is in severe respiratory distress or who has suffered a respiratory arrest</li><li>A more efficient method of respiratory resuscitation than mouth-to-mouth resuscitation</li><li>Decreases rescuer exposure to communicable diseases</li><li>Possible fatigue for rescuer</li></ul>
Laryngeal mask airway	An inflatable silicone mask and rubber connecting tube that is inserted blindly into the airway forming a seal	<ul><li>The airway is introduced into the pharynx and advanced until it meets resistance</li><li>Balloon cuff is then inflated</li><li>Easier insertion than a trachea tube</li><li>Used in unconscious child</li><li>Patient comfort</li></ul>
Tracheal intubation	A plastic tube inserted in the trachea to establish and maintain an airway when the airway cannot be maintained effectively using other measures. For example, nasal trumpet or bag valve mask ventilation	<ul><li>Skilled medical professional (physician, nurse practitioner, respiratory specialist) necessary for insertion</li><li>The nurse acts as a valuable assistant during the intubation procedure</li></ul>

(CPAP: continuous positive airway pressure; PEEP: positive-end expiratory pressure)

Types of ET Intubation

1. Orotracheal
2. Nasotracheal (most beneficial)
3. Tracheostomy (for prolonged ventilation)

Procedure (Assisting with Ventilation)

- Prepare equipment and supplies.
- Draw up medications.
- Turn up the volume on the cardiac monitor so that members of the team can easily hear the audible QRS indication of the child's heart rate and note any bradycardia with the procedure.
- Turn on the suction. Make sure that suction is working by placing your hand over the tubing before you attach the suction catheter.
- Continue to ventilate the child with 100% oxygen.
- When there is no suspected cervical spine injury in the child over age 2 years, place a small pillow under the child's head to facilitate opening of the airway.
- When assisting with the intubation, stand before the patient's head and prepare to assist with suction of oral secretions, applying cricoid pressure during the insertion of tube providing BVM as needed and assisting with suctioning the tube.
- Before the initial intubation attempt and after each subsequent attempt to intubate, provide several inhalations of 100% O_2.
- Administer premedications and medications for sedation.
- Observe whether the healthcare provider who is intubating the child follows the recommended procedure.

Nurse's Responsibility

Ensuring and Maintaining Correct Tube Placement

- Observe for symmetrical chest raise and auscultate over the lung fields for equal breath sounds.
- Inspect the tracheal tube for the presence of water vapor on the inside wall, indicating that the tube is in the trachea.
- To rule out accidental esophageal intubation, auscultate over the abdomen (absence of breath sounds).
- Once the tracheal placement is verified, mark the tube with an indelible pen at the level of child's lip and secure it with tape.
- Document the number on the tracheal tube at the level of child's mouth.
- Anticipate a chest X-ray to confirm correct placement of the tracheal tube.
- After placement is confirmed, the tracheal tube is connected to the ventilator by respiratory personnel for continuous artificial ventilation.
- To avoid expelling of tube:
  - Use soft restraints if necessary to prevent the child from removing the tracheal tube.
  - Provide sedative/paralyzing medication.
  - Use caution when moving the child for X-rays, changing linens, and performing other procedures.

Monitoring the Intubated Child

- Determine adequacy of O_2.
- Auscultate the lungs for equal air entry, determine the HR.
- Perform quick survey of the equipment and look for any disconnected tubes or kinks in the tubing.
- Use the PALS mnemonic "DOPE" for troubleshooting when the status of the child deteriorates.
  - D—displacement
  - O—obstruction
  - P—pneumothorax (decrease breath sounds, decreased chest expansion)
  - E—equipment failure
- Make sure that all equipment are appropriately connected and functioning.
- Suctioning should be done when necessary.

- If displaced, remove the tube from child mouth and begin BVM ventilation.
- *Pneumothorax:* Prepare to assist with needle thoracotomy.
- Assess nutritional status, intake and output (urine output should be at least 2 mL/kg/h for the infant and younger child and 1 mL/kg/h for the older child), and skin integrity especially around the face and lips for the child with ET tube.
- In some cases, there is increase in the amount of oral or nasal secretions, which requires appropriate perioral skin care.
- The child's lips and the mouth may be dry and uncomfortable; therefore provision of oral care and moisture is important.

Weaning and Extubation

- Weaning the patient from a ventilator involves gradual physical and psychological withdrawal from dependence on the mechanical device.
- Criteria for weaning may vary with primary disease.
- If the intubated child is receiving nasogastric feedings and is at risk for aspiration, feedings are usually stopped a few hours before extubation.
- Steroids may be administered before extubation to control laryngeal edema.
- The child should remain on cardio-respiratory monitor.
- Resuscitation and reintubation equipment must be available at bedside.
- Perform chest physiotherapy and suctioning just before removal.
- Administer cool mist or oxygen by nasal cannula or mask after extubation.
- Monitor the child for respiratory distress.
- Observe adequacy of oxygen through ABG measurements or pulse oximeter.

Other care includes:
- Monitoring vital parameters
- Monitoring and care of invasive lines
- Maintenance of fluid and electrolyte balance
- Administration of drugs as prescribed in **Table 8.2**.

Table 8.2: Drugs used in mechanical ventilation.

Name	Dose (mg/kg)	IV infusion
Sedatives		
1. Midazolam	0.05–0.1	Loading: 0.05 mg/kg/IV Maintenance: 0.025 mg/kg
2. Fentanyl	2–10	Loading: 2–10 mg/kg/IV Maintenance: 1–5 mg/kg/h
3. Morphine	0.1	Loading: 0.05 mg/kg/IV Maintenance: 0.02 mg/kg/h
4. Lorazepam	0.05–0.1	
5. Diazepam	0.1–0.2	Loading: 0.1 mg/kg/h Maintenance: 0.3–0.6 mg/kg/h
Muscle relaxants		
1. Pancuronium	0.1	
2. Vecuronium	0.1	
3. Atracurium	0.5	
4. Succinylcholine	1–2	

(IV: intravenous)

Complications

- *Related to immediate intubation:*
  - Hypoxia
  - Bradycardia
  - Sore throat
  - Traumatic laryngitis
  - Infection
  - Glottic edema
  - Mucosal lesions of larynx due to ET tube pressure
  - Subglottic stenosis secondary to fibrosis (severe complication)
- *After extubation:*
  - Airway edema and pain
  - Fatigue
  - Atelectasis
  - Stridor

Highlights

+ Mechanical ventilation can be defined as the technique through which gas is moved toward and from the lungs through an external device connected directly to the patient.
+ Artificial ventilation methods are mainly divided into positive-pressure and negative-pressure ventilations.
+ When assisting with the intubation, stand before the patient's head and prepare to assist with suction of oral secretions, applying cricoid pressure during the insertion of tube providing BVM as needed and assisting with suctioning the tube.
+ Assess nutritional status, intake and output (urine output should be at least 2 mL/kg/h for the infant and younger child and 1 mL/kg/h for the older child), and skin integrity, especially around the face and lips for the child with ET tube.

PULSE OXIMETRY

Definition

Pulse oximetry is a noninvasive method allowing the monitoring of patient's oxygen saturation.

Indications

- High risk for adverse events (respiratory failure/distress)
- Receiving supplemental oxygen administration
- Children who are on patient-controlled anesthesia
- During postextubation period for at least 48 hours
- Children under sedation for procedure or therapeutic purposes
- Children with seizures, postoperative patients
- During transportation of critical/high-risk children

Equipment Needed

- Pulse oximeter monitor
- Probe
- Plaster
- Bedside oxygen delivery system

Sites for Placing Sensor

- *Neonates:* Sole of the foot below toes, palm of the hand, wrist, forehead
- *Infants:* Great toe, ball of foot, palm, wrist
- *Child:* Index finger, forehead
  - The oximeter responds only to pulsations, such as those in pulsating capillaries of the area tested.

Preparation

- Identify the child and explain the procedure to the child and his/her parents as appropriate.
- Assess history, focusing on events that may have precipitated respiratory distress.
- Do respiratory assessment that includes observation of respiratory rate, use of accessory muscles, and auscultation for abnormal breath sounds.
- Ensure that child's fingernail beds are clean and free of nail polish to reduce interference in providing accurate reading.
- Gather necessary equipment and check for working condition.

Procedure

Procedure is tabulated in **Table 8.3**.

Table 8.3: Procedure for pulse oximetry.

Steps	Rationale
Perform hand hygiene	To reduce transmission of microorganism
Select appropriate sensor and attach the cable to the pulse oximeter unit	Base sensor selection on the child's age, size, and preferred site to be used
Attach the sensor to the selected site with the light source on one side of the tissue pad and the sensor on the other, facing each other, for optimal performance; keep the sensor site at the level of heart	Allow measurement of light transmitted through a pulsating arterial vascular bed to calculate the percentage of hemoglobin saturated with oxygen (SaO_2). Avoid placing sensor over thick skin, nail polish, false nails, extremities that are moved excessively by the child, and areas where perfusion is known to be poor
Tape sensor in place, loosely but securely	Failure to position and secure may cause motion artifact and thus incorrect SaO_2 measurement. Taping too tightly may impede circulation, causing an incorrect reading
Cover sensor site with opaque material	Excessive light, such as from phototherapy, direct sunlight or excessive ambient lighting, can interfere with the sensor's ability to produce an accurate reading
Turn pulse oximeter on and verify if the child's apical pulse corresponds to the pulse rate shown on the monitor. If machine has a visual waveform display or other bar graph indicator to indicate that an accurate signal is received, ensure that the reading is present at the highest level	Lack of correlation between the child's actual pulse rates shown on the monitor indicates the unreliability of the SaO_2 findings
Alarm limits should be determined in conjunction with the healthcare prescriber and take into consideration child's age, underlying condition, and past history of normal parameters Set alarm limits as by manufacture's instruction. Set sensitivity by high rate button and low rate button simultaneously. Turn the wheel while depressing buttons to set the desired sensitivity	When alarms are set correctly, the oximeter can detect hypoxemia before the child becomes cyanotic and the nurse can be alerted to a downward trend and deterioration in the child's status. Although oxygen saturation of 95–96% is adequate (i.e., not requiring acute O_2 therapy), these values are associated with higher rates of airway pulmonary or cardiovascular system involvement and should be considered potentially abnormal. O_2 saturation of 97% is on the border of normal. But saturations <97% can occur with airway pulmonary or cardiovascular system involvement or respiratory infections in children
Set low saturation limit and low pulse alarm by simultaneously pushing each button and turning the wheel to the predetermined numeric value	Set low saturation alarm at 92% in most cases. This allows for early intervention and treatment if O_2 is to be delivered once a 90% saturation level is observed. Low-pulse alarms are often set as follows based on the child's age: ■ <1 month: 80 beats/min ■ 1–3 months: 70 beats/min ■ >3 months: 60 beats/min
Determine with the doctor when oxygen is administered or flow rate is increased or decreased	
Document the procedure with date and time and perform hand hygiene	

Limitations

- The pulse oximeter measures solely oxygenation, not ventilation.
- It is not a substitute for blood gases checked in laboratory, because it gives no indication of base deficit, CO_2 levels, blood pH, or HCO_3^- concentration.
- Erroneously low reading may be caused by hypoperfusion of the extremity being used for monitoring; incorrect sensor application, highly calloused skin; or movement especially during hypoperfusion.
- Hb has a higher affinity to carbon monoxide than O_2 and a high reading may occur despite the patient actually being hypoxemic. (In carbon monoxide poisoning, this inaccuracy may delay the recognition of hypoxemia.)
- Cyanide poisoning gives a high reading, because it reduces oxygen extraction from arterial blood.
- Methemoglobinemia characteristically causes pulse oximetry reading in the mid-80s.

Highlights ● ● ● ●

- ✦ Pulse oximetry is a noninvasive method allowing the monitoring of patient's oxygen saturation.
- ✦ Ensure that child's fingernail beds are clean and free of nail polish to reduce interference in providing accurate reading.
- ✦ The oximeter responds only to pulsations, such as those in pulsating capillaries of the area tested.
- ✦ The pulse oximeter measures solely oxygenation, not ventilation.
- ✦ It is not a substitute for blood gases checked in laboratory, because it gives no indication of base deficit, CO_2 levels, blood pH, or HCO_3^- concentration.
- ✦ Erroneously low reading may be caused by hypoperfusion of the extremity being used for monitoring; incorrect sensor application, highly calloused skin; or movement especially during hypoperfusion.

ABDOMINAL PARACENTESIS

Definition

Abdominal paracentesis is the removal of fluid from the peritoneal cavity.

Indications

- To determine the cause of ascites
- To determine if intra-abdominal bleeding is present or if a viscous has ruptured
- For therapeutic removal of fluid when distension is pronounced or there is associated respiratory distress

Contraindications

- Uncooperative patient
- Uncorrected bleeding diathesis
- Acute abdomen that requires surgery
- Intra-abdominal adhesions
- Distended bowel

Equipment Needed

A sterile tray containing:
- Sponge holder
- Syringe (5 mL) with needles
- 20-mL syringe with Luer lock
- Three-way adopter and tubing
- Aspiration needles
- Antiseptic solution
- Gloves, gown, and mask
- Local anesthetic
- Drape or cotton blankets
- Collection bottle/container
- Specimen bottles and laboratory forms
- Sterile dressing towels
- Cotton balls, gauze pieces
- Dressing pads

Preparation

- Explain the procedure to the parents and the child as appropriate.
- Obtain a written consent from the parents.

- It is very helpful to get an ultrasound scan of the ascites before the procedure. The radiologist will mark the spot for paracentesis.
- Record the child's vital signs.
- Have the child void before procedure is begun.
- Position the child in Fowler's position with back, arms, and feet supported.
- Drape the child with sheet exposing abdomen.

Positioning

- *Child with large quantity of ascites:* Supine position with head of bed elevated to 30–45°
- *Patients with less amount of fluid:* Lateral decubitus position.

Site Selection

- Approximately 2 cm below the umbilicus in the midline
- Right or left lower quadrant, approximately 4–5 cm medial to the anterior supine iliac spine (**Fig. 8.9**).

Procedure

- Perform hand hygiene. Don sterile gown, gloves, and mask.

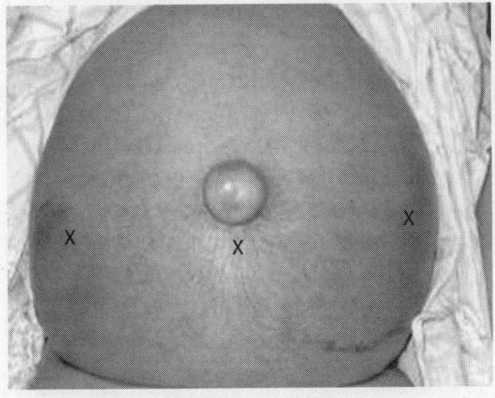

Fig. 8.9: Site for abdominal paracentesis.

- Use skin prep solution to clean skin over the proposed puncture site and drape to define a sterile field.
- Anesthetize the skin over the proposed puncture site with lidocaine drawn up in the 5-cm^3 syringe with the attached 25-G needle. Anesthetize down to the peritoneum. Aspirate periodically, if ascites fluid returns, withdraw the needle slightly to re-enter tissue before further anesthetic is infiltrated.
- Attach 18-G needle to free end of intravenous (IV) tubing, leave capped, and close valve tightly on the tubing.
- Puncture the rubber stopper of the vacuum bottle with the other end of the tubing.
- Insert the 18-G needle perpendicularly through the anesthetized abdominal wall and advance until hub of needle is 5 mm to 1 cm away from the skin surface.
- Open up the tubing clamp. Ascetic fluid should begin to flow into the bottle.
- When paracentesis is done, simply remove needle from abdominal wall.
- Place a small pressure dressing on puncture site.

Postprocedure Care

- Have the patient remain supine for 2–4 hours.
- Monitor vital signs q1/2 hourly for 2 hours, q hour for 4 hours, and every 4 hours for 24 hours.
- Label the specimens and send to laboratory with due form.
- Record the amount and kind of fluid removed, number of specimens sent to laboratory, and the child's condition through treatment.
- Watch for leakage after paracentesis.

Complications

- Hypovolemia leading to shock and collapse
- Infection (peritonitis)

- Injury to the blood vessels and other abdominal organs
- Renal failure due to reduced systemic circulations
- Hypoproteinemia
- Abdominal wall hematoma
- Persistent peritoneal leak

Nurse's Responsibility

- Assist in preparing skin with antiseptic solution.
- Open sterile tray and package of sterile gloves, and provide anesthetic solution.
- Have collection bottle and tubing available.
- Assess the pulse and respiratory status frequently during the procedure; watch for pallor, cyanosis or syncope and faintness.

Highlights ●●●●

> ✦ Abdominal paracentesis is the removal of fluid from the peritoneal cavity.
> ✦ It is child with large quantity of ascites: Supine position with head of bed elevated to 30–45°.
> ✦ It is very helpful to get an ultrasound scan of the ascites before the procedure.
> ✦ The site for abdominal tap/paracentesis are approximately 2 cm below the umbilicus in the midline or right or left lower quadrant, approximately 4–5 cm medial to the anterior supine iliac spine.
> ✦ After the procedure, monitor vital signs q1/2 hourly for 2 hours, q hour for 4 hours, and every 4 hours for 24 hours.

BLOOD TRANSFUSION

Definition

A blood transfusion is the introduction of whole blood or blood components into the venous circulation.

Indications

- *Infants:*
  - Asymptomatic infant with hematocrit <20%
  - Infant with hematocrit <30% and requiring oxygen >35% or requiring CPAP or mechanical ventilation; or having significant apnea or bradycardia; or having heart rate >180/min or respiratory rate >80/min persisting for >24 hours; or having a weight gain <10 g/day observed over 4 days while on >100 cal/kg/day or undergoing surgery
  - Infant with hematocrit <35% if receiving oxygen >35% or getting mechanical ventilation
- *Children:*
  - Hb 4 g/dL or less (hematocrit 12%) irrespective of the clinical condition
  - Hb 4–6 g/dL (hematocrit 13–18%) with features of hypoxia acidotic breathing, dyspnea, or impaired consciousness.
  - Hyperparasitemia in malaria (>20%).
  - Features of cardiac decompensation such as cardiomegaly or CCF.

Classifications

A. *Unmodified:*
  - Cellular: packed RBCs, platelets, granulocytes
  - Plasma: fresh frozen plasma, cryoprecipitate (CRYO), factor components.

B. *Modified:*
  - Irradiated: RBCs, platelets, granulocytes; leukocyte-depleted RBCs, platelets
  - Saline washed: RBCs, platelets

Unmodified Components

a. **Packed RBCs**
Here some of the plasma is removed from whole blood. For improvement of oxygen-carrying capacity in chronic anemia with hypoxic manifestations as also CCF, this is the best product.
Dose: 10 mL/kg over 3–4 hours. A transfusion of 3 mL/kg increases Hb concentration by around 1 g/dL.

Indications

In neonates
- Physiologic anemia of infancy/anemia of prematurity
- Hb < 10 g/dL if symptomatic
- Hb < 13 g/dL in cardiopulmonary disease
- Hb < 10 g/dL in FTT
- Replacement of iatrogenic blood loss
- Situations requiring large volume transfusions, for example, exchange transfusion

Infants and older children
- Hb < 7 g/dL, symptomatic anemia
- Blood loss due to hemorrhage

b. Platelets

Indications
- Decreased platelet count in premature infants
- Decreased platelet count in active bleeding, major invasive or surgical procedure
- Decreased platelet count in bone marrow failure
- Minor surgical procedure
- Cardiovascular bypass/ECMO with excessive hemorrhage
- ITP

Dose: 0.1 U/kg raises platelet counts by 30,000/cmm

c. Granulocytes

Indications
- Neonatal sepsis with meningitis, septic shock, or necrotizing enterocolitis
- Absolute neutropenia

Dose: 10–15 mL/kg every 24 hours

d. Fresh frozen plasma

It is the fluid portion of the blood unit that is centrifuged, separated, and frozen at <–30°C within 6 hours of collection.

Indications
- Severe hemorrhagic disease of the newborn (HDN) with vitamin K–dependent coagulopathy
- Replacement of isolated factor deficiencies in the absence of specific component therapy
- DIC
- Replacement therapy in antithrombin III, protein C or S deficiency
- Reversal of hemostatic disorders in dilutional coagulopathy from massive transfusion
- Reversal of adverse effects in a baby born to the mother on such agent as phenobarbital or phenytoin
- Thrombotic thrombocytopenic purpura (TTP) for therapeutic plasma exchange
- Coagulopathy due to drug (L-asparaginase) therapy
- Invasive procedures provided that prothrombin time (PT) and/or partial PT (PPT) are quite high (1–1.5 times than normal).

Dose: 10 mL/kg BW over 1–2 hours, to be repeated every 0.5 hour until hemorrhage is controlled.

e. Whole blood

Indication: Acute massive blood loss

Dosage: Volume of whole blood = weight (kg) × change in Hct desired × 2

f. Factor VIII (plasma-derived or recombinant)

Indication: Hemophilia A, acquired factor VIII deficiency

Dosage: 1 U/kg, IV of factor VIII = 2% of factor activity

35–50 U/kg, IV of factor VIII every 12–24 hours

g. Factor IX (plasma-derived or recombinant)

Indication: Hemophilia B

Dosage: 1 U/kg of factor IX = 1% of factor activity 30–50 U/kg, IV every 8–24 hours

h. FEIBA (factor eight inhibitor bypass activity)

Indication: Plasma-derived hemophilia A or B with inhibitors (antibodies)

Dosage: 75–100 U/kg, IV every 8–24 hours (max. dose 200 U/kg/day)

i. Factor VIIa (recombinant)

Indication: Hemophilia A or B with inhibitors

Dosage: 90 µg/kg, IV every 2 hours (35–120 µg/kg dosage range)

j. Cryoprecipitate (rarely used)

Indications
- Control bleeding in patients with DIC
- Hypofibrinogenemia

Dosage: Four bags CRYO/10 kg, IV

Equipment Needed

A tray containing:
- Unit of blood or blood components, whichever is ordered
- Blood transfusion set
- IV pole
- Venipuncture set containing a pediatric size gauge needles if one is not already in place
- Antiseptic wipes
- Plaster gloves

Correct Storage Conditions

- *Whole blood/RBCs:* Transfusion should be started within 30 minutes of removing the pack from storage temperature (+2 to 6°C). It should be completed within 4 hours of starting infusion if the hospital temperature is between 22°C and 25°C. In case of high ambient temperature, shorter out of refrigeration times should be used.
- *Platelets:* Transfuse as soon as they have been received and should be completed in about 20 minutes.
- *FFP:* In adult, FFP 1 U 200–300 mL in 20 minutes (start within 30 minutes) and in children depending on the clinical Condition. These products should be infused through a new, sterile blood administration set containing an integral filter and should be changed 12 hourly if multiple transfusions are needed. For platelet transfusion, a fresh set primed with saline should be used. The child should be monitored frequently during infusion of blood or blood products.

Preparation

- Obtain a written consent from the parents (institutional policy).
- Assess vital signs for baseline data.
- Determine any known allergy or previous adverse reactions to blood.
- Note specific signs related to child's pathology and the reason for transfusion.
- Explain the procedure and its purpose to parents as well as child as appropriate.
- If the child has an IV solution infusing, check whether the needle and solution are appropriate to administer blood.
- Obtain the correct blood component for the child.
  - Check the physician's order with the requisition.
  - Check the requisition form with the blood bag label. Specifically check the client's name, identification no., blood grouping and typing, and the expiry date of blood.
  - Observe the blood for abnormal color, gas bubbles, etc.

Procedure

- Perform hand hygiene.
- Set up the equipment.
  - Ensure the blood filter inside the drip chamber is suitable.
  - Attach the blood tubing to the blood filter.
- Put on gloves.
- Close all the clamps on Y set.
- Using a twisting motion, insert the spike into a container on NS.

- Hang the container on the IV pole about 1 m above the planned venipuncture site.
- Prime the tubing.
- Allow a small amount of NS to infuse to make sure there are no problems with the flow or venipuncture site.
- Invert the blood bag gently several times to mix the cells with the plasma.
- Expose the port on the blood bag by pulling back the tabs.
- Insert the remaining Y set spike into the blood bag.
- Suspend the blood bag.
- Open the upper clamp on the Y set arm to the blood, and prime tubing.
- Establish blood transfusion. Adjust the flow rate as prescribed.
- Observe the child closely for the first 5–10 minutes.
- Monitor the vital signs.
- Remove gloves and perform hand hygiene.

Postprocedure Care

- Document the relevant data.
- Monitor the vital signs after blood transfusion.
- If no infusion is to follow, clamp the blood tubing and remove the needle.
- If the primary IV is to be continued, flush the maintenance line with the saline solution.
- Discard the administration set according to agency policy.

Complications

Immediate reactions:
- Serious hemolytic transfusion reaction
- Febrile reactions
- Circulatory overload
- Air emboli
- Hypothermia
- Electrolyte disturbances

Delayed reactions:
Transmission of infections agents, including HIV, HBV, HCV, syphilis, and malaria, and CMV
- *Alloimmunization:* Antibody formation, occurs in patient receiving multiple transfusions
- Delayed hemolytic reaction

Nurse's Responsibility

- *For PRBCs and whole blood:* Regulate infusion rate using microaggregate filter via infusion pump into 5 mL/kg/h over 2–4 hours (usual rate).
  Do not use the tubing to infuse >1 U of blood.
  - Monitor vital signs before transfusion, 15 minutes after initiation, hourly during transfusion, and upon completion of transfusion.
  - Do not refrigerate the blood in the nursing unit. Only the blood bank refrigerator may be used.
  - Ensure that each unit is infused in 4 hours or less. If a longer infusion time is needed, the unit must be divided in the blood bank.
  - Do not infuse solutions other than NS in the line with RBCs.
- *FFP:*
  - Regulate infusion rate using microaggregate filter to 20 mL/min over 1–2 hours every 12–24 hours until hemorrhage stops.
  - Monitor PT and PPT before and after FFP infusion.
  - Monitor levels of other coagulation factors (e.g., fibrinogen, fibrin split product, D-dimer, ATIII, and proteins C and S).
- *Platelets:*
  - Regulate infusion rate to 10 mL/kg/h, IV push over an hour or as patient can tolerate.

- Monitor vital signs before transfusion, 15 minutes after initiation, and at the end of transfusion.
- Obtain platelet count 60 minutes to 24 hours after infusion.
- *Granulocytes:*
  - Monitor vital signs before transfusion, 15 minutes after initiation and at the end of transfusion.
  - Premedicate 1 hour before transfusion, usually with antihistamines, acetaminophen, or steroids infuse at slow rate (2–4 hours) within a 24-hour period.
  - Minimum of 4–6 hours between amphotericin B and granulocyte infusion recommended.
- *Factor VIII:*
  - Use reconstituted factor within 3 hours of mixing.
  - Inject reconstituted factor intravenously over 2–5 minutes.
  - Assess for signs of an adverse reaction such as hives, itchy wheals with redness, and tightness in chest wheezing, low blood pressure (BP), or trouble breathing. Notify healthcare provider immediately if symptoms are present.
- *Cryoprecipitate:*
  - Monitor closely PT/PPT and levels of fibrinogen; fibrinogen split products, D-dimer.
  - Use a filter needle to draw up and administer within 15–30 minutes.

General Instructions

These are applied to all types of transfusions.
- Take vital signs, including BP, before administering blood to establish baseline data for intratransfusion and post-transfusion comparison; 15 minutes after initiation; hourly while blood is infusing; and upon completion of the transfusion.
- Check the blood type and group of the recipient against the donors, regardless of the blood products used.
- Administer the first 50 mL of blood or initial 20% of volume (whichever is smaller) slowly and stay with the child.
- Administer with NS in a piggyback setup or have NS available.
- Administer blood through an appropriate filter to eliminate particles in the blood and prevent the precipitation of formed elements by gently shaking the container frequently.
- Use blood within 30 minutes of its arrival from the blood bank; if it is not used, return it to the blood bank—do not store it in a regular unit refrigerator.
- Infuse a unit of blood (or the specified amount) within 4 hours. If the infusion exceeds this time, the blood should be divided into appropriate-size quantities by the blood bank, with the unused portion refrigerated under the controlled conditions.
- If a reaction of any type is suspected, take vital signs, stop the transfusion, maintain a patent IV line with NS and new tubing, notify the practitioner, and do not restart the transfusion until the child's condition has been medically evaluated.
- Blood usually administered to children by infusion pump; therefore the usual precautions and management related to pumps apply. When the blood infusion is started with a standard transfusion set, the filter chamber is filled to allow the total filter to be used.
- The drip chamber is partially filled with blood to permit counting of the drops.
- When the flow rate is adjusted, it is important to remember that blood administration sets do not use microdrops (60 drops/mL) but regular drops (usually 10–15 drops/mL). Therefore it must be considered when calculating the flow rate.
- Oxygen may be administered to provide optimum environmental conditions for hemoglobin saturations.

- Oxygen administration is of limited value, however, because each gram of hemoglobin is able to carry a limited amount of the gas. In addition, prolonged use of supplemental oxygen can decrease erythropoiesis. Therefore the child is monitored closely for evidence of decreasing benefit from oxygen. One of the first signs of hypoxia is restlessness.

Highlights

- A blood transfusion is the introduction of whole blood or blood components into the venous circulation.
- Whole blood/RBCs: Transfusion should be started within 30 minutes of removing the pack from storage temperature (+2 to 6°C).
- It should be completed within 4 hours of starting infusion if the hospital temperature is between 22°C and 25°C.
- In the case of high ambient temperature, shorter out of refrigeration times should be used.
- Monitor vital signs before transfusion, 15 minutes after initiation, hourly during transfusion, and upon completion of transfusion.
- Use blood within 30 minutes of its arrival from the blood bank; if it is not used, return it to the blood bank—do not store it in a regular unit refrigerator.
- If a reaction of any type is suspected, take vital signs, stop the transfusion, maintain a patent IV line with NS and new tubing, and notify the practitioner.
- Do not restart the transfusion until the child's condition has been medically evaluated.

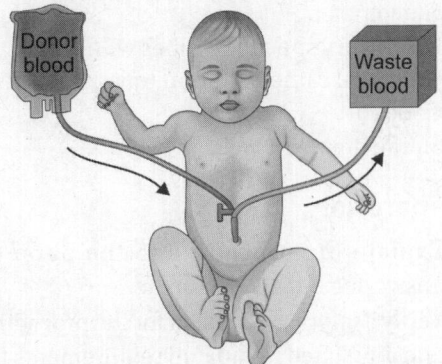

Fig. 8.10: Exchange blood transfusion.

EXCHANGE BLOOD TRANSFUSION

Definition

An exchange transfusion is a medical treatment in which aphaeresis is used to remove one person's RBCs or platelets and replace them with transfused blood products.

It is an introduction of whole blood in exchange for 75–85% of an infant's circulatory blood that is repeatedly withdrawn in small amounts and replaced with equal amounts of donor blood (**Fig. 8.10**).

Indications

- Sickle cell disease
- Thrombocytopenic purpura
- Hemolytic disease of the newborn
- Polycythemia: child's blood is removed and replaced with an NS solution or plasma or albumin
- Severe newborn's jaundice
- Toxic effect of certain drugs
- Severe disturbances in body chemistry

Equipment Needed

- Open bed with radiant heat source (for infant)
- Bed in ICU (for child)
- Cardiopulmonary monitor
- Pulse oximeter
- Noninvasive BP monitor
- Soft restraints
- Fresh whole blood (screened)
- Blood warmer with appropriate tubing
- Blood administration set
- Sterile gown
- Sterile gloves
- Mask and cap
- Exchange transfusion tray with form
- Pretransfusion laboratory results

Chapter 8: Emergency Procedures

- Glucometer
- Laboratory specimen tubes with labels
- Umbilical catheterization tray
- Code cart
- Sterile drapes/towels

Preparation

- Explain the procedure to the parents, answering questions as necessary.
- Verify if informed consent for the procedure and any stated mandated requirements for blood administration have been obtained.
- Arrange for donor blood.
- Obtain preprocedural laboratory tests as ordered.
- Assess the child's history for clinical indications of need for exchange transfusion, history of previous transfusions and relevant laboratory data.
- Ensure that all emergency drugs should be calculated and posted for provision of immediate resuscitation, if necessary.
- Ensure that the infant/child has been NPO for 3–4 hours before procedure to prevent aspiration of stomach contents during the procedure.
- Verify IV fluid orders with healthcare prescriber and ensure separate IV access for fluid, dextrose maintenance, and glucose and medications.

Procedure

The procedure is given in **Table 8.4**.

Table 8.4: Procedure for exchange blood transfusion.

Procedure	Rationale
Perform hand hygiene	Reduces transmission of microorganism
Gather the necessary supplies	Promotes efficient management and provides an organized approach to the procedure
Place the infant supine on radiant warmer in servo control mode, or place the child supine in bed, attach cardiopulmonary monitor and pulse oximeter, and apply noninvasive BP monitor with set time intervals of 3 minutes. For the infant secure arms/legs for procedure	Prevent hypothermia that can result in apnea, increased cardiac and oxygen requirement, acidosis, and stress. The warmer allows for easier access to infant. Monitoring provides for ongoing assessment of the infant. Securing of extremities prevents contamination of sterile field and dislodgement of catheter as the young infant moves
Check blood products with 2 licensed personnel (e.g., 2 RNs, RN/MD), verify crossmatch and child's identification number	Ensure proper identification and crossmatching
Set up blood tubing and warmers as per manufacture's direction. Prime tubing. Temperature of blood should not exceed 98.6°F (37°C)	Ensure appropriate use of equipment
Assist the pediatrician with sterile gown and gloves as necessary. All personnel in the area must wear mask	Minimizes contamination of area. Reduces transmission of microorganisms
Open sterile towel on bedside stand to establish sterile working area for pediatrician	
Open exchange transfusion tray and remove transfusion record form	

Contd...

Contd...

Procedure	Rationale
Document pretransfusion vital signs and laboratory results	Provides baseline data
Connect tubing from exchange transfusion tray: - Attach blood warmer tubing to side port of stopcock - Attach second extension tubing to top port of stopcock and place other end in blood-discard bag - The pediatrician will connect the stopcock to the child's IV access site - Release roller clamp	Decreases chance of dislodgement and therefore contamination of personnel. The waste blood container should be below table level to allow gravity to assist with drainage
Monitor vital signs closely during procedure every 15 minutes. Document temperature, pulse, respiration, blood pressure, oxygen saturation, and blood aliquots in and out, maintaining ongoing total balance	Ensure prompt detection of vital signs instability, which may occur because of too large amount of infusion or rapid speed of withdrawal. Ensures detection of heart failure due to fluid depletion or overload
The pediatrician is responsible for performing aspirations/infusion of blood aliquots, maintaining aseptic technique - Open stopcock to the child, withdraw desired amount of blood, continue monitoring child, and record blood amounts - Assess vital signs to determine infant's tolerance to amount and rate of withdrawal - Rotate stopcock to waste/discard tubing, expel contents of syringe - Rotate stopcock to warm blood tubing, fill with same increment as withdrawal amount - Rotate stopcock to child; infuse blood into child and record "blood in" amount. Repeat above step as needed. Perform procedure over 1–4 hours	Equal amounts of blood in and out in maintaining homeostasis. This process completes one cycle of the exchange process
Obtain laboratory work during the procedure as ordered; monitor blood glucose every 15 minutes or as ordered if there are signs of hypoglycemia	Continuous monitoring is needed due to effects of anticoagulants and other additives used in blood products
During the procedure, gently invert blood bag every 15 minutes	Keep cells and plasma mixed
Assist to obtain postprocedural tests as ordered	Validates the effectiveness of the exchange as well as the need for any adjustment of fluids
Upon completion of procedure, clamp blood tubing and disconnect from catheter. Flush IV line with normal saline and reconnect the ordered IV solution	Maintain the line patency
Dispose of equipment and waste in appropriate receptacle. Remove gloves and perform hand hygiene	Standard precautions reduce transmission of microorganism

(BP: blood pressure; IV: intravenous)

Nursing Considerations

- 160 mL/kg (double the normal volume of 80 mL/kg) blood is used for exchange blood transfusion.
- The donor blood is checked to make certain that it is not >48 hours old.
- If fresh whole blood is not used, stored blood is mixed in amounts as ordered with frozen plasma or human plasma protein fraction.
- Unless contraindicated the infant's parents may be present.
- The integrity of all blood tubing connection is inspected periodically.
- Notify the physician when each 160 mL of blood has been exchanged.
- The patient's blood is slowly withdrawn (usually 5-10 mL at a time, depending on patient's size and severity of illness).

Postprocedure Care

- Monitor for complications.
- Maintain neutral thermal environment.
- Handle the infant minimally and gently for next 24 hours.
- Monitor cardiac and respiratory rates every 15 minutes for 4 hours, then every 30 minutes for 24 hours, and hourly for 48 hours or as ordered.
- The axillary temperature is checked every 1-3 hours for 48 hours.
- The cord is observed for bleeding every 5-15 minutes for 1-2 hours after the procedure.
- Feeding by gavage or bottle with soft nipple with a large enough hole to ensure that adequate intake is initiated 4-6 hours after the transfusion is ordered.
- The infant is fed slowly and repositioned after each feeding.
- Fluid intake and output are measured and ongoing care is provided as for all high-risk infants.

Complications

- Thrombocytopenia
- Hypocalcaemia
- Metabolic acidosis
- Hypoglycemia
- Catheter malfunction
- Apnea
- Bradycardia
- Hypotension
- Hyperkalemia
- Hypomagnesaemia
- Hypertension
- Respiratory distress
- Vessel thrombosis
- Seizures
- Sepsis
- Renal failure
- Omphalitis (neonate)
- Necrotizing enterocolitis (neonate)
- Jitteriness
- Cyanosis
- Bleeding from the cord
- Metabolic alkalosis

Highlights

- An exchange transfusion is a medical treatment in which aphaeresis is used to remove one person's RBCs or platelets and replace them with transfused blood products.
- It is an introduction of whole blood in exchange for 75-85% of an infant's circulatory blood that is repeatedly withdrawn in small amounts and replaced with equal amounts of donor blood.
- Ensure that all emergency drugs should be calculated and posted for provision of the immediate resuscitation, if necessary.
- Ensure that the infant/child has been NPO for 3-4 hours before procedure to prevent aspiration of stomach contents during the procedure.
- 160 mL/kg (double the normal volume of 80 mL/kg) blood is used for exchange blood transfusion.
- Monitor cardiac and respiratory rates every 15 minutes for 4 hours, then every 30 minutes for 24 hours, and hourly for 48 hours.

GASTRIC LAVAGE

Definition
Gastric lavage means washout or irrigate the stomach with solution.

Indications
- Accidental poisoning (except corrosives and hydrocarbons)
- Management of upper GI bleeding
- For collecting samples of gastric juice for the diagnosis of acid-fast bacilli

Equipment Needed
A clean tray containing:
- Ryle's tube
- Suction apparatus
- Liquid paraffin
- Mouth gag
- Saline or plain water
- Specific antidotes (if the poison is identified)

Preparation
- Obtain vital signs.
- Explain the procedure to the parents.
- Place the child supine with head hyperextended and supported underneath by a hand. Restrain the conscious child to prevent injury.
- Ensure adequate airway protection.
- Have all the equipment ready.

Procedure
- Wash hands and don gloves.
- Open the mouth and use the mouth gag.
- After lubricating the tube with liquid paraffin (avoid it in a neonate), advance the tube over the tongue toward the back of the throat.
- Keep advancing the tube until the mark on the tube reaches the tip.
- Confirm that the tube is in the stomach by pushing air through the tube and auscultating over stomach.
- Bubbling of air when the outer end is placed in a cup of water indicates that tube is in trachea rather than stomach.
- Fix the tube securely on the face with adhesive tape.
- Gently suction the gastric contents.
- Perform lavage of stomach using aliquots of NS (10–100 mL/kg/cycle). The fluid may be infused by gravity or with a syringe, but rapid, forceful fluid injection should be avoided, as this may force stomach contents out of pylorus.
- The lavage fluid is drained by gravity (by holding the end of the tube below the level of the stomach) or removed by syringe aspiration.
- Keep repeating the cycle till the color of the returning fluid is the same as that of the lavage fluid.
- While removing the tube, always pinch its end to prevent spilling of the contents into the trachea.

Postprocedure Care
- Keep the child in comfortable position.
- Monitor the vital parameters, including level of consciousness.
- The child should be observed for any respiratory symptoms that might indicate pulmonary aspirations.
- Send the specimen to laboratory (as necessary).
- Document the procedure in record—type of fluid used, total amount, and sequence of procedure with date and time.

General Instructions
- The tube may be inserted well through the nostrils.
- Do not use excessive force while passing the tube.
- Watch out for laryngeal spasm and bradycardia during the procedure.

- Monitor the vital signs every 15 minutes during the procedure.
- Avoid introducing air into the stomach.
- Ensure that the amount of fluid returned should approximate the amount infused.
- If concretions are suspected (e.g., aspirin), it may be helpful to flex the child's hips and gently massage the stomach.
- When using dual-plunger system, the simultaneous inflow of lavage fluid and outflow of stomach contents tend to better aspirate stomach contents, yielding more efficient lavage.
- Retching or vomiting commonly occurs when the tube is removed.
- When the lavage has been completed, the same Ryle's tube may be used for installing activated charcoal before withdrawal.

Complications

- Pulmonary aspiration
- Laryngospasm
- Respiratory insufficiency
- Hypoxia
- Cardiac dysrhythmias
- Trauma to oral mucosa
- Esophageal lacerations/perforations
- Esophageal spasm
- Electrolyte imbalance
- Hypothermia (in the case of cold lavage)
- Petechiae of head, neck, chest, and small subconjunctival hemorrhages (when lavage is overzealous or child is agitating)

Nurse's Responsibility

- Give careful attention to airway/respiratory status, accurate tube placement, and proper position of the child (left lateral, head down).
- Ensure adequate lubrication of tube to prevent complications such as injury and spasm.
- Use warmed saline for lavage.
- In the case of tube obstruction due to food materials or other solid particles, manipulate the fluid flow to keep the system patent.
- Discontinue the procedure when the child is forcefully gagging or vomiting around the tube.

Highlights ● ● ● ●

- Gastric lavage means washing out or irrigating the stomach with solution.
- It is commonly done in the management of accidental poisoning (except corrosives and hydrocarbons) and upper GI bleeding.
- Perform lavage of stomach using aliquots of NS (10–100 mL/kg/cycle). The fluid may be infused by gravity or with a syringe.
- Rapid, forceful fluid injection should be avoided, as this may force stomach contents out of pylorus.
- The lavage fluid is drained by gravity (by holding the end of the tube below the level of the stomach) or removed by syringe aspiration.
- Keep repeating the cycle till the color of the returning fluid is the same as the lavage fluid.
- While removing the tube, always pinch its end to prevent spilling of the contents into the trachea.
- Watch out for laryngeal spasm and bradycardia during the procedure.
- Monitor the vital signs every 15 minutes during the procedure.
- Give careful attention to airway/respiratory status, accurate tube placement, and proper position of the child (left lateral, head down).

UMBILICAL VEIN CATHETERIZATION

Definition

A lifesaving procedure in which a radio-opaque catheter is passed through an umbilical vein of a newborn to obtain blood samples, for an exchange transfusion or for emergency administration of drugs, fluids, etc.

Indications

- For exchange blood transfusion
- Rapid replacement of blood or fluids
- Setting up of infusion when other sites fail
- To monitor central venous pressure

Contraindications

- Infected stump
- Contemplated abdominal surgery
- Omphalitis
- Omphalocele
- Necrotizing enterocolitis
- Peritonitis

Equipment Needed

A sterile tray containing:
- 7–8 Fr size catheter
- 10-mL syringe with heparinized saline
- Sterile slit towels
- Mosquito forceps, antiseptic solution—spirit, Betadine
- Cotton balls in a bowl
- Prescribed fluid
- Kidney tray
- Pair of gloves
- Suture material

Preparation

- Restrain the infant by using a padded crucifix splint for fixing all four limbs.
- The infant should be placed under the radiant warmer in the servo mode to maintain skin temperature around 36.5°C.
- Site should be prepared aseptically using spirit—Betadine—spirit.
- Drape the area using sterile towels.

Procedure

- Sterilization of cord area and then cutting the cord 2 cm from the skin junction, that is, close to the base of the stump.
- With edge gripped with mosquito forceps, three blood vessels are seen at the base. Two are umbilical arteries with regular outline and thick walls. The umbilical vein has irregular outline and thin collapsed wall.
- After clearing the vein of any clot, etc., the catheter is advanced gently into its lumen for 5–7 cm.
- As soon as the blood begins to flow freely into the catheter, it fills the catheter completely.
- The catheter should be connected to the drip set or the syringe.
- At the end of the procedure, a sterile polyvinyl marker is required to be inserted in the orifice of the umbilical vein.
- It should be tried to facilitate a subsequent catheterization.

Complications

- Thrombosis of blood vessels
- Embolization
- Perforation of vessel
- Air embolism
- Misplacement of catheter into the portal venous system
- Bleeding
- Infection
- Necrotizing enterocolitis
- Extrahepatic portal hypertension (rare)
- Liver necrosis
- Pericardial effusion or tamponade
- Arrhythmias
- Hydrothorax

Highlights ●●●

> ✦ Umbilical vein catheterization is a lifesaving procedure in which a radio-opaque catheter is passed through an umbilical vein of the newborn.
> ✦ It is done to obtain blood samples, for an exchange transfusion or for emergency administration of drugs, fluids, etc.

THORACENTESIS

Definition
Thoracentesis refers to the puncture by needle through the chest wall into the pleural space for the purpose of removing pleural fluid.

Indications
- To remove pleural fluid or air (both for diagnostic and therapeutic purposes)
- To induce pneumothorax
- To inject antibiotics in the case of empyema

Equipment Needed
- *A sterile tray containing:*
  - Sponge-holding forceps
  - Syringes with needles
  - Three-way stopcock with tubing
  - Small bowl with antiseptic solution
  - Specimen bottles and slides
  - Gown, mask, and gloves
  - Sterile dressing towels/slit
  - Cotton swabs, gauze pieces, and pads
  - 20-mL syringe with Luer lock (as necessary)
- *A clean tray containing:*
  - Mackintosh and towel
  - Kidney tray
  - Tincture benzoin
  - Procaine 1%
  - Suction apparatus (if needed)

General Instructions
- Sedation may be given in anxious child to prevent movement during procedure.
- The three-way stopcock should be fitted with needle before it is introduced into the chest cavity.
- The bevel of aspiration needle should be short to prevent pricking of the lungs.
- Remain with the child and watch his general condition during the procedure.
- Monitor vital signs during the procedure.
- Follow strict aseptic technique during the procedure.
- If any signs of complications are noted such as respiratory distress, excessive coughing, crepitus, and hemoptysis, the aspiration is discontinued.

Preparation
- In order to know the exact position of effusion, an X-ray chest should be done before thoracentesis.
- Explain the procedure to the parents and the child as appropriate.
- Get a written consent (hospital policy).
- Check vital signs.
- Make the child sits back on the bed and lean forward against a stool or chair back.

Procedure
- Perform hand hygiene and don gloves, mask, and gown.
- Prepare the chosen area (8th and 9th intercostal spaces in the posterior axillary line, or the area of maximum dullness) with antiseptic wipes.
- The area is infiltrated with 1% procaine down to the pleura.
- A large-bore needle with a syringe is inserted in the space along the upper edge of the lower rib. This is important to avoid injury to the intercostal nerves and blood vessels.

  Note: Entry into the pleural cavity is indicated by a feeling of "give."
- With suction, the fluid begins to flow into the syringe.
- Not >100–500 mL should be removed at a time.
- When the needle is withdrawn, the skin puncture site should be sealed with tincture benzoin.

Postprocedure Care
- Apply a sterile dressing and pressure bandage on the site.
- Position the child comfortably on the bed with the affected side up.

- Monitor the child for complications.
- Auscultate the lungs for breath sounds.
- Compare the chest movements on both sides.
- Check the puncture site for leakage of fluids.
- Monitor the vital parameters.
- If a water seal drainage system is used, the care should include as that of a client with under water seal drainage system.
- In older children, deep breathing exercises can be encouraged.
- Send the specimen for laboratory investigation as prescribed.
- Arrange for X-ray chest if indicated.
- Document the procedure in nurse's record.

Complications

- *Pneumothorax:* Due to entry of air
- *Hemothorax:* Due to injury to the blood vessels
- *Pulmonary edema:* Due to reaccumulation of fluid
- Infection
- *Mediastinal shift:* Due to large amount of fluid withdrawn or due to a tension pneumothorax

Highlights ●●●●

+ Thoracentesis refers to the puncture by needle through the chest wall into the pleural space for the purpose of removing pleural fluid.
+ The three-way stopcock should be fitted with needle before it is introduced into the chest cavity.
+ The bevel of aspiration needle should be short to prevent pricking of the lungs.
+ Not >100–500 mL should be removed at a time.
+ If any signs of complications are noted such as respiratory distress, excessive coughing, crepitus, and hemoptysis, the aspiration is discontinued.
+ After the procedure, position the child comfortably on the bed with the affected side up.

MEMORY EXERCISE

1. **The first response to unwitnessed unresponsive infant is to:**
   a. Activate emergency response system
   b. Check pulse
   c. Start rescue breathing
   d. Start chest compression

2. **An appropriate nursing action for a 12-month-old child with complaints of chocking with a candy is to:**
   a. Open airway and give rescue breathing
   b. Give five back blows
   c. Give five chest thrusts
   d. Give a series of five back blows and chest thrusts

3. **The amount of blood needed for exchange transfusion procedure is:**
   a. 80 mL/kg
   b. 160 mL/kg
   c. 240 mL/kg
   d. 200 mL/kg

4. **The amount of fluid to be used for gastric lavage is:**
   a. 10–50 mL/cycle
   b. 20–50 mL/cycle
   c. 10–100 mL/cycle
   d. 50–100 mL/cycle

5. **The following are the appropriate nursing actions when a child develops blood transfusion reaction,** *except:*
   a. Continue blood transfusion in slow rate
   b. Take vital signs
   c. Maintain a patent IV line with NS and new tubing
   d. Notify the practitioner

CHAPTER 9

Safety and Recreation

LEARNING OBJECTIVES

After reading this chapter, the readers should be able to:
- Recognize the importance of play therapy among hospitalized children.
- Select age-appropriate play materials for sick children.
- Incorporate dramatic play and therapeutic play in nursing care activities.
- Handle the children gently during restraint procedure.

Keywords: play, communication, restraint, therapy, time-out, medications

PLAY THERAPY

Introduction

Play is the universal language of children. It is one of the most important forms of communication and can be an effective technique to relate with them.

Goals of Play Therapy

- To maintain normal living pattern
- To minimize psychological trauma
- To provide optimal growth and development of the child

Functions of Play in Hospital

- Provides diversion and relaxation
- Helps the child feel more secure in a strange environment
- Lessens the stress of separation and feeling of homesickness
- Provides a means for releasing of tension and expression of feelings
- Encourages interaction and development of positive attitudes toward others
- Provides an expressive outlet for creative ideas and interests
- Provides a means for accomplishing therapeutic goals
- Places the child in an active role, providing the opportunity to make choices and to be in control

Classification of Play Therapy

Therapeutic play

It is a nondirected play technique and focuses on helping the child to cope with his or her feelings and fears. Supervised play with medical equipment in the hospital environment can help children work through their feelings about what happened to them.

Dramatic Play

It is a well-recognized technique for emotion release, allowing children to reenact frightening or puzzling hospital experience. It enables the children to learn about procedures and events that are of concern to them and to assume the roles of the adults in the hospital unit.

Types of Play Materials That can be Used in Hospital

Simple craft material	Toys, doctor and nurse dolls
Blocks	Play syringes
Puzzles	Stethoscopes
Story books	Old cloth to restrain the toys, make bandage
Walls	Puppets
Doll houses	Music
Phonograph records	Electronic games
Clay and play dough	Push–pull toys
Paints	Picture books
Pounding boards	Paper and pencil for drawing
Tricycles	Crayons
Carts and wagons	Rocking horse
Surprise boxes	Squeezing balls

Types of Bedside Play

1. Storytelling—imaginative or anecdotal
   - Children <5 years: Stories with themes about people who shut their eyes and ears, things that are missing, change in appearance, etc.
   - Children between 5 years and 10 years: Stories with themes about making things that last, acquiring competitive skill, pleasing adults, role model, triumph over danger, being ashamed or losing face, and patterns of living with friends.
2. Water play during bath
   - Blowing soap bubbles, filling and squeezing a bath sponge, bathing a doll, and playing with boats.
3. Television
   - Telling about programs, commercials, etc., and use of closed-circuit television to present health-teaching films and to provide lessons in finger crafts.
4. Needle play
   - Handling empty syringes (without sharp needles), intravenous (IV) tubing, etc. and pretending to give shots to a doll, stuffed animal, parent, or nurse. The nurse can demonstrate the method of giving an injection by drawing up the solution or water and squirting a bit into the air.
5. Pre- and postoperative teaching
   - Handling operating room mask, cap, gown, etc. and any material relevant to care.
6. Art
   - Drawing with crayons or blank paper followed by discussion of what is drawn.

Nurse's Responsibilities

- The nurse must consider the age, interest, diagnosis, and limitations imposed by the illness when planning activities for any child.
  For example, an acutely ill child can enjoy storytelling.
- Avoid the term "play room" when caring for older aged children and adolescents, instead call it the "activity room" or social room. Ideally adolescents should have their room space.
- Use play as appropriate while providing routine nursing care to the child, for example, to encourage deep breathing, encourage the child to blow bubbles or blow a whistle.

- Award the child a sticker, special pencil, or any small gift if he or she reaches a certain level of performance.
- When using play as a part of nursing care, it is important to evaluate the outcome of play. For example, for the child blowing bubbles, determine whether this activity enhanced coughing and deep breathing.
- Special consideration must be given to the children who are isolated and have limited movements or restricted extremities.

  Note: Toys for children in isolation unit must be disposable or be disinfected after use. Stuffed animals should not be used in this unit.
- Have parents provide the child with a shoe box, a small suitcase, or backpack for easy storage to prevent small play items from becoming lost in the sheets or under the bed.
- Providing space for special needs of children in age-group can be difficult. Hence, play room schedules can be structured to allow one age-group at a time.

  For example, adolescents can use the facilities in the afternoon when younger children are asleep.
- When supervising play for children who are ill or convalescing, it is best to select activities that are simpler than would normally be chosen according to children's developmental level.
- Incorporate opportunity for musical expression into routine nursing care, for example, dance or movement suggestions may encourage a child to ambulate.
- Avoid doing any painful procedures in play room whenever possible.
- Teach the child to take care of toys.

Play Activities for Special Procedures

- *Fluid intake*:
  - Make ice pops using child's favorite juice.
  - Cut gelatin into funny shapes.
  - Use small medicine cups, decorate the cups.
  - Color the water with permitted food coloring or powered drink mix.
  - Let the child fill a syringe (without needle) and squirt it into the mouth or use it to fill small decorated cups.
  - Cut straws into half and place in a small container (much easier for child to suck liquid)
  - "Make a progress poster." Give rewards for drinking a predetermined quantity.
- *Deep breathing*
  - Blow the bubbles with a bubble blower or straw.
  - Blow on a pinwheel, feather, whistle, and balloon.
  - Practice band instruments such as flute.
  - Have blowing contest using balloons, cotton balls, etc. among children.
  - Suck and leave the paper or cloth from one container to other using a straw.
  - Take a deep breath and blow out the candles on a birthday cake.
  - Use a little paint brush to paint nails with water and blow nails to dry.
- *Range of motion and use of extremities*
  - Play pretend and guessing games (e.g., imitate a bird, butterfly, horse).
  - Have tricycle or wheelchair race in safe area.
  - Play video game (fine motor development).
  - Play "hide and seek", hide toys some where in bed (or room if ambulatory) and have child find it the using specified hand or foot.

- Provide clay to mold with fingers.
- Paint or draw on large sheets or papers placed on floor or walls.
- Encourage the child to comb own hair.
- Pretend to teach aerobic exercises or dancing.
- Position bed so that child must turn to view television or doorway.
- Soaks
  - Play with small toys or objects (cups, soap dishes) in water.
  - Wash dolls.
  - Pick up coins from bottom of bath container.
  - Make designs with coins on bottom of container.
  - Pretend a boat is a submarine by keeping it immersed.
  - Sitz bath: Give the child something to listen to or look at (e.g., music).
  - Punch holes in bottom of plastic cup, fill with water, and let it rain on child.
- Injection
  - Let, child handle syringe, vial, and swab and give an injection to doll or stuffed animals.
  - Draw a magic circle on area before injection, draw smiling face in circle after injection but avoid drawing on puncher site.
  - Have child count numbers during injection.
  - Give rewards for successful cooperation.
- Ambulation
  - Give the child something to push, for example, toddler—push–pull toys; school age—wagon or decorated IV stand.

Guidelines for Infection Control in Play Therapy

Play materials are the source of potential infection. Hence, infection control in play area can be maintained by the following measures:

- Do not allow stuffed or nonwashable play materials in the play room.
- All the toys should be washed with soapy warm water after use. Special care should be taken when it is used by children who are having infectious diseases or drooling problems, the materials should not be used by others without washing.
- Clean the toys using cloth immersed in disinfectant if they cannot be washed.
- Encourage handwashing of personnel/caregiver accompanying the children before entering play room.

Highlights ● ● ● ●

- ✦ Play is the universal language of children. It is one of the most important forms of communication.
- ✦ The goals of play therapy are to maintain normal living pattern, to minimize psychological trauma, and to provide optimal growth and development of the child.
- ✦ Play therapy for hospitalized children is mainly classified into: (1) therapeutic play and (2) dramatic play.
- ✦ The nurse must consider the age, interest, diagnosis, and limitations imposed by the illness when planning activities for any child.
- ✦ When using play as a part of nursing care, it is important to evaluate the outcome of the play. For example, for the child blowing bubbles, determine whether this activity enhanced coughing and deep breathing.
- ✦ Toys for children in isolation unit must be disposable or be disinfected after use. Stuffed animals should not be used in this unit.
- ✦ Avoid the term "play room" when caring for older children and adolescents, instead call it the "activity room" or social room. Ideally adolescents should have their room space.
- ✦ Play materials are the source of potential infection. Hence, infection control in play area should be maintained.

RESTRAINTS

Definition
"Restraints are the measures used to limit the child's ability to move around freely or reach normal body parts."

Types of Restraints
1. Environmental
2. Physical
3. Mechanical
4. Chemical

Environmental: Environmental restraint limits the area where the child can move freely and may refer to a time-out or seclusion.

Physical: Physical restraint involves having one or more persons restraining the child through body contact alone.

Mechanical: Mechanical restraint refers to the use of devices placed on the wrists, ankles, or chest, for example, arm boards and cloth boards.

Chemical: Any medicines that help child to calm down and relax.

Indications
- When child's behavior is out of control and puts himself or others in danger, for example, drug use, head injury, or mental disorder
- While doing the procedures, for example, venipuncture
- After surgery, for example, wrist restraints to prevent the child from pulling out tubes or other medical devices

Principles
- The institution should have the policy in place to satisfy the reason for restraint.
- When determining the need for restraining a child, the nurse needs to consider the child's growth and developmental level, mental status, and significant others and self.
- Apply the principle of atraumatic care, the nurse uses a restraint only when necessary and for the short duration of time as possible.
- Use of at least one alternative method for restriction before using a restraint.
- Various restraints to facilitate examination or maintain safety are essential in the care and treatment of pediatric patients.
- Restraints are used only when necessary.
- Improperly applied restraints can cause skin irritation and can impair circulation.
- Free movement facilitates growth and development.

Guidelines for Use of Restraints
- At least two caregivers are needed to physically restrain the child.
- Physical restraint should be used in a quiet environment away from other children.
- Mechanical restraints to be used must be easy to remove in the case of an emergency.

Types of Mechanical Restraints

Clove Hitch Restraint

Purpose
Wrist or ankle restraint to prevent the range of motion of extremities (**Fig. 9.1**)

Nurse's responsibilities
- Check wrist or ankle for any sign of circulatory or neurologic compromise.
- The ends of the restraints are never tied to the side rails and should be tied on the bed frame.
- The part must be padded to prevent undue pressure, constriction, or tissue injury.

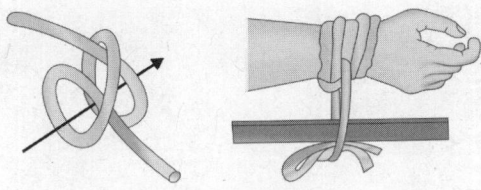

Fig. 9.1: Application of clove hitch restraint.

Elbow Restraints

Made up of a piece of muslin long enough to reach comfortably from just below the axilla to the wrist, with a number of vertical pockets into which tongue blades are inserted.

The restraint is wrapped around the arm and secured with tapes or pins. Pin the top of the restraint under the shirt sleeve to prevent restraint from slipping (**Fig. 9.2**).

Purpose

- To prevent the child from the reaching the head or face (e.g., after lip surgery, scalp vein infusion).
- To prevent scratching in the case of skin disorders.

Nurse's responsibilities

- Position the restraint so it does not rub against axilla.

- Check pulse, temperature, and capillary refill of the extremity.

Mummy Restraint

A blanket or sheet is opened on the bed with one corner folded to the center. The infant is placed on the blanket with shoulders at the fold and feet toward the opposite corner with infant's right arm straight down against the body. The right side of the blanket is pulled firmly across the right shoulder and chest and secured beneath the left side of the body. The left arm is placed straight against the infant's side and the left side of the blanket is brought across the shoulder and chest and tucked beneath the infant's body of the right side. The lower corner is folded and brought over the body and fastened securely with safety pins (**Figs. 9.3A to C**).

Purpose

- Short-term restraint of infant for examination or treatment that involves the head and neck, for example, venipuncture, throat examination, and gavage feeding.

Nurse's responsibilities

- Ensure that all extremities are secured within the sheets.

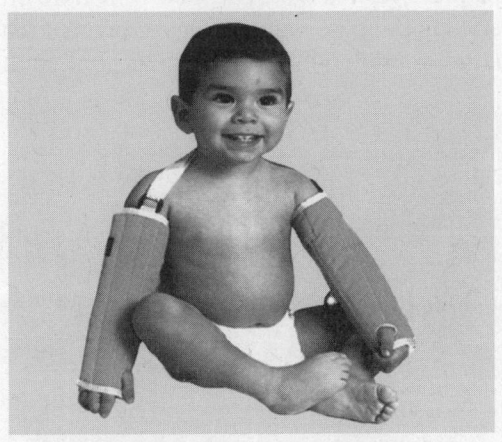

Fig. 9.2: Elbow restraints.

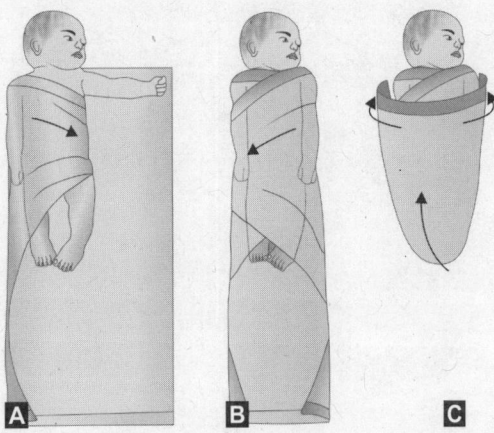

Figs. 9.3A to C: Steps in applying a mummy restraint.

- For chest examination, the folded edge of the blanket is brought over each arm and under the back, after which the loose edge is folded over and secured at chest.

Jacket (Vest Restraint)
- The jacket is put on the child with the ties in the back so that the child is unable to manipulate them.
- The long tapes are secured to the under-structure of the crib or chair (**Fig. 9.4**).

Purpose
Used to keep the child flat in the bed, in situations such as after surgery or safe in chair.

Nurse's responsibilities
- Ensure that the child can turn the head to side and that at the head-end, the bed is elevated.
- Place the ties in the back so the child cannot manipulate.

Crib Top Bubble Restraint
Placing clean plastic cover over the bed

Purpose
To prevent infants or young children from falling out of bed

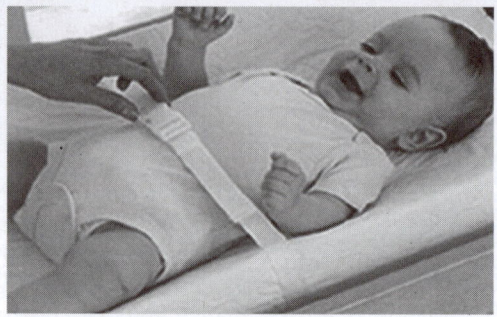

Fig. 9.5: Abdominal belt.

Nurse's responsibility
Ensure that there are no tears or loose plastic.

Abdominal Restraint
This is used to hold the infant in a supine position on the bed, by using abdominal binder or belt and the strips are tied with the side of the cot (**Fig. 9.5**).

Crib Net Restraint
This is a net or dome used to cover the child's cot (**Fig. 9.6**).
It is used to prevent the child from climbing the side rails of the cot.

Safety Belts
These are made up of electrically non-conductive materials. These belts are used on stretcher and operation tables to prevent the children from falling. These belts go around

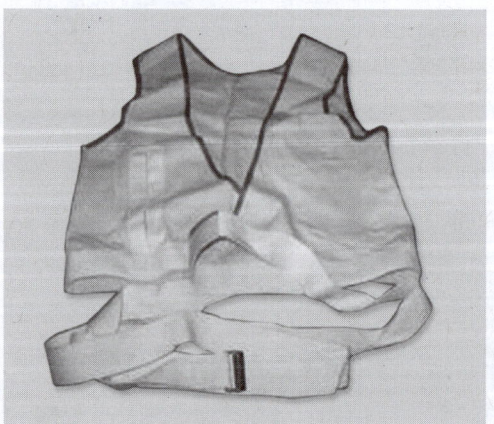

Fig. 9.4: Jacket restraint.

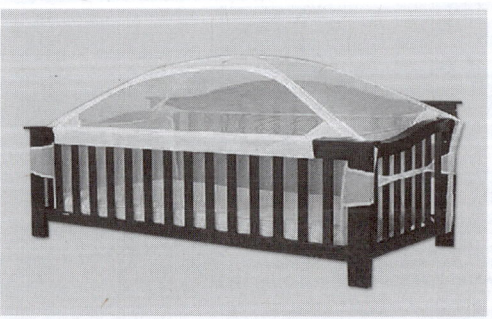

Fig. 9.6: Crib net restraint.

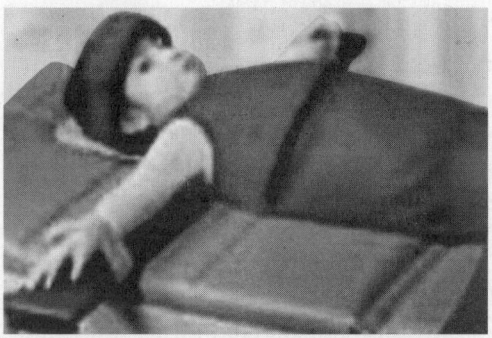

Fig. 9.7: Safety belt.

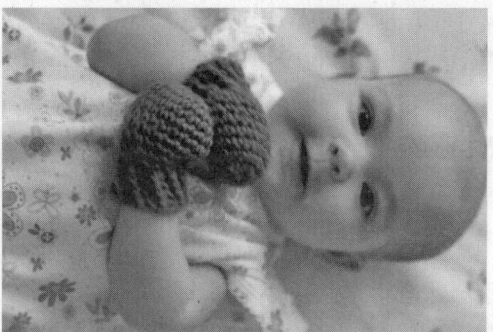

Fig. 9.9: Mittens.

the child's wrist and head to the frame of the bed under the mattress (**Fig. 9.7**).

Side Rails

It is to prevent children falling from bed and can be used along restraints (**Fig. 9.8**).

Mitten

The hand is inserted in a bag-like pouch (mitten) and tied properly around the wrist.

The mitten covers the hand and restricts the movement of the fingers (**Fig. 9.9**).

Purpose

It is used in the case of facial surgeries, burns, IV infusion, and any skin lesion of the face and body parts to avoid scratching.

Splints

Splints are made up of cardboard, plastic, cotton, and gauze pad to restrict the movement of the extremity (**Fig. 9.10**).

Hazards of Restraints

- If restraint is too tight, it can cause obstruction in blood circulation, tissue damage, redness, scar formation, discoloration of the skin, etc.
- Nerve damage
- Psychological disturbance
- Alteration in body image
- Disturbance in normal development
- Accidental or intentional removal of restraints may result in possible removal of tubes, IV lines, injury, etc.
- Injury to restrained extremity
- Fracture or muscle strains during application with violent patient

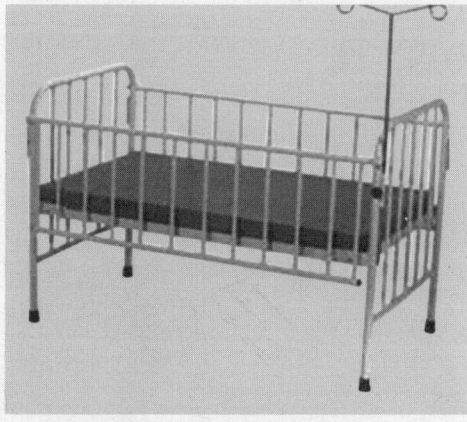

Fig. 9.8: Side rails of the cot.

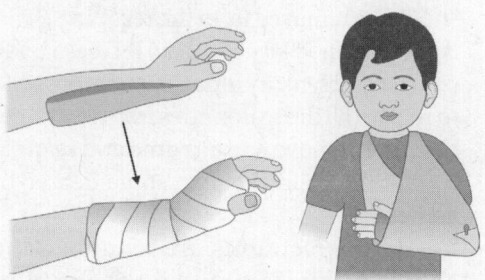

Fig. 9.10: Splints for supporting upper limb.

- Dislocation or contusion of extremity
- Numbness and tingling in restrained extremity

Nurse's Responsibilities in Restraining a Child

- The reason for applying restraints must be explained to both the child and the parents.
- While applying the restraint and periodically during the period of restraining, the nurse should talk smoothly to the child to provide stimulation and diversion. Such interaction increases the child's sensory input and tends to relieve the sense of helplessness and loneliness.
- When restraints are applied, they should be put on effectively yet as loosely as possible to prevent interference with restraints and circulation so that the child can move safely to some degree.
- Sufficient padding must be used under the extremities restraints to prevent skin irritation.
- The ties on restraints should be attached to crib frame instead of side rail to prevent the traction on the restraint or injury to the child when the side rail is raised or lowered.
- Restraints must be checked every 15–30 minutes to determine whether they are achieving their purpose and whether constricting the respirations or circulation in any way.
- Periodically at least every 2 hours the child should be removed from the restraints, held if possible and played with, to increase body contact and sensory input. If it is impossible to release all the extremities from restraints at a time, remove one at a time and reapply so that the child can gain some degree of activity.
- Before the restraints are reapplied the child's position should be changed to improve the physiologic functioning.

In the Case of Chemical Restraints

- Check the medicines the child currently takes. Make sure that these medicines are safe to take along with medicines used for chemical restraint.
- Medicines used for chemical restraint are commonly offered to the child in pill form first. If the child refuses, medicines may be given as a shot or in an IV.
- After the medicine is given, the child should be constantly monitored. Vital signs should be checked often until the medicine wears off.

In the Case of Environmental Restraints

- Make sure that the room used for seclusion is calm and safe. There should be windows with unbreakable glass so that the caregivers can monitor the child. There should be no exposed wiring, nails, or screws that may be used as weapons.
- The child must be observed constantly by caregivers. This may be done in person or with a video camera.
- Caregivers have to review the need for seclusion every 2 hours. Seclusion will end as soon the child behaves as caregivers have requested. This may include stopping violent behavior that puts others at risk.

Highlights ● ● ● ●

> - Restraints are the measures used to limit the child's ability to move around.
> - Environmental restraint: Environmental restraint limits the area where the child can move freely and may refer to a time-out or seclusion.
> - Physical restraint: Physical restraint involves having one or more persons restraining the child through body contact alone.
> - Mechanical restraint: Mechanical restraint refers to the use of devices placed on the wrists, ankles, or chest, for example, arm boards and cloth boards.

Contd...

Chapter 9: Safety and Recreation

Contd...

- Chemical restraint: Any medicines that help the child to calm down and relax.
- Apply the principle of atraumatic care, the nurse uses a restraint only when necessary and for the short duration of time as possible.
- Various restraints to facilitate examination or maintain safety are essential in the care and treatment of pediatric patients.
- If restraint is too tight, it can cause obstruction in blood circulation, tissue damage, redness, scar formation, discoloration of the skin, etc.
- While applying the restraint and periodically during the period of restraining, the nurse should talk smoothly to the child to provide stimulation and diversion.
- Restraints must be checked every 15–30 minutes to determine whether they are achieving their purpose and whether constricting the respirations or circulation in any way.
- When the medicine is given for sedation, the child should be constantly monitored. Vital signs should be checked often until the medicine wears off.

MEMORY EXERCISE

1. **The type of play that can be used to teach deep breathing exercise is:**
   a. Hide and seek
   b. Doctor–nurse kit
   c. Blowing wheel
   d. Moving wagon

2. **Type of restraint that can be used for preventing scratching in a child with scabies is:**
   a. Clove hitch restraint
   b. Elbow restraint
   c. Mummy restraint
   d. Mittens

3. **The nurse should release the restraints once in:**
   a. 15 minutes
   b. 1 hour
   c. 2 hours
   d. 30 minutes

4. **Which of the following is environmental restraint?**
   a. Time-out
   b. Locking in separate room
   c. Tie the baby on chair
   d. Sedation

5. **The types of the play materials used for play therapy should be all of the following, *except*:**
   a. Stuffed toys
   b. Blunt ended
   c. Washable
   d. Large size

CHAPTER 10

Care of Child with Fracture

LEARNING OBJECTIVES

After reading this chapter, the readers should be able to:
- Explain the purpose of different types of traction.
- Identify the needs of child with traction.
- Perform nursing care to prevent complications.
- Assist in application of plaster cast.
- Assess the condition of casted extremity.
- Educate the parents regarding home care of child with cast.

Keywords: fracture, immobilization, traction, weight, plaster cast, numbness, hollow sound.

TRACTION CARE

Definition

Traction is a method of immobilization, which may be used to reduce mobility and to immobilize the fractured part, to align an injured extremity, and to allow the extremity to be restored to its normal length.

Purposes

- To realign bone fragments
- To provide rest for an extremity
- To help prevent or improve contracture deformity
- To correct a deformity
- To treat a dislocation
- To allow preoperative or postoperative positioning and alignment
- To provide immobilization of specific areas of the body (**Table 10.1**)
- To reduce muscle spasms (rare in small children)

Equipment Needed

- *Skin cleansing supplies:*
  - A basin
  - Jugs with hot and cold water separately
  - Soap in a soap dish
  - Sponge clothes
  - Bath towel
  - Talc powder
- Skeletal pin site cleansing supplies:
  - Sterile gauze pieces in a bowl
  - Sterile surgical pad
  - Antiseptic solution and ointment for topical application

Chapter 10: Care of Child with Fracture

Table 10.1: Types of traction.

S. no.	Type	Indications	Nurse's responsibility
1.	Cervical skin	Neck sprains/strains, torticollis, cervical nerve injury, nerve root compression	There is a 2- to 3-kg limit of weights. Avoid compressing the throat or ears with the chin strap
2.	Sidearm 90–90	Fracture and dislocation of the upper arm or shoulder	Hand may feel cold because of its elevation. Hand can be covered with sock or mitten if desired
3.	Dunlop sidearm 00–90	Supracondylar elbow fracture of the humerus	Avoid pressure over bony prominences or nerves
4.	Pelvis sling	Pelvic fracture	There is a 4- to 10-kg limit of weights. Ensure proper size of belt and apply it just over iliac crest
5.	Bryant's traction	Infant with a femur fracture or developmental dislocation of hip	Supply plenty of diversional activities. If child flips over, a sheet or Posey restraint may be used. Avoid pressure over dorsum of foot and heel
6.	Buck's traction	Hip and knee contracture, Legg–Calvé–Perthes disease, SCFE	Remove boot every 8 hours and assess skin. Legs may be slightly abducted
7.	Russell's traction	Supracondylar femur fracture, hip and knee contractures	Sling may need to be repositioned often; mark leg to ensure proper placement
8.	Split Russell's traction	Femur fracture, SCFE, Legg–Calvé–Perthes disease	Avoid pressure over bony prominences or nerves. Weights are not added or removed without order
9.	90–90 traction	For femur fracture reduction when skin traction is inadequate. Skeletal traction with force applied through pin in distal femur	A foam boot may be used for suspension of the lower leg. Force of traction applied to femur via the pin. The amount of weight used is just enough to hold lower limb suspended
10.	Cervical skeletal tongs	Tongs attached to skull via pins. Used with fractures or dislocations of the cervical or high thoracic vertebrae	Assess frequently for increased pain, respiratory distress, and cranial nerve or brachial plexus injury. Place on striker frame or a specially equipped bed to ease positioning without disruption of alignment
11.	Halo traction	Metal halo attached to skull via pins. Used for cervical or high thoracic vertebrae fracture or dislocation and for postoperative immobilization following cervical fusion	Tape small wrench in front of a brace so that front panel can be quickly removed in an emergency. May become ambulatory in this type of traction; will be top-heavy so may need assistance with balance
12.	Balanced suspension traction	Used for femur, hip, or tibial fracture. Thomas splint suspends the thigh while the Pearson attachment allows knee flexion and supports the leg below the knee	Avoid pressure to popliteal area

(SCFE: slipped capital femur epiphysis)

- Kidney tray
- Pair of sterile gloves
- Plaster
- Scissor
- Sterile sponge holder
- Pillows
- Pressure-reducing mattresses (e.g., water mattress)
- Foot board
- Vital signs tray

Preparation

- Assess for the following:
  - Type of fracture/surgery that the child sustained.
  - Physical condition and integrity of skeletal system.
  - Purpose and type of traction being used.
  - Age and weight of child, traction weight ordered by orthopedician.
  - Presence of possible latex allergies.
  - Check vital signs to identify signs of infection such as fever.
- Perform range of motion exercises to all extremities, unless contraindicated every shift.
- Explain child and family members about the care.
- Encourage parents to stay with child during traction care.
- Have the child to assist in the examination according to his/her developmental level.

Procedure

Steps	Rationale
Elevate head end of bed to the angle ordered	When the head of bed is maintained at the proper angle, it provides adequate counteraction. If the force of pull of traction is more than the counteraction supplied by the body, the child will slide toward the traction force or the traction splint may impinge on the traction pulley
Apply trapeze for convenience in moving in bed (if not contraindicated)	Children in lower extremity traction can be turned to one-quarter to the uninvolved side to enable back care. This turn will not result in misplacement and is important for reclining pressure
Ensure the traction apparatus is properly secured to the bed. Assess the traction setup, including the amounts of weight ordered	
Full inspection of traction apparatus: verify the alignment of traction cards, integrity of tape, and tightness of knots securing of tapes should not interfere with the line of traction	For traction to work effectively, counteraction must be maintained. There must be a reasonable balance between traction and counteraction forces to achieve optimal healing and patient comfort
Ensure that weights are hanging free from bed and floor while that the correct amount of weights are used. Reposition weights as needed at a reasonable level from the floor, a considerable distance from the pulley, hanging free of bed, and always away from the child	Balanced traction is designed to maintain a constant pull on child and adequate weight provides counteraction needed to keep bones aligned for optimal healing. Weights should never be removed or added without specific orders

Contd...

Contd...

Steps	Rationale
Perform neuromuscular assessment	Promotes early identification of neuromuscular problems and prompt interventions to diminish compromised circulation and oxygenation of tissues
Perform skin assessment and provide skin care: - Provide pressure-reducing mattress - Make total body skin checks for redness or breakdown, especially over areas that receive greatest pressure - Wash and dry skin at least daily - Stimulate circulation with gentle massage only over healthy skin - Avoid skin friction with bed linens or traction device - Keep skin dry and free from moisture such as sweat or urine - Change position at least every 2 hours to relieve pressure	Promotes early identification of skin problems and prompt interventions to diminish disruptions to skin integrity Helps to maintain muscle tone. Venous thrombus is a serious complication of immobility Ongoing assessment and implementation of a variety of nursing interventions will assist to prevent skin breakdown, infection, and pain
Assist child to perform passive and active range of motion of all extremities at least every shift	

Complete intervention to prevent complications of immobility and promote healing:
- Check pulse in affected areas
- Assess circular dressings for an excessive tightness
- Assess restrictive devices such as splints or braces
  - Be sure that they are not too loose or too tight
  - Remove periodically and check for pressure areas
- Encourage deep breathing, coughing, and use of incentive spirometry
- Note any neurovascular changes such as the following: color in skin and nail beds, capillary refill, alteration in sensation, increased pain, alterations in motor ability, skin temperature, and presence or absence of pulses
	Early identification is the key to prevention and treatment of complications of fracture. Subtle findings will often indicate impending complications at the earliest stage

Notify the doctor of any abnormal findings Care of skin traction: - Replace nonadhesive straps or elastic bandage on skin traction when permitted or absolutely necessary, but make certain that traction on limb is maintained by someone during procedure	

Contd...

Contd...

Steps	Rationale
■ Assess bandages to ascertain if they are correctly applied (diagonal or spiral), not too tight, which could cause slippage and malalignment of traction	
Care of skeletal traction: ■ Check pin sites frequently for signs of bleeding, inflammation, and infection ■ Cleanse and dress pin sites as per protocol ■ Apply antiseptic or antibiotic daily as per protocol ■ Cover ends of pin with protective padding to prevent child's being scratched by pin ■ Note pull of traction on pin; pull should be even ■ Check pin screws to be certain that screws are tight in metal clamp that attaches traction apparatus to pin	

CAST CARE

Definition

Casts are constructed of a hard material (traditionally plaster), which is used to immobilize a bone that has been injured or a diseased joint.

Materials Used for Cast Application

- Gauze strips and bandages impregnated with plaster of Paris
- Synthetic lightweight, water-resistant materials (e.g., fiber glass and polyurethane resin)

Types of Casts (10.1)

- Long leg cast (LLC)
- Short leg cast (SLC)
- Bilateral LLC
- Full spica cast
- 11/2 spica cast
- Single spica
- Short arm cast (SAC)
- Long arm cast (LAC)

Preparation

- Before cast application, perform baseline neurovascular assessment for comparison after immobilization. Following are to be included:
  - Color (note cyanosis or other discoloration)
  - Movement (note inability to move fingers or toes)
  - Sensation (note whether loss of sensation is present)
  - Edema
  - Quality of pulses.
- Obtain cooperation from the child and reduce his/her anxiety by showing the child the cast materials and using an age-appropriate approach to describe cast application.
- Premedicate as ordered to reduce pain when manual traction is applied to align the bone.

Chapter 10: Care of Child with Fracture

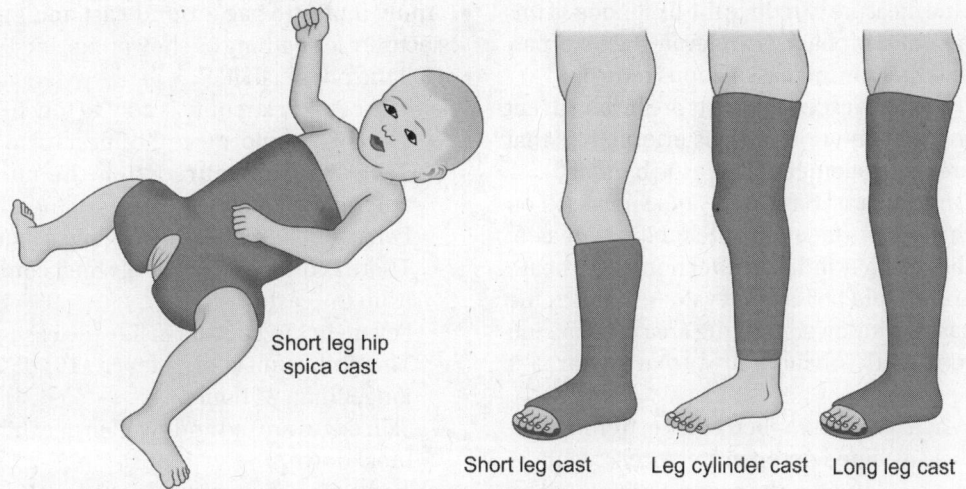

Fig. 10.1: Types of cast.

Procedure

- A nurse may assist in cast application by holding the extremity in alignment.
- A tube of stockinette is stretched over the area to be casted and bony prominences are padded with soft cotton sheeting.
- Dry rolls of gauze impregnated with the open end of the roll angled downward to allow soaking of the bandage.
- The wet plaster rolls are applied in bandage fashion and molded to the extremity.
- A heat-producing chemical reaction occurs between the plaster and water as plaster becomes a crystalline gypsum.
- During application of the cast, the underlying stockinette is pulled over the raw edges of the cast and secured with a layer of wet plaster 1–2.5 cm below the rim to form a smooth, padded edge to protect skin.

Postprocedure Care

- The cast must remain uncovered to allow it to dry from the inside out.
- Turning the child in a plaster cast at least every 2 hours will help to dry a body cast evenly and prevent complications related to immobility.
- Position the child with casted extremity elevated on pillows.
- Use of a regular fan or a hair dryer on the cool setting to circulate air may be helpful when the humidity is high.
- A wet plaster cast should be handled using the palms of the hands to prevent indenting the cast and creating pressure areas and should be supported by a pillow covered with plastic.
- The cast and involved extremity are observed frequently to assess neurovascular integrity and detect any signs of compromise.
- Teach the child to use crutches in case of lower extremity immobilization so that the child can maintain mobility.

Nursing Considerations

- A dry plaster of Paris can produce a hollow sound when tapped with the finger.
- During the first few hours after a cast is applied, the chief concern is that the extremity may continue to swell to the extent that the cast becomes a tourniquet, shutting off circulation and producing neurovascular complications.

- One measure to reduce the likelihood of this potential problem is to elevate the body part and thereby increase venous return.
- If edema is excessive, casts are bivalved (cut to make anterior and posterior halves that are held together with elastic bandage).
- Once the cast has dried, "hot spots" felt on the cast surface or foul-smelling areas of the cast may indicate infection underneath and should be further evaluated. Often the cast is windowed over the area of suspicion to directly observe and treat the area if necessary.
- When a cast is applied to an extremity that has sustained an open fracture, a window is often left over the wound area to allow for observation and dressing of the wound.

Assisting with Cast Removal

Children may be frightened by cast removal. Prepare the child using age-appropriate terminology:

- The cast cutter will make a loud noise.
- The skin or extremity will not be injured (demonstrate by touching the cast cutter lightly to your palm).
- The child will feel warmth or vibration during cast removal.

Home Care Management of Child with Cast

- For the first 48 hours, elevate the extremity above the level of the heart and apply cold therapy for 20–30 minutes, then after 1 hour and repeat.
- Assess for swelling and have the child wiggle the fingers or toes hourly.
- For itching inside the cast:
  - Never insert anything into the cast for the purposes of scratching.
  - Blow cool air in from a hair dryer set on the lowest setting.
  - Do not use lotions or powders.
  - Check the skin at the cast edges daily for irritation.
- Protect the cast from wetness.
- Apply a plastic bag around cast and tape securely for bathing or showering.
- Call the physician if:
  - The casted extremity is cool to touch.
  - The child cannot move the fingers or toes.
  - Severe pain occurs when the child attempts to move the fingers or toes.
  - Persistent numbness or tingling occurs.
  - There is drainage or a foul smell comes from the cast.
  - Severe itching occurs inside the cast.
  - The child runs a high fever >101°F for longer than 24 hours.
  - Skin edges are red and swollen or exhibit breakdown.
  - The cast gets wet or cracked, split or softened.

Highlights

- Traction is a method of immobilization, which may be used to reduce and or immobilize the fractured part, to align an injured extremity, and to allow the extremity to be restored to its normal length.
- Casts are constructed of a hard material (traditionally plaster), which is used to immobilize a bone that has been injured or a diseased joint.
- Obtain cooperation from the child and reduce his/her anxiety by showing the child the cast materials and using an age-appropriate approach to describe cast application.
- Premedicate as ordered to reduce pain when manual traction is applied to align the bone.
- A dry plaster of Paris can produce a hollow sound when tapped with the finger.
- If edema is excessive, casts are bivalved (cut to make anterior and posterior halves that are held together with elastic bandage).
- When a cast is applied to an extremity that has sustained an open fracture, a window is often left over the wound area to allow for observation and dressing of the wound.
- For the first 48 hours, elevate the extremity above the level of the heart and apply cold therapy for 20–30 minutes, then after 1 hour and repeat.
- Encourage the child with cast to wiggle the fingers or toes hourly.

MEMORY EXERCISE

1. **90–90 traction is used for:**
   a. Cervical problems
   b. Fracture of humerus
   c. Hip fracture
   d. Femur fracture
2. **Nursing care of child with skeletal traction includes all, *except*:**
   a. Keeping skin dry and free from moisture
   b. Changing position at least every 2 hours
   c. Ensuring the weight hang freely
   d. Keeping child in same position to prevent complications of traction
3. **Which of the following is incorrect about nursing care of child with cast?**
   a. The cast must remain covered for 48 hours.
   b. Position the child with casted extremity elevated on pillows.
   c. Fan or dryer can be used to dry the cast.
   d. The plaster cast should be handled with the palms.
4. **If a child complains of itching inside the cast, we can:**
   a. Insert a thin stick or pencil to scratch
   b. Blow cool air from hair dryer
   c. Apply lotions or talc powder
   d. Wet the cast with some water
5. **Which of the following is abnormal in a child with plaster cast?**
   a. The extremities are warm to touch.
   b. Mild edema will be present for first 48 hours.
   c. Persistent numbness.
   d. The cast produces hollow sound.

CHAPTER 11

Care of Child Undergoing Surgery

LEARNING OBJECTIVES

After reading this chapter, the readers should be able to:
- Provide perioperative care of children undergoing surgery.
- Assess the children for complications of surgery.
- Perform dressing of surgical wound.
- Assist in suture removal.

Keywords: surgery, nursing care, preparation, monitoring, wound, dressing, materials, dehiscence, suture

PRE- AND POSTOPERATIVE NURSING CARE

Surgery either planned or unplanned is a potentially stressful experience for children. Hence, the children and their caregivers need adequate information about the child's condition, surgical procedure, and various phases of care. Facilities should be provided to make children and their family to be comfortable during the hospital stay.

The care of child undergoing surgery involves mainly three phases:
1. Preoperative care
2. Intraoperative care
3. Postoperative care

Preoperative and postoperative care are discussed in the following sections.

Principles of Perioperative Nursing Care

- To care and treat children in a safe manner, as close to home as possible, in an environment that is suitable to their needs
- To Involve parents in decision-making relevant to the child care
- To deliver quality of care through adequate training and providing essential support

Preoperative Care

Equipment needed:
- Identification (ID) band
- Surgical clothing
- Vital signs tray
- Pulse oximeter (if needed)
- Weighing scale
- Preoperative check list

- Razor (if needed)
- Premedications (as prescribed)

Preparation of child and family

It involves three kinds of preparation:
- *Psychological preparation*:
  - Discuss surgical procedure with parents and child and evaluate their level of understanding (**Table 11.1**).
  - Discuss limitations on diet if appropriate, depending on the orders of anesthesiologist.
  - Explain what nil per os (NPO) sign is; stress that child will be fed again as soon as fluid and food can be tolerated.
  - Discuss about preoperative injections honestly; the injections do cause discomfort. Explain that medications will make the child drowsy.
  - Discuss means of transportation to operating room; and appearance of operating room personnel (colored caps and clothing, masks, gloves, etc.)
  - Encourage the child to play with caps, gowns, masks, gloves, and with appropriately dressed dolls.
  - Discuss anesthesia as a different kind of sleep or a special sleep.
  - Demonstrate postoperative procedures (deep breathing, coughing, and use of blow bottles, turning) and have return demonstrations.
  - Demonstrate the equipment to be used postoperatively; e.g., arm boards, tubes, bandages, restraints, oxygen tent, or mask.
  - Discuss postoperative discomfort and the relief available with medicines.
  - Explain about the child care in the recovery room until awake or in the intensive care unit until well enough to return to the pediatric unit.
  - Secure a favorite blanket, toy, or other objects to the bed or stretches when the child is taken to the operating room.
  - Assure child that parents will be hereby waiting for him or her after the operation is over. Tell the parents where to wait during surgery.

Table 11.1: Age-specific considerations in preparation of child.

Age-group	Preparation guidelines
Infants	Do not make any changes in baby's daily routine prior to surgery (sleeping, feeding) unless contraindicated Keep familiar people and familiar items around the infant to maintain calmness and avoid cranky
Early childhood	Allow time to ritualism in play and other activities Use dramatic play during explanation about the procedure Dispel if there is any misconception Use simple words Assure the child that his/her parents will be present with him/her
Middle childhood	Provide detailed explanation using simple words Encourage peer involvement Have a hospital tour to introduce to equipment and places Provide reading materials, if needed Provide privacy
Adolescents	Encourage peers to visit, communicate with the client. Even phone communication can be facilitated to reduce the child's anxiety Can use media such as videos and slides in explaining about the procedure Provide privacy Emphasize on positive aspects during explanation as adolescent children are concerned about their body image
Children of all age-group	Provide diversional activities, such as watching TV, play materials, and books, if children are stable

- *Physical preparation:*
  - Monitor vital signs; if any abnormality report to surgeon and record it in chart.
  - Give NPO for the period prescribed prior to the surgery (**Table 11.2**).

  Note: Traditionally, solid foods and semi-liquids were withheld from the midnight before surgery, with clear liquids withheld from 4 to 8 hours before the procedure, depending on the child's age.

  However, research indicates that clear liquids given up to 2 hours before elective surgery for children of any age do not present any additional risk for pulmonary aspiration.

  New guidelines can be summarized as 8-6-4-2 (i.e., 8 hours—solid, 6 hours—formula, 4 hours—breast milk, and 2 hours—clear liquids). This results in children who are less anxious are better hydrated and fewer headaches and less nausea postoperatively.

  - If the child is ambulatory, take the child away from the area while other children eating breakfast.
  - Ensure that good hydration is essential before period of NPO.
  - Make certain that all other prescribed preoperative procedures have been completed (enema, insertion of nasogastric tube, etc.).
  - Prepare operative site as per institutional policy. Shaving may not be necessary for children.
  - Bathe the child; give mouth care the evening before or the morning of the surgery.
  - Remind the child not to swallow the rinse water.
  - Check the child's body for rashes, scratches, bruises, or other skin lesions. These should be noted in the child's chart preoperatively.
  - Dress the child in clean hospital gown or other attire according to institutional procedures.
  - If the child's underpants or other clothing are permitted to wear, label them so they are not lost.
  - Observe for loosened teeth, dental appliances such as partial plates or braces and report if present.
  - Dental appliances are removed if possible and given to the parents. Presence of loose teeth is reported to the anesthetist.
  - Remove makeup and nail polish. Adolescents especially should be told not to apply makeup and nail polish preoperatively.
  - Urge child to urinate immediately before medication is given preoperatively.
  - Prepare preoperative medications before surgery as ordered. Inform the child that it is ready to give it immediately.
  - Encourage the child to scream if the injection is uncomfortable.
  - Chat with older child while giving the injection.
- *Protective measures:*
  - Ensure that a consent form for the anesthetic and surgical procedure has been signed correctly and witnessed by child's parents or legal guardian.
  - Adolescents old enough according to law can sign consent forms themselves prior to medication.
  - Ensure that all laboratory reports (urine, blood and other, radiological report,

Table 11.2: Recommended fasting hours for children.

Ingested material	Minimum fasting period (hours)
Clear fluids	>2
Breast milk	4
Infant formula	6
Nonhuman milk	6
Light meal	6

Chapter 11: Care of Child Undergoing Surgery

and the results of any other tests) are included in chart.
- Administer correct dosage of preoperative medication (**Table 11.3**).
- Fasten side rails of crib or bed securely after preoperative medication has been given.
- Make certain that child's ID band is securely attached.
- Record complete notations on nurse' notes regarding preoperative procedures and child's emotional and physical state before surgery.
- Have a familiar person stay with the child to provide explanations of strange events and places and to protect him or her physically while awaiting surgery.
- Children should not be left alone.

Postoperative Nursing Care of Child

Equipment needed
- Gloves
- Vital signs tray
- Fluids as prescribed
- Bedpan/urinal
- Blankets
- Warming devices
- Incentive spirometer
- Pillow for splinting
- Emergency drugs
- Resuscitation and intubation equipment

Table 11.3: Commonly used premedications.

Drug	Route	Dose
Atropine	IM, PO	0.02 mg/kg, min: 0.15 mg, max: 0.5 mg
Glycopyrrolate	IM, PO	0.01 mg/kg, max: 0.35 mg
Phenobarbital	IM	3.0 mg/kg
Morphine	IM	0.05–0.10 mg/kg
Meperidine	IM, PO	1–2 mg/kg
Diazepam	PO	0.2 mg/kg

[IM: intramuscular; PO: per oral (by mouth)]

- Oxygen and oxygen delivery system
- Cardiopulmonary monitoring equipment
- Ventilator

Preparation
- Prepare postanesthetic bed prior to shifting from operation theater (OT).
- Assess the child for developmental stage and level of cognitive functioning.
- Assess OT and recovery room records for the type of anesthesia, medicines administered vital signs, blood loss, fluid and blood replacement, and procedural information and complications.
- Determine whether the family members would like to visit the child.
- Respect the child's feelings.

Care during postoperative period
- *Activity level*
  - Assess the child's activity.
  - Constant nursing attention or restraint may be necessary to prevent dislodging intravenous infusion lines, dressings, drains, or chest tubes.
- *Vital signs and skin color*
  - Vital signs are taken as often as necessary depending on the child's condition and the policy of the hospital.
  - Generally, they are taken q15 minutes for first 1 hour, q30 minutes for second 1 hour, and every hour until the vital parameters are stabilized.
  - Keep the blood pressure cuff on the child's arm, and inflate it only when necessary to prevent disturbing the child.
  - Report signs of shock immediately.
  - Keep the child warm.
  - Place the child in a supine position with legs elevated slightly.
- *Adequacy of ventilation*
  - Place O_2, resuscitative, and suction equipment near the bed and use as necessary.

- Have the child deep breathe, turn, and cough.
- Splint operative site with pillow or hand before doing these procedures to minimize discomfort.
- Teach older children to learn to splint themselves.
- Administer medications for pain, if necessary.
- If the child cannot breathe deeply, he or she may use equipment, such as Uniflo inspirometer.
- *Level of consciousness (LOC) and feeding*
  - Assess LOC.
  - Child should be on NPO until completely awake.
  - Determine the ability to swallow.
  - Begin feedings with bits of chipped ice or sips of water.
- *Pain management*
  - Attempt to alleviate pain through nursing measures such as turning the child on the side, repositioning extremities, massaging aching muscles, and talking soothingly to the child.
  - If these measures fail, give pain medications as prescribed.
- *Intake and output*
  - Rate and kind of fluid being given should be accurate according to prescription.
  - Assess for infiltration, and if present notify to physician.
  - Apply arm board, reposition, and retape the arm.
  - Notify the physician if child has not voided (time depends on surgical procedure and postoperative order).
- *Dressing*
  - Assess for evidence of dark blood or bright red blood (new) observed after surgery.
  - Report signs of shock, if present.
  - Notify physician of bleeding or drainage; change bed linen if soiled.
- *Anxiety*
  - Reunite parents and child as early as possible postoperatively.
  - Decrease parental anxiety by answering any questions they may ask.
- *Complications*
  Assess for immediate complications and continued nursing assessment is imperative to identify signs and symptoms of possible postoperative complications.

Common Postoperative Complications

a. Shock
b. Hemorrhage from wound
c. Nausea and vomiting
d. Distention of abdomen
e. Hypoxia
f. Atelectasis
g. Hypostatic pneumonia
h. Retention of urine.
i. Infection of wound
j. Thrombophlebitis

Highlights

- Surgery either planned or unplanned is a potentially stressful experience for children. Hence, the children and their caregivers need adequate information about the child's condition, surgical procedure, and various phases of care.
- Ensure that a consent form for the anesthetic and surgical procedure has been signed correctly and witnessed by child's parents or legal guardian.
- Adolescents old enough according to law can sign consent forms themselves prior to medication.
- Make attempt to alleviate pain through nursing measures such as turning child on the side, repositioning extremities, massaging aching muscles, and talking soothingly to the child.
- Assess for immediate complications and continued nursing assessment is imperative to identify signs and symptoms of possible postoperative complications.

SURGICAL DRESSING

Definition
Surgical dressing is a sterile protective covering, applied to a surgical wound/incision using aseptic techniques with or without medication.

Purposes
- To promote granulation and healing of surgical wound
- To prevent the entering and growth of microorganisms
- To apply medications
- To immobilize and support the wounds
- To remove dead tissues
- To minimize discomfort to the child who underwent surgery

Types of Surgical Dressing
Selection of surgical dressing is based on the site, size, condition, and type of the wound:
1. **Dry dressings:** Tend to absorb wound moisture, for example, gauze bandages, membranes and foils, and foams. These dressings may tightly adhere to granulation and will break up during removal. Children also feel less discomfort.
2. **Moisture keeping dressings:** These dressing help the wound to heal faster and do not breakup during removal, for example, pastes, creams, and ointments; hydrocolloids and hydrogels; and nonpermeable membranes or foils.
3. **Bioactive dressings:** Enhance granulation tissue formation, reduce slough formation, and inhibit growth of microorganism thereby promote wound healing, for example, antimicrobial and interactive dressings.
4. **Skin substitutes:** These are heterogeneous type of wound coverings that help in closure of wound and replace the function of the skin as well, for example, epidermal substitutes, autologous and allogenous skin.

Commonly Used Dressing Materials
- Foams
- Gauzes
- Polymeric films
- Hydrocolloids
- Hydrogels
- Debriding agents
- Enzymatic dressings
- Human amniotic membrane
- Porcine skin
- Tulles: Light thin net-like gauze cloth impregnated with paraffin and antibiotics, which helps for nontraumatic removal (**Fig. 11.1**).

Equipment Needed
A sterile tray containing:
- Small bowls—two
- Sterile glove—one pair
- Cotton swabs
- Artery forceps
- Dissecting forceps
- Scissor
- Gauze pieces and gauze pad

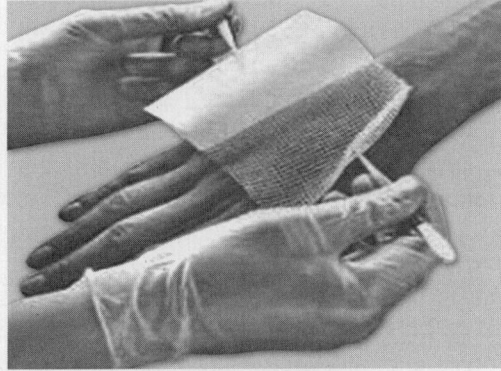

Fig. 11.1: Tulles.

An unsterile tray containing:
- Adhesive tape
- Betadine solution
- Normal saline solution
- Kidney tray (small size)—one
- Medications as prescribed
- Mackintosh and towel

Preparation
- Explain the parents and the child about the procedure. Use dramatic play; use doctor and nurse toy kit to minimize anxiety.
- Provide comfortable position to the child.
- Arrange articles near the client.

Procedure
- Wash hands and wear gloves (surgical asepsis).
- Remove the old dressing and discard it in kidney tray.
- Observe the condition of wound.
- Take the cotton swab and soak swab with Betadine solution.
- Clean the affected area from the center outward in a circular pattern.
- Clean only in circular pattern and do not use back and forth motion.
- When the Betadine solution is dry, in about 30 seconds, use another cotton swab soaked in the normal saline solution and repeat the procedure, cleaning from center outward.
- Apply the medication ointment (if prescribed) using sterile cotton applicators.
- Pick up two outer corners of the sterile gauze with your fingers. (Do not touch the gauze anywhere else to avoid the contamination that may cause wound infection.)
- Apply adhesive tape all around edges of gauze to keep wound clean and dry.

Aftercare
- Discard the waste as per hospital policy of biomedical waste management.
- Clean and replace the articles.
- Perform hand hygiene.
- Document the procedure in nurses record with observation made:
  - Condition of wound (color, any foul smelling, any discharge)
  - Technique followed in dressing
  - Solutions and medication used (if any)

Nursing Considerations in Surgical Dressing
- Follow strict aseptic technique.
- Wound cleansing should not be undertaken to remove normal exudates.
- Cleaning should be performed in a way that minimizes trauma to the wound.
- Wounds are best cleaned with sterile isotonic saline or water.
- Fluids should be warmed to 37°C to support cellular activity.
- Skin and wound cleansers should have a neutral pH, if it is altered then resistance to bacteria decreases.
- Antiseptics are not routinely recommended for cleansing and should only be used sparingly for infected wounds.

REMOVAL OF SUTURES

Equipment Needed
- A sterile tray containing:
  - Suture cutting scissors—one
  - Toothed dissecting forceps—one
  - Gauze pieces
  - Gloves
- A clean tray containing:
  - Mackintosh and towel
  - Kidney tray

Preparation of Child
- Explain the child that he/she may feel little discomfort such as pulling sensation or stinging.

Chapter 11: Care of Child Undergoing Surgery

- Position the child
- Wash hands and wear clean gloves
- Inspect the wound for edge approximation and signs of infection
- Remove the gloves

Procedure

- Wash hands and wear sterile gloves.
- Wet the dried crusts using normal saline.
- Clean the suture line with an antimicrobial solution.

Plain, Interrupted Suture

- Gently grasp the knot with forceps and raise it slightly.
- Place the curved tip of the suture scissors directly under the knot or on the side, close to the skin.
- Gently cut the suture and pull it out with the forceps (**Fig. 11.2**).
- Make sure that you remove all suture materials and place the suture on clean gauze.
- Remove alternate sutures. Assess the wound for dehiscence; if none occurs, remove the remaining sutures.

Removal of Staples

- Place the lower jaw of the remover under a staple.
- Squeeze the handles completely to close the device.

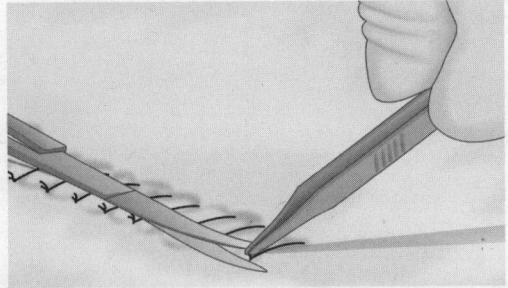

Fig. 11.2: Removal of plain sutures.

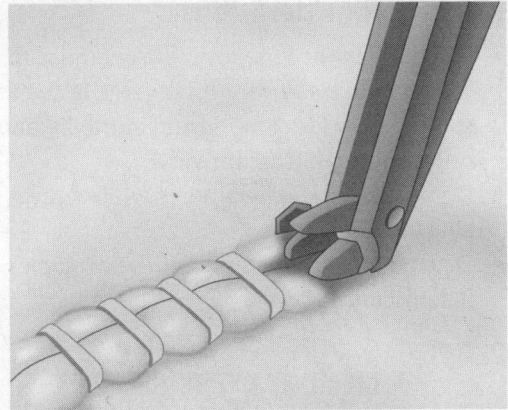

Fig. 11.3: Removal of staple.

- This bends the staple in the middle and pulls the edges out of the skin (**Fig. 11.3**).
- Clean the suture line with normal saline.
- Cover the wound with sterile wound strips.

Aftercare

- Clean and replace the articles.
- Discard the wastes.
- Wash hands.
- Document the date and time of suture or staple removal, the number removed, dressings or adhesive wound strips applied, child's response, and the appearance of the incision.

Highlights ●●●●

- ✦ Surgical dressing is a sterile protective covering, applied to a surgical wound/incision using aseptic techniques with or without medication.
- ✦ There are four types of dressings: (1) dry dressings, (2) moisture keeping dressings, (3) bioactive dressings, and (4) skin substitutes.
- ✦ Skin and wound cleansers should have a neutral pH, if it is altered then resistance to bacteria decreases.
- ✦ Antiseptics are not routinely recommended for cleansing and should only be used sparingly for infected wounds.

Nursing Considerations

- If dehiscence occurs, cover the wound with sterile gauze saturated with sterile 0.9% sodium chloride solution and immediately notify the healthcare provider.
- Do not lift the staple remover while squeezing the handle.
- Do not remove remaining sutures or staples if dehiscence occurs.

MEMORY EXERCISE

1. The psychological preparation of a school-age child includes all, *except:*
   a. Allowing time to ritualism in play and other activities
   b. Using dramatic play during explanation about the procedure
   c. Dispelling if there is any misconception
   d. Informing the child that his/her parents will be not be present with him/her
2. Antibacterial and interactive dressings are examples of:
   a. Wet dressing
   b. Bioactive dressings
   c. Dry dressing
   d. Skin substitutes
3. In an infant posted for surgery, breastfeeding should be stopped before:
   a. 8 hours
   b. 6 hours
   c. 4 hours
   d. 2 hours
4. Light thin net-like gauze cloth impregnated with paraffin and antibiotics are called:
   a. Enzymatic dressings
   b. Tulles
   c. Human amniotic membrane
   d. Porcine skin
5. Which of the following is incorrect about nurse's responsibility in suture removal:
   a. Assess for wound dehiscence before removing all sutures.
   b. Do not apply any solution before removing the sutures.
   c. Inspect the wound for edge approximation before complete removal.
   d. Apply plain sterile dressing over the wound after the suture removal.

CHAPTER 12

Meeting Children's Hygiene Needs

LEARNING OBJECTIVES

After reading this chapter, the readers should be able to:
- Identify the hygienic needs of hospitalized children.
- Demonstrate basic hygiene procedures.
- Incorporate dramatic play in meeting needs.

Keywords: neglected mouth, self-image, comfort, infection, thermoregulation, cleanliness

Hygiene is one of the fundamental requirements of any child in any educational establishment, at home, or in hospital.

The skin has many different functions and therefore it is imperative that it is cared for and kept clean. The functions of skin are given below:
- Protects deeper and more delicate organs
- Acts as a barrier against invasion of microorganisms
- Regulates temperature
- Produces sweat when body temperature rises.

BENEFITS OF GOOD HYGIENE

- Makes the child feel good, giving a positive self-image.
- Washing is like a tonic, making the child feel healthy.
- Prevents infection and infestation by parasites.
- Promotes independence, forming good habits later on in life.
- Stimulates the physical, emotional, and cognitive areas of development by involving pouring games.
- Treats skin problems such as eczema, sweat, rash, and sore skin, which can make the child irritable.

MAIN AREAS FOR CONSIDERATION

When meeting hygiene need, the main areas for consideration are:
- *Skin:* Some cultures use certain moisturizer creams to soften the skin.
- *Nail:* Keep short and cut horizontal, not digging into the corners.
- *Genitalia:* Do not push back the foreskin, simply wash the glans.
- *Hair:* Comb with a soft brush.
- *Mouth:* Brush teeth as soon as teeth are apparent and avoid sugary drinks to prevent tooth decay.

- *Eyes:* Use clean cotton wool balls and clean water; clean eyes from edge of nose outward, using two clean pieces for each eye and clean, dry pieces for drying.
- *Ears:* To prevent perforation of eardrums and pushing wax further down the ear, do not use cotton buds to clean ears.
- *Umbilicus:* Use clean water or prescribed cream to clean.

ORAL HYGIENE

Indications
- Children receiving:
  - Chemotherapy
  - Corticosteroids
  - Antibiotics
  - Oxygen therapy
- Child requiring oral suction
- Intubated child
- Fluid restricted or nil by mouth (NBM)
- Dehydrated child

General Principles
- Inspect the mouth at least daily, noting the presence of *Candida*, ulcers, breaks in oral mucosa, saliva consistency, condition of teeth, tongue, gingival, and lips.
- Note pain or difficulty in using voice or swallowing.
- Consider using an assessment tool.
- Commence brushing routine with eruption of first teeth.
- Brush child's teeth at least twice a day.
- Help and supervision will be required until around the age of 7 years.
- Antibacterial mouthwashes and antifungal preparations may be necessary for some children.

Equipment Needed
A clean tray containing:
- Soft pediatric toothbrush
- Fluoride toothpaste
- Jug with water
- Sterile water (for <1 year baby)
- Gauze pieces in bowl
- Glycerin
- Torchlight to assess the condition of oral cavity
- Kidney tray

Preparation
- Explain the procedure to the child.
- Assess the condition of the mouth and need for care.
- Encourage the involvement and self-care where appropriate.

Procedure
- Perform hand hygiene.
- Gently brush teeth and gums with pediatric toothbrush and fluoride toothpaste for at least 2 minutes; use tiny smear of toothpaste and pea-sized amount for children.
- Encourage the child to spit after brushing; if they are able to, do not swallow.
- Rinse mouth with water (use sterile water for babies <1 year); if child is unable to spit, gauze or swab may be used for this purpose, or moisturizing the mouth.
- Orally intubated children should, where possible, have endotracheal (ET) tube moved to alternate side of the mouth daily.
- Apply emollient to lips.

Postprocedure Care
- Praise the child for cooperation.
- Replace the articles and discard the wastes.
- Record the procedure with date and time and observations made in oral cavity.

EYE CARE

Indications
- Infection
- Immune suppression

- Congenital abnormalities
- Postoperative surgical requirement
- Poor blinking reflexes
- Inability to close the eyes completely
- Newborns and infants are prone to get sticky eyes because they have underdeveloped lacrimal drainage system. Therefore they also need eye care.

Purposes

- Help to maintain hygiene
- Prevent drying of the cornea
- To treat infection, administer required medications

Equipment Needed

A sterile tray containing:
- Sterile cotton swabs
- Sterile water
- Small bowls—two (one for swab and the other one for sterile water)
- Kidney tray
- Medications if any

Preparation

- Explain the procedure to the child and the parents as appropriate.
- Assess the condition of the eye.
- Check the doctor's order for any specific instructions.

Procedure

- Swaddle the babies and toddlers in a blanket; position with head/back supported, either lying or sitting.
- Perform hand hygiene with alcohol-based solution.
- Prepare surface. Open sterile dressing pack.
- Dip cotton swab into sterile water and gently wipe along closed eyelid from inner to outer canthus.
- Discard the swab and repeat if necessary by using a new swab each time.
- Wash hands, reapply alcohol-based solution, and repeat procedure on the other eye.
- If eye drops and ointment are required, wash hands, gently retract lower eyelid, and apply one drop and make sure that the dropper should not touch the eyes.
- Dab away any excess medications from the skin.

Postprocedure Care

- Reposition the baby.
- Replace the articles.
- Perform hand hygiene and record the procedure in nurse's chart.

EAR CARE

General Instructions

- It is advisable to keep children's ears dry, when washing their hair, showering, or swimming, especially if they are known to have ear problems.
- The use of swimming plugs or cotton balls, which are smothered in Vaseline, will keep the ear canals dry.
- Some wax in the ears is normal.
- Glands in the inner one-third of the ear canal produce wax as the squamous cells in the ear canal migrate toward from the eardrum; wax is normally shed with these cells.
- It is not advisable to use cotton buds, matches, or hairpins to clean or to dry the child's ear. These items can damage the linings of ear canal and if pushed in far enough, can also damage the child's eardrum.
- Never put any small materials that may cause ear problems.
- Some children do have a buildup of wax, for example, those wearing hearing aids; olive oil can be used to keep the wax soft, in the hope that it will be expelled naturally. If the child needs to have the wax removed, it is advisable to see an experienced practitioner.

- Refer to doctor if any discharge or bleeding is seen from child's ear.
- Please remember to apply sunscreen to the ears when the child is exposed to sunlight.
- Exposure to excessive sunlight can lead to basal cell carcinoma.
- It is also advisable to wear a cap during sunlight.
- Avoid spraying anything into the ears, for example, hair spray or any other cosmetic preparations.
- Always protect against and preferably avoid exposure to loud noise.

BATHING

Special Considerations

Infants

Use a sponge bath or tub bath to bathe young infants who cannot sit unaided. Support the infant's body at all times. Ensure appropriate water temperature. Avoid use of talcum powder.

Toddler

Bathe older infants and toddlers at the bedside or in a regular bathtub depending on their health condition.

School-age Children and Adolescents

Older children may prefer a shower if available and acceptable for their health condition.

Assess whether a shower would be safe and provide privacy.

General Instructions

- Adhere to safety principles to prevent falls, burns, and aspiration of water.
- Never leave a child alone in a bathtub.
- Use a gentle, pH-balanced soap with moisturizer if there is a need to rehydrate the skin.
- Note any condition that might require special consideration or further assessment, such as paralysis, loss of sensation, surgical incisions, skin traction/cast, external lines (intravenous lines, urinary catheter, or feeding tube) or other alteration in skin integrity.
- Pay special attention to the ears, between skinfolds, the neck, the back, and the genital area for alterations in skin integrity.

Equipment Needed (for Sponge Bath)

A trolley containing:
- Two jugs with hot and cold water
- Bath towels
- Sponge clothes (soft)
- Basin
- Mild alkaline soap
- Bath thermometer
- Kidney tray
- Clothing
- Comb
- Talcum powder (older child)
- Bucket
- Bath blanket

Preparation

- Explain the procedure to the child and the parents as appropriate.
- Check the doctor's order for any special instructions.
- Assess the skin condition of the child for any changes in color, ulcer, etc.
- Allow the child to play in bathwater with water toys.
- Make sure that the room is warm without draught (75°F).
- Provide privacy.

Procedure

- Perform hand hygiene.
- Mix hot and cold water in a basin.
- Check the temperature of the water.
- Undress the baby.
- Place the baby (if small) on a thick bath towel.

- Keep the child covered with a towel or bath blanket.
- *Start with the baby's face:* Use one moistened, clean cotton ball to wipe each eye from inner to outer canthus.
- Wash the rest of the face with a soft, moist washcloth without soap.
- Clean the outside folds of the ears with a soft washcloth.
- Add a small amount of baby soap to the washcloth and gently bathe the rest of the body from neck down.
- Uncover only one area at a time.
- Rinse with a clean washcloth.
- Wrap the child with dry towel.
- Put on dress.

Postprocedure Care

- Comb the hair.
- Apply talcum powder if not contraindicated.
- Praise the child for cooperation.
- Replace the articles.
- Perform hand hygiene.
- Document the procedure in the nurse's record.

Highlights ● ● ● ●

> - The common indications for oral care are children receiving chemotherapy, corticosteroids, antibiotics, oxygen therapy, child requiring oral suction, intubated child, and fluid restricted or NBM.
> - Inspect the mouth at least daily, noting the presence of *Candida*, ulcers, breaks in oral mucosa, saliva consistency, condition of teeth, tongue, gingival, and lips.
> - Orally intubated children should, where possible, have ET tube moved to alternate side of the mouth daily.
> - Apply emollient to lips for maintaining moisture.
> - Newborns and infants are prone to get sticky eyes because they have underdeveloped lacrimal drainage system. Therefore they also need eye care.

Contd...

Contd...

> - It is not advisable to use cotton buds, matches, or hairpins to clean or to dry the child's ear. These items can damage the linings of ear canal and if pushed in far enough, can also damage the child's eardrum.
> - While giving bath, pay special attention to the ears, between skinfolds, the neck, the back, and the genital area for alterations in skin integrity.
> - Use a gentle, pH-balanced soap with moisturizer for giving bath.
> - Make sure that the child is not left alone in a bathtub.

MEMORY EXERCISE

1. **Brushing of teeth should be initiated from which age-group?**
   a. 6 months
   b. As soon as the first tooth eruption occurs
   c. 1 year
   d. 2.5 years
2. **The type of soap to be selected for bathing children:**
   a. Soap with mild acidic pH
   b. Soap with mild alkaline pH
   c. pH-balanced soaps
   d. Do not use soap at all
3. **In an intubated child, the ET tube should be moved to alternative side once in:**
   a. Each shift
   b. Each day
   c. Alternative days
   d. 3 days
4. **which of the following is incorrect about ear care?**
   a. Cotton balls smothered in Vaseline can keep the ear canals dry
   b. Can use olive oil in the case of buildup of wax
   c. Use cotton buds to remove wax
   d. Do not use hairpins to remove wax

CHAPTER 13

Recent Advances in Prenatal, Neonatal, and Pediatric Care

LEARNING OBJECTIVES

After reading this chapter, the readers should be able to:
- List the recent technologies used in care of children.
- Describe the functions of each equipment.
- Operate the equipment as per manufacturer guidelines.
- Provide technology-based care to newborn and children.

Keywords: HEPA filter, contamination, fetal heart rate, uterine contractions, hyperbilirubinemia, neonatal environment, family-centered neonatal care, noninvasive ventilation, therapeutic hypothermia, hypoxic–ischemic encephalopathy

LAMINAR FLOW HOODS

Definition: A laminar flow hood is a carefully enclosed bench designed to prevent the contamination of semiconductor wafers, biological samples, or any particulate-sensitive materials. Air is drawn through high-efficiency particulate air (HEPA) filter and blown in a very smooth, laminar flow toward the user (**Fig. 13.1**).

Purposes

- To provide clean air in the working area
- To provide a constant flow of air out of the working area to prevent room air from entering
- To suspend and remove contaminants from the working area

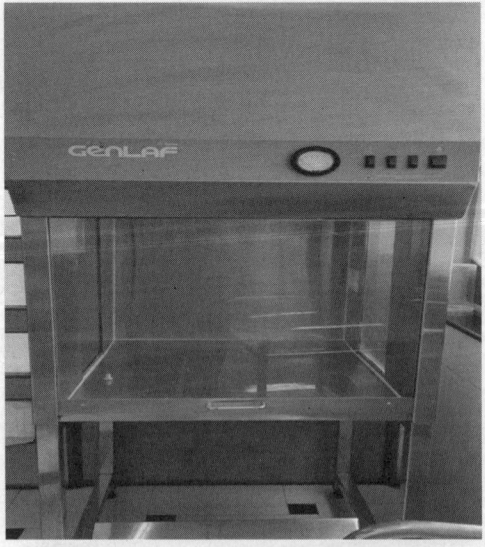

Fig. 13.1: Laminar flow hood.

Mode of Action

The laminar flow hoods take in room air and pass it through a prefilter to remove the dust and other contaminants. Then the air is compressed and channelized through the HEPA filter in a laminar flow fashion, that is, pure air flows out over the entire work surface in parallel lines at a uniform velocity.

Types

Based on the direction of airflow, laminar flow hoods are divided into two types:
1. Vertical laminar flow hoods and
2. Horizontal laminar flow hoods

Advantages

It is one of the most effective methods for reducing the incidence of infection associated with medication administration. The HEPA filter removes nearly all bacteria from the air.

Disadvantages

- There is a chance to reintroduce contaminants into the working area if the correct technique is not followed.
- It must be on 24 hours a day to maintain its purpose.

Guidelines

- If the equipment is switched off for any reason, it must be switched on within half an hour.
- It also should be cleaned thoroughly before reusing.
- A direct path must be maintained between the filter and the area inside the hood.

Highlights ●●●

+ A laminar flow hood is a carefully enclosed bench designed to prevent the contamination of semiconductor wafers, biological samples, or any particulate-sensitive materials.

Contd...

Contd...

+ Air is drawn through high-efficiency particulate air filter and blown in a very smooth, laminar flow toward the user.
+ It is one of the most effective methods for reducing the incidence of infection associated with medication administration.
+ There is a chance to reintroduce contaminants into the working area if the correct technique is not followed.
+ A direct path must be maintained between the filter and the area inside the hood.

NONINVASIVE FETAL ELECTROCARDIOGRAPHY MONITORING

Definition

Noninvasive fetal electrocardiography (NI-FECG) monitoring is a technique carried out during antenatal period or labor to measure the fetal heart rate (FHR) and electrical activity of the fetal heart and associated uterine contraction using surface electrodes placed on the maternal abdomen.

Purposes

- To assess the FHR
- To monitor morphological information of FECG such as PR, ST, and QT intervals
- To note the abdominal contraction of mother
- To count the fetal movements
- To assess the fetal position

Indications

Noninvasive fetal electrocardiography is commonly indicated in the following situations:
- Maternal anemia
- History of heart disease, diabetes mellitus, or hyperthyroidism
- Oligohydramnios
- Obesity

- Multiple pregnancies
- Preterm labor
- Post-term labor
- Malpositioning and malpresentation of fetus

Parts of Noninvasive Fetal Electrocardiography

- Tocodynamometer pads
- Belt to secure the pads
- Probe to count the uterine activity
- Monitor
- ECG recorder

Advantages

- This device can provide more accurate FHR estimation than Doppler ultrasound.
- NI-FECG gives an opportunity to enable the morphological analysis of the FECG, which is vital for determining whether an observed FHR event is normal or abnormal.
- NI-FECG is a noninvasive technique and can be used in earlier stages of pregnancy also.
- This technique is suitable alternative to Doppler cardiotocography in the case of high-risk pregnancies.

Disadvantages

- This technique has the problem of low signal-to-noise ratio of the FECG signal on the abdominal mixture signal, which consists of a dominant maternal ECG component, FECG, and noise.
- Due to the presence of vernix caseosa, NI-FECG cannot be performed effectively due to nonconductivity.
- Fetal movements can interfere with reading.

Preparation

- *Articles*:
  - Assemble articles needed for the procedure.
  - Check the working condition of the machine.

  Articles needed
  - NI-FECG machine
  - Disposable gloves to prevent cross infection
  - Gel to apply on pads
  - Cotton pad or tissue paper to clean the abdomen after the procedure
  - Antiseptic solution to clean the pads (according to manufacturer's instruction)
- *Client*:
  - Explain the procedure to the expectant mother to win confidence and cooperation.
  - Provide privacy.
  - Loosen the clothes over abdomen.
  - Elevate the head end to 45° to enhance comfort.

Steps in Procedure

1. Perform hand hygiene.
2. Wear the gloves.
3. Connect the monitor to the electric outlet.
4. Switch on the monitor button.
5. Clean the tocodynamometer pads with prescribed antiseptic swabs.
6. Apply gel over the pads.
7. Place the pads on the mother's abdomen, one just above the umbilicus and the other on midway between umbilicus and right iliac fossa (placement may vary based on fetal presentation and position).
8. Note the readings on monitor.
9. Secure the pads with belts.
10. Provide left lateral position to the mother.
11. Switch on the ECG recorder.
12. Give the probe to mother and instruct her

to press it whenever she feels fetal movements.
13. Continue to assess the readings for a prescribed period of time.
14. Switch off the device after a prescribed time.
15. Loosen the belt and remove the pads from abdomen.
16. Clean the area with tissue paper or cotton.

Aftercare

- Assist the mother to adjust her clothing.
- Clean the pads and keep it in its box.
- Replace the articles.
- Document the procedure.
- Notify to the senior staff or the doctor if there are any abnormal findings.

Highlights

- Noninvasive fetal electrocardiography monitoring is a technique carried out during antenatal period or labor to measure the fetal heart rate and electrical activity of the fetal heart and associated uterine contraction using surface electrodes placed on the maternal abdomen.
- The pads should be placed on the mother's abdomen, one just above the umbilicus and the other on midway between umbilicus and right iliac fossa.
- Placement may vary based on fetal presentation and position.
- Instruct her to press the probe whenever she feels fetal movements.
- Assess the readings for a prescribed period of time.

TRANSCUTANEOUS BILIMETER

Definition

Transcutaneous bilimeter or bilirubinometer is a device that is used to measure bilirubin level.

Unit of Measurement

The bilirubin level will be measured using this device by mg/dL or mol/L.

Purpose

To assess the risk of hyperbilirubinemia among newborns

Mode of Operation

Bilimeter works by directing white light into the skin of the neonate and measuring the intensity of the specific wavelengths that are returned (**Fig. 13.2**).

Advantages

- It is a noninvasive technique that uses light instead of needle to assess serum bilirubin; hence, there is no pain for newborns.
- The measurement of bilirubin by this device is within a clinically beneficial range that has been correlated with total serum bilirubin concentration measured by high-pressure liquid chromatography.
- This device can be used by healthcare professionals at all levels of healthcare system: physician clinics, hospitals, as well as community health centers.
- No need to wait for the results.
- Easy to operate and carry from place to place.

Disadvantages

- Use of bilimeter is limited to the routine screening of all newborns for hyperbilirubinemia.
- The measurement of bilirubin mainly depends on the extravascular level of bilirubin present in the body.

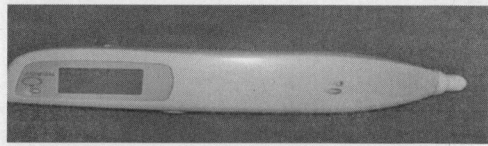

Fig. 13.2: Bilimeter.

- There is less evidence for its effectiveness in assessing bilirubin level in preterm neonates and dark-skinned babies.

Sites
- Forehead
- Sternum (most preferable site)

Steps in Procedure
1. Wash hands.
2. Wear disposable gloves.
3. Calibrate the device by pushing the button.
4. Place the bilimeter on forehead or sternum.
5. Press the measurement button (the number of time of pressing will vary depending on the manufacturer) and the result will appear on the screen immediately.
6. Dispose the calibration tip.

Guidelines
- The healthcare personnel must undergo training for the technique of using this device.
- Cleaning of the device is based on the manufacturer guidelines.
- This device should be charged using batteries.

Highlights ●●●

> ✦ Transcutaneous bilimeter or bilirubinometer is a device that is used to measure the bilirubin level.
> ✦ It is a noninvasive technique that uses light instead of needle to assess serum bilirubin; hence, there is no pain for newborns.
> ✦ To check press the measurement button (the number of time of pressing will vary depending on the manufacturer) and the result will appear on the screen immediately.
> ✦ This device should be charged using batteries.

GIRAFFE INCUBATOR

Definition
The Giraffe incubator is a state-of-the-art neonatal environment that promotes natural, peaceful healing while fostering a close bond between families and their babies and at the same time enhancing access to care by healthcare personnel.

Purposes
- To promote neurodevelopmental care and growth
- To enhance the care continuum
- To provide controlled environment through continuous warmthness
- To foster speedy recovery and early discharge of newborns

Advantages
- *Family-centered care:* The equipment is designed in such a way to accommodate the healthcare providers as well as the family members who are seated. Side doors can be removed completely for greater access of the parents and promote parent–baby bonding (**Figs. 13.3A and B**).
- *Thermoregulation:* It provides the warming touch of care by bidirectional airflow through double walls. Preheat mode with silenced alarms can be used for admission procedure.
- *Less chance for infection:* Servo-controlled humidity system designed in such a way that enhances easy cleaning and reduce infection.
- *It has a mechanism for heat loss prevention:* Even if the door panel is opened for any reason, air boost can be easily enabled to protect the baby from heat loss and support thermal stability.

Chapter 13: Recent Advances in Prenatal, Neonatal, and Pediatric Care

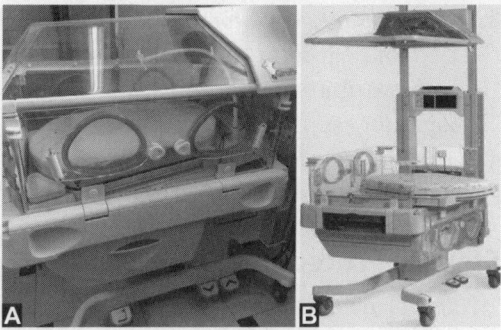

Figs. 13.3A and B: Giraffe incubator: (A) When closed; (B) When open.

Highlights

- The Giraffe incubator is a state-of-the-art neonatal environment that promotes natural, peaceful healing while fostering a close bond between families and their babies and at the same time enhancing access to care by healthcare personnel.
- The rotating mattress helps the healthcare providers to reposition the newborn without any difficulty.
- There is a provision for connecting this device with hospital information system and electronic health records. So, baby's medical history can be updated.

- The rotating mattress helps the healthcare providers to reposition the newborn without any difficulty. This in turn reduces the negative touch and stimulation, while improving procedural success. Moreover the pressure diffusing ability of this mattress adjusts according to the baby's condition and thereby reduces stress and improves comfort.
- There is a provision for connecting this device with hospital information system and electronic health records. So, baby's medical history can be updated.
- The touch screen display helps the healthcare providers to streamline the information and control the baby's environment. It also displays the important information readily available for family members. The large color display aides in initial setting of air temperature thus individualizing care according to the baby.
- The presence of hands: free alarm silence function in this equipment made it easier quickly silence alarms by waving hand. This helps to provide immediate attention and care to the baby, while maintaining calm, soothing environment for the baby.

BUBBLE CPAP

Definition

A bubble continuous positive airway pressure therapy (CPAP) system is a noninvasive ventilation method in which CPAP is delivered to a spontaneously breathing newborn to maintain lung volume during expiration. In this, blended and humidified oxygen is delivered via short binasal prongs or nasal mask. Pressure in the circuit is maintained by immersing the distal end of the expiratory tubing in water. The depth to which the tubing is immersed underwater determines the pressure generated in the airways of the infant. As the gas flows through the system, it bubbles out and prevents buildup of excess.

Purposes

- To maintain positive airway pressure
- To provide optimum humidification
- To increase functional residual capacity of neonate's lung
- To improve oxygenation
- To prevent atelectasis

Mechanism of Action

The bubble CPAP system helps in breathing of infants requiring respiratory support. It is incorporated with unique feature of humidification technology and air/oxygen blender (**Fig. 13.4**). CPAP works by maintaining positive pressure in the airway during spontaneous breathing, thereby increasing functional residual capacity and improving oxygenation in infants with RDS. CPAP does this by stabilizing airspaces that have a tendency to collapse during expiration due to surfactant deficiency.

Salient Features of Bubble CPAP

- Consistent and accurate delivery of CPAP
- Servo-controlled humidifier
- Bubble generator
- Easy to operate

Types of CPAP Device

1. *The F&P Bubble circuit:* Preferred for infants of all gestations and for all causes of respiratory distress.
2. *The Drager Babylog 8000 ventilator:* Used for near-term and term babies with a birth weight >1,250 g.
3. *The Stephanie ventilator with Argyle prongs:* Used for near-term/term babies who have been extubated and continue to need respiratory support.
4. *The EME Flow Driver:* Used for babies who have birth weight of <1,250 g.

Steps in Procedure

1. Perform hand hygiene.
2. Wear gloves.
3. Set the gas supply flow rate as required in the flowmeter.
4. Set the FiO_2 percentage on the dial knob (21–100%).
5. Set the humidifier by selecting desired mode using mode key. Select the heater wire *on/off* by using heater wire key.
6. Set the positive end expiratory pressure (PEEP) at the positive airway pressure (PAP) valve. Adjust PEEP knob clockwise or anticlockwise to the desired PEEP level in the PAP valve.
7. Remove the lid from the jar and fill the water reservoir. Fill the jar to the fill line with sterile water. Replace the lid to close the jar.

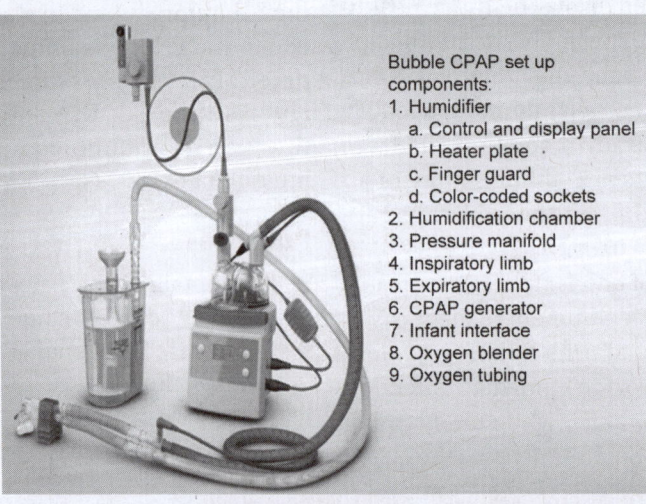

Bubble CPAP set up components:
1. Humidifier
    a. Control and display panel
    b. Heater plate
    c. Finger guard
    d. Color-coded sockets
2. Humidification chamber
3. Pressure manifold
4. Inspiratory limb
5. Expiratory limb
6. CPAP generator
7. Infant interface
8. Oxygen blender
9. Oxygen tubing

Fig. 13.4: Bubble CPAP unit.

8. To attach the PAP valve to a mounting clam, slide the equipment into the corresponding equipment mount holder. This will help to keep the device in vertical position.
9. Connect the exhalation port by rotating the PAP adjustment lever to the full anticlockwise position. Adjust the gas flow to the desired level and connect the expiratory end of the breathing circuit to the gas inlet connector.
10. PAP should be set using clockwise rotation, adjust the device to the desired back pressure.
11. Fix the patient interface.
12. Confirm the circuit is correctly set up.
13. Turn on the gas flow.
14. Choose the appropriate hat size (22–25, 25–29, 29–36, and >37 cm) to provide snug fit. Select an appropriate size prongs and connect it to the circuit. Position the prongs gently in the nares and secure with lateral tapes to the hat. The prongs should rest approximately 2–3 mm from the nares and should not be in contact with the columella (end of septum).

Nurse's Responsibility in Caring Neonates with Bubble CPAP

- *Observation and documentation:* Monitor the heart rate, respiratory rate, SpO_2 percentage, axillary temperature as per protocol and record it nurse's chart. Mention whether nasal prongs/mask are used, its size, water level, suction, etc. in nurse's chart. Neonate's condition, including response to handling and changes in skin also, should be documented.
- *ABG analysis:* Arterial blood sample should be collected and the results should be notified to the neonatal intensivist.
- *Medications:* Administer the medications round the clock; maintain fluid and electrolyte balance.
- *Airway management:* Ensure that gases are delivered at core temperature (37°C) with adequate humidification. This will facilitate mucociliary action, clear secretions, optimize gas exchange, and reduce the chance for infection. Confirm the patency of nasal prongs, humidification, infant position, feeding techniques, etc.
- *Suction:* Suctioning may be done when there is severe apnea, less response to tactile stimulation, or increase in oropharyngeal secretions.
- *Positioning:* The newborn should be positioned to facilitate comfort and optimize respiratory effort. Prone, supine, and lateral positions can be used alternately to promote upper airway stability, reduce work of breathing, facilitate physiological flexion of the trunk and limbs, and enhance normal growth and development.
- *Skin care and prevention of injury:* Provide meticulous skin care, oral care, and umbilical cord care. Skin-to-skin contact (kangaroo mother care) can be facilitated once the condition of baby is stable.
- *Family-centered care:* The parents should be kept informed about the infant's progress from time to time. When the infant is able to tolerate minimal handling, involve the parents in daily care. Demonstrate and discuss the common NICU procedures in care of newborns to the parents.
- *Prevention of complications:* (1) Pneumothorax: Assess the infant for signs of pneumothorax such as respiratory distress, increased work of breathing, severe apnea, desaturation of oxygen, decreased air entry, and asymmetrical movement. If suspected, support the baby and inform the neonatal intensivist. (2) Retinopathy of prematurity

(ROP): Judiciously use oxygen therapy and comply with oxygen protocols. Ensure that oxygen saturation and transcutaneous monitor alarms are set at correct limits. (3) Gastric distension: All infants who are on CPAP require nasogastric (NG) tube insertion (size—6 Fr) to prevent over distension of the stomach. Always check for the positioning of NG tube. Feeding should be given as per order. Gastric decompression can be done to enhance venting of air from the stomach. (4) Injury to nasal septum and nares: To prevent friction injury to the nasal septum and nares, we must limit excessive movement of the nasal prongs through good positioning and alignment of prongs. Always use appropriate size prongs or mask. Do not use any lubricants except normal saline for insertion of prongs. Ensure that the hat remains fitted over the glabella to anchor prongs/mask effectively. Release the prongs/masks as well as chin strap every 2 hours and gently massage the nares, cheeks, and chin. If there is any redness or injury to nares, mask can be used alternatively.

- *Monitor the oxygen concentration using calibrated oxygen measuring unit.*
  - Maintain the water level between minimum and maximum lines without the drop tube beneath the surface of the water. Adjust the water level through water level adjustment port. Remove the Luer cap and connect a syringe to the port for adding or removing water as required.
  - Airway pressure should be monitored continuously using a manometer and adjust the device accordingly.
  - Regularly monitor the humidification chamber for water level. Replace the chamber if water level exceeds.
  - Check whether all the connections are tight before use and after adjustment.
  - Ensure that airflow is present at all times if there is an interruption in airflow.
  - Constantly observe the circuit for condensate, drain as needed.
  - Regularly assess the PAP valve for bubbling.
  - Check for any leakage of air in the system as well as at the patient end. If air leaks are minimized, increase the airflow to maintain continuous bubbling.
  - Monitor the newborn's oxygen level.
  - Check the water level in the PAP valve, refill it if it drops below the minimum level.
  - Verify whether the baby is receiving prescribed CPAP level.

Managing the Troubleshooting and Maintenance of Bubble CPAP

- *Loss of bubbling:* If there is regular/intermittent loss of pressure, reposition the baby and use a chin strap to achieve optimal seal.
- Clean the outer sides of bubble CPAP and gas supply line using damp cloth and mild soap and water or isopropyl alcohol. Dry all the surfaces with soft cloth or paper towel.
- Follow operational safety measures as per manufacturer guidelines.
- Check the working condition of the device after cleaning and before using for patients.
- Humidifier can be autoclaved to prevent infection.
- Other parts of the equipment should be disinfected using prescribed disinfectant agents. Dry the parts before reassembling them.

Chapter 13: Recent Advances in Prenatal, Neonatal, and Pediatric Care

Highlights ●●●

- A bubble CPAP system is a noninvasive ventilation method in which CPAP is delivered to a spontaneously breathing newborn to maintain lung volume during expiration.
- In this, blended and humidified oxygen is delivered via short binasal prongs or nasal mask.
- It is incorporated with unique feature of humidification technology and air/oxygen blender.
- For effective delivery of oxygen, choose the appropriate hat size (22–25, 25–29, 29–36, and >37 cm) to provide snug fit. Select an appropriate size prongs and connect it to the circuit.
- Airway pressure should be monitored continuously using a manometer and adjust the device accordingly.
- Take appropriate measures to prevent complications.
- Ensure that gases are delivered at core temperature (37°C) with adequate humidification.

BODY COOLING

Aim
To reduce the temperature of the vulnerable deep brain structures to 33–34°C.

Purposes
- To protect the neurons by reducing cerebral metabolic rate
- To attenuate the release of excitatory amino acids such as glutamate and dopamine and improve the uptake of glutamate
- To lower the production of toxic nitric oxide and free radicals.

Types
- Whole-body hypothermia
- Selective head cooling

Eligibility Criteria for Therapeutic Hypothermia

- *Gestational age:* The newborn should be ≥35 weeks of gestation.
- *Time:* <6 hours post-birth.
- *Evidence of asphyxia as defined by the presence of at least two of the following criteria:*
  1. Apgar score <6 at 10 minutes or continued need for resuscitation with positive pressure ventilation with or without chest compression
  2. Any acute perinatal event that may result in hypoxic–ischemic encephalopathy (HIE) such as placental abruption, cord prolapse, and severe abnormal FHR.
  3. Cord pH <7 or base deficit 12 or more
  4. Arterial pH <7
- Clinically defined moderate or severe HIE (stage II or III based on modified Sanart's classification).
- Moderate to severe abnormal background activity on amplitude-integrated electroencephalogram (EEG) (i.e., discontinuous, burst suppression, or low voltage with or without seizure activity.

Classification of Hypoxic–Ischemic Encephalopathy

Clinical features	Moderate HIE	Severe HIE
Level of consciousness	Lethargic	Stuper/coma
Spontaneous activity	Decreased	Nil
Posture	Distal flexion, full extension	Decerebration
Tone	Hypotonia	Flaccid
Primitive reflexes	Weak suck, incomplete Moro	Sucking and Moro reflexes

Contd...

Contd...

Clinical features	Moderate HIE	Severe HIE
Autonomic system Pupil	Constricted	Dilated/nonreactive
Heart rate	Bradycardia	Variable heart rate
Respiration	Periodic breathing	Apnea

(HIE: hypoxic–ischemic encephalopathy)

Phases of Cooling

Phase 1: Active cooling, it is for 72 hours from the initiation of cooling

Phase 2: Rewarming, 12 hours of active gradual rewarming after completion of 72 hours of cooling. In this phase, the temperature will be increased by 0.5°C every second hourly as per the order.

Side Effects

- Delayed intracardiac conduction with sinus bradycardia
- Prolonged QT interval
- Ventricular arrhythmias
- Reduced cardiac output
- Hypotension
- Reduction in surfactant production
- Increase pulmonary vascular resistance
- Increase oxygen consumption and oxygen requirement
- Affects coagulation cascade and viscosity—coagulopathy that may be complicated by thrombus or hemorrhage
- Anemia
- Thrombocytopenia
- Leukopenia—increased risk of sepsis
- Renal impairment
- Metabolic and lactic acidosis
- Hypokalemia
- Hypoglycemia
- Impaired liver function

Equipment Needed

- Medi-therm III hyper/hypothermia system (**Figs. 13.5A and B**)
- Rectal temperature probe

Nurse's Responsibilities

- *Maintaining oxygenation:* Babies who are on body cooling will be put on ventilator

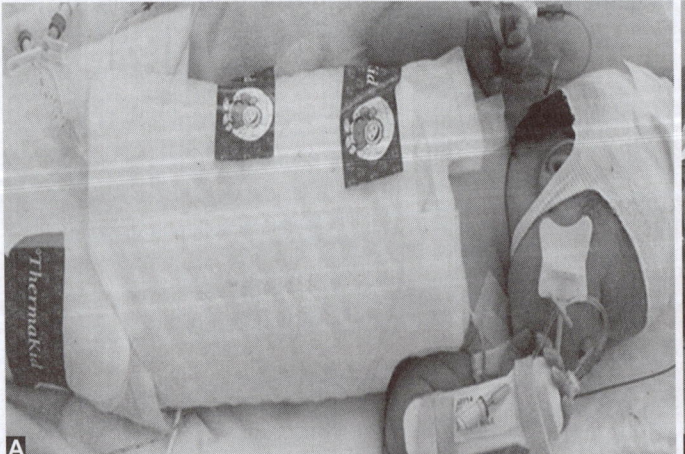
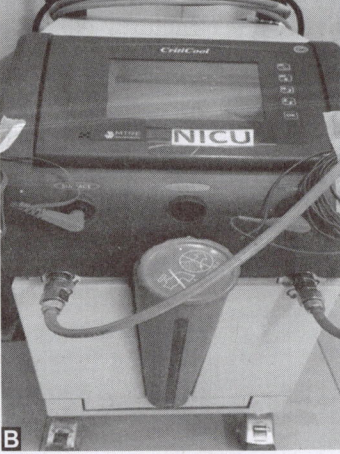

Figs. 13.5A and B: Body cooling: (A) HIE baby on body cooling therapy; (B) Cooling system. (HIE: hypoxic–ischemic encephalopathy)

support to maintain adequate oxygenation and ventilation. Because hypothermia shifts the oxyhemoglobin curve and can result in a decreased oxygen delivery. If the baby is not ventilated the metabolic rate may increase without increase in oxygen supply.
- *Maintaining perfusion:* Peripheral IV line should be started before the initiation of cooling procedure as there will be vasoconstriction of peripheral vessels and hence poor perfusion.
- *Constant monitoring:*
  - The baby's cardiopulmonary status should be constantly monitored. The newborn may go for hypovolemia and hypotension. Monitor BP and heart rate; watch for arrhythmias. Check the rectal temperature and CO_2 level should be corrected based on temperature.
  - 43–56% of newborns with HIE on undergoing body cooling therapy get seizures. So, they must be assessed for pupil reaction, level of consciousness, and signs of increased intracranial pressure. EEG should be monitored constantly during cooling. Also, they have to undergo formal EEG and magnetic resonance imaging (MRI) after 3–7 days of rewarming. At times, there is a need for MRI earlier to make decision regarding palliative care.
  - Note the doctor if any side effects arise.
- *Sedation:* Sedation with low dose of morphine infusion may be needed to provide optimal comfort and enhance the efficacy of cooling procedure. Inadequate sedation may result in increased metabolic rate.
- *Fluid and electrolyte:*
  - Serum electrolytes need to be monitored on admission, prior to the initiation of cooling then at 4, 8, 12, 24, and 72 hours.
  - May need to restrict the fluid to avoid fluid overload and cerebral edema.
  - Sodium and magnesium levels should be maintained at upper limit of normal to prevent the risk of cerebral edema and has neuroprotective effect, respectively.
- *Skin care:*
  - Assess the skin at frequent interval for color, perfusion, any breakdown, and signs of subcutaneous necrosis. Subcutaneous necrosis is characterized by indurations, erythematous nodules, and plaques over bony prominence such as back, arms, buttocks, thighs, and chest. It may be due to the sensitivity of brown fat to hypoxia and made worse by cooling.
  - Repositioning of baby should be done at frequent interval.
- *Family-centered care:*
  - Explain the family members about body cooling procedure, that is, its benefits, risks, complications, and expected duration of therapy.
  - Reassure the parents that their newborn will be kept comfortable during the therapy.
  - Promote parent–child bond through changing nappy, touch, etc.

Highlights ●●●●

+ Body cooling is a procedure that is aimed to reduce the temperature of the vulnerable deep brain structures to 33–34°C to protect the neurons by reducing cerebral metabolic rate.
+ There are two types: Whole-body hypothermia and selective head cooling.

Body cooling has two phases:
+ Phase 1: Active cooling, it is for 72 hours from the initiation of cooling.

Contd...

APPENDIX
Normal Values in Children

Blood volume	
Male	52–83 mL/kg
Female	50–75 mL/kg
Plasma volume	
Male	25–43 mL/kg
Female	28–45 mL/kg
Total red blood cell (RBC) count	
Cord blood	$3.9–5.5 \times 10^{12}$ cells/L
1–3 days	$4.0–6.6 \times 10^{12}$ cells/L
1 week	$3.9–6.3 \times 10^{12}$ cells/L
2 weeks	$3.6–6.2 \times 10^{12}$ cells/L
1 month	$3.0–5.4 \times 10^{12}$ cells/L
2 months	$2.7–4.9 \times 10^{12}$ cells/L
3–6 months	$3.1–4.5 \times 10^{12}$ cells/L
0.5–2 years	$3.7–5.3 \times 10^{12}$ cells/L
2–6 years	$3.9–5.3 \times 10^{12}$ cells/L
6–12 years	$4.0–5.2 \times 10^{12}$ cells/L
Total white blood cell (WBC) count	
Birth	$9.0–30 \times 10^{9}$ cells/L
24 hours	$9.4–34 \times 10^{9}$ cells/L
1 month	$5.0–19.5 \times 10^{9}$ cells/L
1–3 years	$6.0–17.5 \times 10^{9}$ cells/L
4–7 years	$5.5–15.5 \times 10^{9}$ cells/L
8–13 years	$4.5–13.5 \times 10^{9}$ cells/L

Differential count
Mean percentage

	Neutrophils	Lymphocytes	Eosinophils	Monocytes
Cord blood	61	31	2	6
2 weeks	40	48	3	9
3 months	30	63	2	5
6 months to 6 years	45	48	2	5
7–12 years	55	38	2	7

Total neutrophil count bands	150–400 × 10⁶ cells/L
Segmented	3,000–5,800 × 10⁶ cells/L
Total lymphocytic count	150–3,000 × 10⁶ cells/L
Total monocyte count	285–500 × 10⁶ cells/L
Total eosinophil count	50–150 × 10⁶ cells/L
Total basophil count	15–50 × 10⁶ cells/L
Total myelocyte count	Nil
Reticulocyte count 1–7 days Children	 0.4–6% of erythrocytes 0.5–1.5% of erythrocytes
Platelet count <7 days >7 days	 84–478 × 10⁹ cells/L 150–400 × 10⁹ cells/L
Hematocrit 1–3 days 2 months 6–12 years Adolescent male Adolescent female	 45–75% 28–42% 35–45% 37–49% 36–46%
Hemoglobin 1–3 days 2 months 6–12 years Adolescent male Adolescent female	 14.5–22.5 g/dL 9.0–14.0 g/dL 11.5–15.5 g/dL 13.0–16.0 g/dL 12.0–16.0 g/dL
Hemoglobin A	>95% of total hemoglobin
Hemoglobin A2	1.5–3.5% of total hemoglobin
Fetal hemoglobin Newborn 3 months 6 months >1 year	 60–90% of total hemoglobin 1–59% of total hemoglobin 2–9% of total hemoglobin <2% of total hemoglobin
Glycohemoglobin Total A1c	4–16 years 6–10% of total hemoglobin 1–5 years 2.1–7.7% of total hemoglobin 5–16 years 3–6.2% of total hemoglobin
Methemoglobin	0.06–0.24 g/dL
Red cell volume Male Female	 20–36 mL/kg 19–31 mL/kg

Expressions like 10^6, 10^9 indicate scientific notation for cell counts.

Appendix: Normal Values in Children

MCH	
0–3 days	31–37 pg
1 month	28–48 pg
3 months	25–35 pg
1 year	23–31 pg
2–6 years	24–30 pg
6–12 years	25–33 pg
MCHC	
All ages	30–37
MCV	
0–3 days	95–121 fL
6 months to 2 years	70–86 fL
6–12 years	77–95 fL
Adolescent	80–100 fL
ESR	
Westergren method	0–10 mm/h
Wintrobe method	0–13 mm/h
Measures of coagulation	
Clotting time	5–8 min/glass tube
Bleeding time	2–7 minutes (normal)
	7–11 minutes (borderline)
PT	
Newborn	13–18 seconds
Older children	11–15 seconds
PTT	
Nonactivated	60–85 seconds
APTT	25–35 seconds
Infant	<90 seconds
TT	
Control time	±2 seconds
Fibrinogen	
Newborn	1.25–3.00 g/L
Children	2.00–4.00 g/L
FDP	<10 mg/L
Coagulation factor	
Factor I	(As above, see fibrinogen)
Factor II	60–150% of normal or accepted units
Factor V	60–150% of normal or accepted units
Factor VII	65–135% of normal or accepted units
Factor VIII	60–145% of normal or accepted units
Factor VIII antigen	50–200% of normal or accepted units
Factor IX	60–140% of normal or accepted units
Factor X	60–130% of normal or accepted units
Factor XI	65–135% of normal or accepted units
Factor XII	65–150% of normal or accepted units

(APTT: activated partial thromboplastin time; ESR: erythrocyte sedimentation rate; FDP: fibrin degradation product; MCH: mean corpuscular hemoglobin; MCHC: mean corpuscular hemoglobin concentration; MCV: mean corpuscular volume; PT: prothrombin time; PTT: partial thromboplastin time; TT: thrombin time)

SERUM BIOCHEMISTRY

Serum Proteins (g/dL)

	Total	Albumin	α1 Globin	α2 Globin	β Globin	γ Globin
Preterm	4.3–7.6	3.0–4.2	0.1–0.5	0.3–0.7	0.3–1.2	0.3–1.4
Newborn	4.6–7.4	6.3–5.4	0.1–0.3	0.3–0.5	0.2–0.6	0.2–1.0
Infant	6.1–7.9	4.0–5.0	0.2–0.4	0.5–0.8	0.5–0.8	0.3–1.2
Thereafter	6.4–8.2	3.5–5.0	0.2–0.3	0.4–1.0	0.5–1.1	0.7–1.2

Plasma albumin
Preterm — 1.8–3.0 g/dL
Term newborn — 2.5–3.4 g/dL
<5 years — 3.9–5.0 g/dL
5–19 years — 4.0–5.3 g/dL

Serum bilirubin (mg/dL)

	Term	Preterm
Cord blood	<2.0	<2.0
0–1 day	<6.0	<8.0
1–2 days	<8.0	<12.0
2–7 days	<12.0	<16.0
>7 days	0.2–1.0	<2.0

Conjugated bilirubin — 0–0.2 mg/dL

Serum urea
Cord blood — 21–40 mg/dL
Preterm — 3–25 mg/dL
Term newborn — 5–18 mg/dL
<1 year — 7–18 mg/dL
>1 year — 7–20 mg/dL

Serum creatinine
Cord blood — 0.6–1.2 mg/dL
Neonate — 0.3–1.0 mg/dL
<1 year — 0.2–0.4 mg/dL
2–12 years — 0.3–0.7 mg/dL
Adolescent — 0.5–1.0 mg/dL

Serum glucose
Cord blood — 45–96 mg/dL
Newborn — 40–90 mg/dL
Children — 60–100 mg/dL

Serum cholesterol
1–3 years — 45–182 mg/dL
4–6 years — 109–189 mg/dL
6–9 years — 122–209 mg/dL
10–14 years — 124–217 mg/dL

Appendix: Normal Values in Children

Serum Ammonia:	
Newborn	90 to 150 µg/dL
Child	40 to 80 µg/dL
Serum phospholipids	
Newborn	75–170 mg/dL
Infant	100–275 mg/dL
Child	180–295 mg/dL
Iron	
Newborn	100–250 µg/dL
Infant	40–100 µg/dL
Child	50–120 µg/dL
Older age	
Male	50–160 µg/dL
Female	40–150 µg/dL
Serum zinc	64–118 µg/dL
Serum magnesium	
0–6 days	1.2–2.6 mg/dL
7 day to 2 years	1.6–2.6 mg/dL
2–14 years	1.5–2.3 mg/dL
Serum amylase	35–127 U/L
Serum alkaline phosphatase	
1–9 years	145–200 U/L (male and female)
10–11 years	130–560 U/L (male and female)
12–13 years	200–495 U/L (male), 150–420 U/L (female)
14–15 years	130–520 U/L (male), 70–230 U/L (female)
16–19 years	65–260 U/L (male), 50–230 U/l (female)
Serum glutamic oxaloacetic transaminase (SGOT)	35–140 U/L
0–5 days	1–55 U/L
1–9 years	5–45 U/L
10–19 years	
Serum glutamic pyruvic transaminase (SGPT)	
0–5 days	6–50 U/L
1–19 years	5–45 U/L
Creatine kinase	
Cord	70–380 U/L
Newborn	87–1,200 U/L
Adult	5–130 U/L
Lactate dehydrogenase (LDH)	
<1 year	170–580 U/L
1–9 years	150–500 U/L
10–19 years	120–330 U/L

PaO$_2$	
Birth	8–24 mm Hg
5–10 minutes	33–75 mm Hg
30 minutes	31–85 mm Hg
More than 1 hour	55–80 mm Hg
1 day	54–95 mm Hg
Thereafter	83–108 mm Hg
SaO$_2$	
Newborn	85–90%
Thereafter	95–99%
PaCO$_2$	
<1 year	27–40 mm Hg
Thereafter	32–48 mm Hg
HCO$_3$	
Arterial	21–28 mmol/L
Venous	22–29 mmol/L
pH	
Birth	7.1–7.36
30 minutes	7.2–7.38
1 day	7.3–7.45
Older children	7.35–7.45
Serum osmolality	275–295 mOsm/kg H$_2$O
Serum sodium	
Newborn	134–146 mmol/L
<1 year	139–146 mmol/L
Children	138–145 mmol/L
Serum potassium	
<2 years	3.0–6.0 mmol/L
2–12 years	3.0–6.0 mmol/L
>12 years	3.5–5.0 mmol/L
Serum calcium	
Newborn	9.0–12.0 mg/dL
Child	8.8–10.8 mg/dL
Serum chloride	
Newborn	96–110 mmol/L
Child	98–106 mmol/L
Inorganic phosphorus	
Newborn	4.8–8.2 mg/dL
1–3 years	3.8–6.5 mg/dL
4–11 years	3.7–5.6 mg/dL
12–15 years	2.9–5.4 mg/dL
Normal urinary values	
Volume	
Neonate	50–300 mL
Infant	350–550 mL
Child	500–1,000 mL
Adolescents	700–1,400 mL

Specific gravity	1.015–1.025
pH	
Newborn	5–7
Children	4.5–8 (avg 6)
Cell count	
Red blood cells	0–2/hpf
White blood cells	0–5/hpf
Epithelial cells	Few
Bacteria	0–20 in centrifuged specimen
Protein	
Total (24 hours)	50–80 mg/24 hours or 1–14 mg/dL
Albumin	37.9%
Globulin (α1)	27.3%
Globulin (α2)	19.5%
Globulin (β)	8.8%
Globulin (γ)	3.3%
Urinary creatinine	
Preterm	8–15 mg/kg/24 hours
Term	10.4–19.7 mg/kg/24 hours
1–7 years	10–15 mg/kg/24 hours
7–15 years	5.2–41 mg/kg/24 hours
Ammonia nitrogen	50–120 mg/24 hours
Amniotic fluid	
Alpha fetoprotein	
Gestational age (in weeks)	
15	13.5 ± 3.42 µg/mL
16	11.7 ± 3.38 µg/mL
17	10.3 ± 3.03 µg/mL
18	9.5 ± 3.22 µg/mL
19	7.1 ± 2.85 µg/mL
20	5.0 ± 2.45 µg/mL
Lecithin	>0.10 mg/dL indicates lung maturity
Lecithin/sphingomyelin ratio (L/S)	2–5 indicates fetal lung maturity

Index

Page numbers followed by *f* refer to figure and *t* refer to table.

A

Abdomen 15, 70
Abdominal girth 58, 59*f*
   general instructions 59
   indications 58
   postprocedure care 59
   preparation 58
   procedure 58
Abdominal paracentesis 214, 216
   complications 215
   contraindications 214
   indications 214
   positioning 215
   postprocedure care 215
   preparation 214
   procedure 215
   site for 215*f*
Accidental tube expulsion 128
Acetic acid 203
Achilles' tendon 77
Adequate feeding, signs of 119
Admission
   procedure 37
   types of 36
Advanced life support 200
Air emboli 219
Airway 198, 199
   edema and pain 212
   management 269
   opening 200
   patency 200
Allen's cards 66*f*
Allen's test 66, 86, 87*f*
Alloimmunization 219
Amiel-Tison method 72
Amplatzer septal occluder 105
Anal reflex 77
Anemia, chronic 216
Anesthesia bag 209
Anoxia 140

Antecubital fossa 85*f*
Anthropometric measurements 51
Anthropometry 57, 60
Antibodies 217
Anus 15, 70, 71
Anxiety 252
Aorta
   coarctation of 105
   recurrent coarctation of 105
Aortic stenosis 105
Apgar score 5, 8*t*, 40
Apnea 200, 224
   monitor 33, 33*f*, 34
      monitor, indication 33
      parts of 33
      purpose 33
Appendages 60
Arm recoil 9
   sign 11*f*
Arterial blood gas 5
   analysis 86, 269
Arterial catheterization 104
Arterial puncture 86, 87
   sites for 86
Artificial feeding 123
Artificial sphincter 179
Artificial ventilation methods 209
Asepto syringe 129*f*
Aspiration 149
Aspirin 226
Assessment procedures 36
Assist-control ventilation 207
   advantage 207
   disadvantages 207
   indications 207
Asthma 136
Atelectasis 212
Atracurium 211
Atrial septal defect 105
Atropine 251

Auscultation 8, 60, 69, 70
Automated external defibrillator 200
Axillary temperature 45

B

Babinski sign 77
Baby bath 20, 24
   purposes 20
   type of 24
Baby's cardiopulmonary status 273
Baby's face 261
Back blow 195
Bag valve mask device 209
Balanced suspension traction 241
Balloon
   atrioseptostomy 105
   dilation 105
Bandages 249
Bangle test 57
Baroda developmental screening test 72
Barotrauma 150
Basic life support 200
   component of 197
Bathing 260
   adolescents 260
   infants 260
   postprocedure care 261
   preparation 260
   procedure 260
   school-age children 260
   special considerations 260
   toddler 260
Bayley scales 72
Bedside oxygen delivery system 212
Betadine 227
   swabs 202
Bilevel positive airway pressure 141

Bilimeter 265f
Bilirubinometer 265
Binet-Kamath and Weshler intelligence scale 72
Biopsy, site for 101
Birth
    asphyxia 5, 40
    history 39
    injuries, medications 2
    order 40
    weight 40
Bladder location 183
Bleeding disorders 86
Blocked ducts 119
Blood
    administration 221, 222
    collection tubes, type of 84t
    gas analysis 88, 90
        aftercare 89
        complications 90
        contraindications 88
        equipment 88
        general instructions 89
        normal values 90
        preparation 88
        procedure 88
        purposes 88
        sites 88
    pressure 48, 50, 223
    sample, collection of 83
    transfusion 216, 221
        classifications 216
        indications 216
        reaction 229
    vessels, thrombosis of 227
Blow bottles, use of 249
Body
    bluish discoloration of 40
    build 60
    cooling 271, 272f
        purposes 271
        therapy 272f
        types 271
    temperature 189
Bolus feedings 125
Bone marrow aspiration 102, 103f, 104
    indications 102
    position 103
    postprocedure care 104
    procedure 103
    sites for 102

Brachial artery 86
Brachioradialis tendon 77
Bradycardia 212, 224
Brain injury 76
Brazelton neonatal behavioral scales 72
Breast 14
    abscess 119
    care of 118
    engorgement 119
    injury 119
    milk 115
        general guidelines for storage of 120
        storage 120t
        type of 118, 120
    pain, deep 119
    problems 119
    surgery 119
Breastfeeding 115, 116, 119
    advantages of 115
    assisting in 115
    exclusive 24
    positions for 117f
Breath sounds
    absence of 210
    classification of 69
Breathing 200
    deep 232
    difficulties 40
    warm 137
Bronchiolitis, acute 136
Bronchitis 136
Bronchospasm 149
    exacerbation of 150
Bronchus
    anterior 147
    apical 147
Brudzinski's sign 77
Bryant's traction 241
Bubble continuous positive airway pressure 267
    salient features of 268
    unit 268f
Bubbling, loss of 270
Buccal mucosa 14
Buck's traction 241
Burping technique 118, 118f

■ C

Cancer 119
Cannula, length of 164, 165

Capillary blood sampling 90, 92
    aftercare 92
    equipment 90
    preparation 90
    procedure 91
    types 90
Cardiac anomalies 2
Cardiac catheterization 104, 106f, 107
    indications 104
    postprocedure care 106
    preprocedural care 105
    procedure 106
    purposes 104
Cardiac monitor 110
Cardinal signs 44
Cardiopulmonary injury 205
Cardiopulmonary resuscitation 197, 200
    indications for 197
    procedure 197
Cardiorespiratory monitor 211
Cast
    application, materials for 244
    care 244
        nursing considerations 245
        postprocedure care 245
        preparation 244
        procedure 245
    removal, assisting with 246
    types of 244, 245f
Catheter 177t
    duration of changing 184
    malfunction 224
    selection 178
    size 2
    type of 133, 134
Central venous catheter 132, 134
Cerebella assessment 78
Cerebrospinal fluid 99
    normal values of 98
    pressure 98
Cervical
    skeletal tongs 241
    skin 241
Chemical restraint 238, 239
Chest 14, 68
    circumference 55, 56, 56f
    compression 201
    site for 199f

Index

percussion 148
physiotherapy 146, 149
  contraindications 146
  duration of 149
  indications 146
  timing of 149
thrust 195
Child abuse, documentation of 81
Citrate-phosphate-dextrose solution with adenine 84
Clean technique 204
Clove hitch restraint 234
  application of 235f
  purpose 234
Coil occlusion 105
Colonic irrigation 189, 190, 194
  complications 189
  general instructions 189
  indications 189
  postprocedure care 189
  preparation 189
  procedure 189
  purposes 189
Color vision 67, 79
Colostomy 188f
  care 187
    complications 187
    equipment needed 187
    indications 187
    preparation 187
    procedure 187
    purposes of 187
  procedure 194
Colostrum 118
Commercial kangaroo mother care bags 25f
Community setup 72
Complete blood count 84
Conduction hearing loss 68
Consanguinity, degree of 41, 41t
Consciousness, level of 77, 252
Continuous feeding 125
Continuous positive airway pressure 6, 141, 209
  device, types of 268
  mechanism of action 268
  purposes 267
  steps in procedure 268
  therapy 267
Control mechanical ventilation 207
  disadvantages 207
  indications 207
Cooling, phases of 272
Cough stimulation 148
Cover test 65
Cradle position 116
  modified 116
Cranial nerve 79
  assessment 79
Cranial surgery 76
Creatinekinase 279
Cremastericreflex 77
Crib net restraint 236, 236f
Crib top bubble restraint 236
Cricoid cartilage injury 205
Croup 136
Cryoprecipitate 218, 220
  indications 218
Cuff
  bladder 49f
  size of 49t
Curved catheters 178, 178f
Cyanosis 62, 224
Cystic fibrosis 136

D

Deep tendon reflexes, elicitation of 60
Deformities 198
Delivery
  mode of 40
  place of 40
Denver developmental screening test 72
Developmental assessment
  general guidelines for 72
  type of 72
Diabetes mellitus, history of 263
Diagnostic cardiac catheterization, type of 104
Diagnostic procedures, assisting in 83
Diazepam 211, 251
Digital thermometer. 44, 44f
Diphtheria 43
Disposable thermometer strips 45
Distal tracheal granuloma 206
Doll's eye 17
Donor blood 224
Dorsum hand 85f
Double diapering 190
  indication 190
  procedure 190
  purposes 190
Drip method 127
Drug calculations 152
Dry dressings 253
Dysrhythmias 149

E

Ears 13, 67, 258
  care 259
  drops 169
  nose and throat 60, 61
Ecchymoses 62, 63
Elbow restraints 235, 235f
  purpose 235
Electrocardiogram 6, 108, 109, 109f, 112
  drawbacks of 108
  function 108
  leads, placement of 109
  working principles of 108
Electrolyte
  daily requirements of 167t
  disturbances 219
  imbalance, correction of 163
Electronic monitor 49
Electronic weighing machine 52f
Emergency procedures 195
Emphysematous lungs 150
Encephalitis 76
Endotracheal tube 6
  selection of 2t
  size 2
Enema 185
  general instructions 185
  indications 185
  position 186
  postprocedure care 186
  preparation 186
  procedure 186
Enterostomy care 193
  aftercare 194
  indications 193
  procedure 193
Epiglottis 200
Epispadias exstrophy 179
Equipment failure 210
Erythema 62
Erythematous nodules 273

Ethylenediaminetetraacetic acid 84
Exchange blood transfusion 221, 221f, 224
   complications 224
   indications 221
   postprocedure care 224
   preparation 222
   procedure 222, 222t
Expressing breast milk 119
   methods of 120
Exstrophy, classic 179
External cardiac massage 5
   methods of 7f
Extremities 71
   use of 232
Extrusion 16
Eye 14, 60, 64, 258
   care 258
      postprocedure care 259
      preparation 259
      procedure 259
      purposes 259
   drops, instillation of 169f
   medication 168

■F

Face 13, 60
Facial skin 14
Fainting 175
Family pedigree chart 41f
Fatigue 150, 212
Febrile reactions 219
Feeding 12, 122
   articles
      cleaning of 121
      sterilization of 121
   history 42
Femoral artery 86
Fentanyl 211
Fever 175
Fine needle aspiration 112, 113
   general instructions 113
   indications 112
   postprocedure care 113
   preparation 113
   procedure 113
Finger stick 90
   site for 91f
Fistula, bronchopleural 206
Flow rate 164, 165
Flow ventilation systems 209

Fluid
   daily requirements of 167t
   intake 232
   less amount of 215
Flushing jejunal feeding tubes, guidelines for 131
Foley's catheter 179
   three-way 178
   two-way 178, 178f
Food, type of 194
Foreign body
   aspiration 197
      signs of 195
   from airway, manual removal of 195
   procedure 195
   removal of 195, 196, 196f
Foremilk 119
Formula feeding 121
Fowler's position 122
Frankfurt plane 53
Frenulum 14
Fresh frozen plasma 217
   indications 217
Fresh whole blood 221
Fundus examination 9

■G

Gastric lavage 225
   indications 225
   postprocedure care 225
   preparation 225
   procedure 225
Gastrocnemius muscle 78
Gastrostomy 157
   feeding 126, 128
      complications 128
      contraindications 126
      indications 126
      methods of 126
      preparation 127
      procedure 127
Gavage feeding 123
   indications 123
   postprocedure care 124
   preparation 124
   procedure 124
Genitalia 70, 257
   female 15, 70
   male 15
Genitals and sexual maturity stages 61

Gesell development evaluation 72
Gestational age 2, 9, 40
   assessment of 10f
   clinical assessment of 9
Giraffe incubator 266, 267f
   advantages 266
   purposes 266
Glabellar reflex 17
Glasgow coma scale 78t
Glass thermometer 44, 44f
Glottic edema 212
Glucose 98
Gluteal folds 15
Glycol electrolyte lavage solution 186
Glycopyrrolate 251
Granulocytes 217, 220
   indications 217
Great arteries, transposition of 105
Gum 68

■H

Haemophilus influenzae type B 44
Hair 61, 257
Halo traction 241
Hard palate 14
Hardy-Rand-Ritter test 67
Head 60, 63
   boxes 143
   circumference 55, 55f, 56
   symmetry 13
   tilt-chin lift 198, 198f
Health education 107
Heart 69
   disease
      congenital 111
      history of 263
   failure, congenital 146
   rate 5, 6, 8, 272
Heel puncture, deep 86
Heelstick 90
   procedure 92f
   site of 91f
Heimlich maneuver 196, 196f, 197f
Hemolytic transfusion reaction 219
Hemophilia
   A 217

B 217
Hemorrhage 205, 206, 229
Hemorrhagic disease, severe 217
Heparin flush guidelines 134t
Hepatitis B 43
High-efficiency particulate air 262
Hind milk 119
Hips 15
Hirschberg test 65
Holtan stadiometer 53
Home care management 107
HOTV chart 66, 66f
Hudson masks 142
Human immunodeficiency virus infection 119
Hydration 12
Hymen 15
Hyperkalemia 224
Hypertension 224
Hyperthyroidism, history of 263
Hyperventilation 150
Hypocalcemia 224
Hypoglycemia 2, 224
Hypomagnesaemia 224
Hypoperfusion 214
Hypotension 149, 224
Hypothermia 219
Hypoxemia 140, 149
   recognition of 214
Hypoxia 140, 200, 206, 212
   signs of 221
Hypoxic-ischemic encephalopathy 272
   classification of 271

■ I

Immunization procedure 173
Incentive spirometer 150f
Incentive spirometry 149
   complications 150
   contraindications 150
   indications 149
   preparation 150
   procedure 150
   purposes 149
Incubator 31, 33
   care of newborn in 32f
   functions 31
   parts of 32
   types 32

Indian Academy of Pediatric Vaccination Schedule 43t
Indwelling catheter 180
   removal of 181
   short-term 176
   three-way 178f
Infection 212
   less chance for 266
Infrared thermometers 45, 45f
Infusion pump 220
Injury 149
Insertion of suppository 192, 193f
   aftercare 193
   indication 192
   procedure 192
Inspiratory pressure 207
Instillation 168, 169f, 170
Intensive care unit 106
Interventional cardiac catheterization procedure, type of 105
Intracardiac shunt 206
Intracranial bleeding 76
Intracranial pressure 96, 146
Intracranial tumors 76
Intradermal injection 160
   indications 160
   preparation 160
   procedure 160
Intramuscular injection 158, 159
   advantages 158
   postprocedure care 159
   preparation 159
   procedure 159
   site for 158
Intravenous cannula, size of 164t
Intravenous catheterization sites 132f
Intravenous fluid
   maintenance, indications for 163
   type of 164, 164t
Intravenous medication, administration of 167
Intravenous pyelogram 61
Intravenous therapy 162
   care during 166
   indications 162
Invasive blood pressure monitoring 86

Iron 279
Isolation room, indications for admission to 36

■ J

Jacket restraint 236f
Japanese encephalitis 44
Jaundice 62
Jaw thrust 198
   maneuver 198f
Jejunostomy feeding 129, 130f, 131
   complications 130
   disadvantages 129
   indications 129
   procedure 130
   purposes 129
Jejunostomy tubes 157
Jitteriness 224
Joints 61
   mobility 9

■ K

Kangaroo mother care 24, 26
   components 24
   duration of 26
   positioning 25f
   prerequisites 24
   uses of 24, 26
Karaya paste 188
Kernig's sign 77
Kidney biopsy 101, 101f, 102
   complications 102
   contraindications 101
   indications 101
   postprocedure care 102
   procedure 101
Kidney tray 185, 228
Knee-chest position 186f

■ L

Lactate dehydrogenase 279
Lactation 115, 120
Laminar flow hood 262, 262f
   advantages 263
   disadvantages 263
   guidelines 263
   mode of action 263
   purposes 262
   types 263

Language development 75
Laryngeal mask airway 209
Laryngoscope blades 209
Laryngotracheal stenosis 206
Leukocytes 99
Lidocaine gel, instillation of 180
Lips 14, 68
Liver biopsy 99, 100
   complications 100
   contraindications 99
   indications 99
   needle, site for insertion of 100f
   postprocedure care 100
   preparation 99
   procedure 100
Lorazepam 211
Low-birth-weight infant 24
Low-flow delivery system 141
Lukewarm water 192
Lumbar puncture 96, 97f, 99
   contraindications 96
   indications 96
   preparation 96
   procedure 97
Lung 69
   compliance 206, 207
   disease, unilateral 206

M

Magnimeter 53
   classification of degree of 54
   formula for calculating degree of 54
Mandatory breaths 207
Mask 249
Mastitis 119
Maternal diseases 40
Mature milk 119
Measles 43
Mechanical restraint 238
   types of 234
Mechanical ventilation 206
   contraindication 206
   drugs used in 211t
Mechanical ventilator 203
Meconium aspiration syndrome 2
Mediastinal shift 229
Medication
   administration of 152
      general principles in 152
      management 157
      ointment 254
      rights in administration of 152
      subcutaneous administration of 161
Meeting children's hygiene needs 257
Memory exercise 194, 229
Meningitis 76
Meperidine 251
Metabolic abnormality 2
Metabolic acidosis 224
Metabolic alkalosis 224
Methemoglobinemia 214
Methods over enema 186
Mid-arm circumference 56, 57
   assessment of 56f
Midazolam 211
Mission Indradhanush 42, 44
Mitten 237, 237f
   purpose 237
Moisture keeping dressings 253
Monitor vital signs 219, 223
Monitoring electrocardiogram 110
Monitoring intubated child 210
Moro reflex 9
Morphine 211, 251
Mouth 14, 68, 257
Mouthwashes, antibacterial 258
Multiple pregnancy 40
Mummy restraint 235, 235f
Muscle 149
   relaxants 211
   strength 77
   tone 8, 9
   symmetry 12
Myelodysplastic children 178

N

Nail 60, 257
Nasal cannula 143
Nasal drops 169
Nasal prongs 141, 143, 143f, 144
Nasal spray, instillation of 170
Nasogastric tube, measuring length of 124f
National Immunization Schedule 43t
Nebulization 137, 140
   complications 137
   contraindication 137
   indications 137
   purposes 137
   therapy 139
      drugs used for 137
Nebulizer
   care of 140
   parts of 138, 138f
Necessitate neonatal resuscitation 1, 2
Neck 14, 60, 64
Necrotizing enterocolitis 224
Needle play 231
Neonatal examination 7, 11
Neonatal resuscitation 1, 6f, 7
   indications 1, 1t
   preparation 2
   purpose 1
Neurologic reflexes 8
Neurological abnormalities 2
Neurological examination 76
Neuromuscular maturity 9
Nevus flammeus 63
New Ballard
   chart 10f
   scale 9
Newborn
   care 1
   drying of 3f
   intensive care unit 5
   positioning of 3f
   reflexes 15t
Nipples 14
Nomogram 153f
Nonbreathing mask 142, 142f
Noninvasive fetal electrocardiography monitoring 263
   advantages 264
   aftercare 265
   disadvantages 264
   indications 263
   preparation 264
   purposes 263
   steps in procedure 264
Noninvasive fetal electrocardiography, parts of 264
Nonlatex catheter 178
Normal electrocardiogram 111f
Normal saline 203
   simple irrigation with 184
Nose 14, 67

Nutrition 60
Nutritional support 135

O

Obstructive lung disease 206
Odorous gas 194
Old catheter 185
Omphalitis 224
Open care system 26
Open stopcock 223
Operation theater 251
Oral administration, precautions for 157
Oral cavity 68
Oral hygiene 258
  equipment needed 258
  general principles 258
  indications 258
  postprocedure care 258
  preparation 258
  procedure 258
Oral medications 154
  administration of 156
  delivery 144
    method, selection of 144
Oxygen 202, 220
  saturation 6, 86
  tent 249
Oxygen therapy 140, 145
  methods of administration 141
  principles 140
  purposes 140
Oxygenation, maintaining 272
Oxyhood 141, 143*f*

P

Pain 149, 175
  management 252
Paladai 122*f*
Palate 68
Pallor 62
Palmar grasp 17
  reflex 14
Pancuronium 211
Paper bag 185
Partial thromboplastin time 84
Patent ductus arteriosus 105
Pelvis sling 241
Perfusion, maintaining 273
Periodical leads 109

Perioperative nursing care
  preoperative care 248
  principles of 248
Peripherally inserted central catheter 132
Peritonitis 215
Periurethral glands 181
Persistent pulmonary hypertension 2
Pertussis 43
Petechiae 63
Phosphorus, inorganic 280
Phototherapy 28, 31
Physical examination 59
  positions 60
  setting 59
Physical restraint 238
Physiotherapy 149
Placing sensor, sites for 212
Plain sutures, removal of 255*f*
Plantar grasp 17
Plasma 216
  albumin 278
  derived 217
Platelets 217–219
  indications 217
Play in hospital, functions of 230
Play materials, types of 231
Play therapy 230
  classification of 230
  goals of 230
  infection control in 233
  nurse's responsibilities 231
  play activities 232
Pneumomediastinum 205
Pneumothorax 205, 206, 210, 211, 229
Polio 43
Polyethylene glycol electrolyte lavage solution 186
Popliteal angle 9
  sign 11*f*
Positive pressure ventilation 6
Positive-end expiratory pressure 208, 209
  advantages 208
  ventilation methods 209
Posterior bronchus 147
Posterior iliac crest 103*f*
Postpyloric feeding 129
Postresuscitation care 5

Postural drainage 147
  positions for 147*f*
Precolostrum 118
Pregnancy-induced hypertension 1
Prematurity 2
Premedications 251*t*
Preschooler and school aged 177
Pressure support ventilation 208
Preterm milk 119
Procaine 228
Protein 99, 281
  energy malnutrition 61
Prothrombin time 84
Psychological preparation 249
Pulmonary edema 229
Pulmonary hemorrhage 149
Pulse 47
  oximeter 5
Pulse oximetry 212
  equipment needed 212
  limitations 214
  preparation 212
  procedure for 213, 213*t*
Pump method 126*f*
Pupil 272
Purpura 63
P-wave amplitude 112

Q

Q waves 112
QRS
  amplitude 112
  axis 110
  duration 111
QT interval 111
Quadriceps skinfold thickness 57, 57*f*

R

Radial artery 86
Radiant warmer 26, 26*f*, 28
  care of 28
  parts of 26
  preparation 27
  procedure 27
  purpose 26
Radiofrequency ablation 105
Range of motion 232

Rectal temperature 46
Red blood cells 7
Reflex 8, 15
   abdominal 77
   assessment 77
   elicitation of 10
Reintubation equipment 211
Removal of sutures 254
   aftercare 255
   equipment needed 254
   nursing considerations 256
   preparation of child 254
   procedure 255
   removal of staples 255
Renal failure 224
Rescue breathing 199*f*
Respiration 48
Respiratory care 136
Respiratory distress 224
Respiratory effort 8, 198
Respiratory failure, diagnosis of 86
Restraining child, nurse's responsibilities in 238
Restraints 234, 238, 249
   guidelines for use of 234
   hazards of 237
   indications 234
   principles 234
   types of 234
Resuscitation
   initial steps in 3
   procedure 4
Retention catheter 178
Rhythm 110
Rib 149
   cage 196
Rooting reflexes 14
Rotate stopcock 223
Rubber catheter, single-use 178*f*
Russell's traction 241

■ S

Safety and recreation 230
Safety belt 236, 237*f*
Saliva consistency 258
Scalp cradle cap, condition of 13
Scalp vein 85*f*
   site, care of 167
Scarf sign 9, 11*f*
Scrotum 15
Sechrist 207

Seizures 224
Selecting indwelling catheter 178*t*
Sensorineural hearing loss 68
Sepsis 224
Serum
   alkaline phosphatase 279
   ammonia 279
   bilirubin 278
   biochemistry 278
   calcium 280
   chloride 280
   cholesterol 278
   creatinine 278
   electrolytes 273
   glucose 278
   magnesium 279
   phospholipids 279
   potassium 280
   sodium 280
   urea 278
Servo controlled incubator 32
Sexually transmitted diseases 71
Shakir's tape method 56, 57*t*
Short-term enteral feeding 123
Shout and tap 197
Sickle cell disease 221
Side rails 237, 237*f*
Silastic tubes 203
Simple craft material 231
Simple language 72
Simple mask 141, 141*f*, 144
Sims' lateral position 186*f*
Single ureterostomy 191
Sinus 110
Skeletal pin site cleansing 240
Skill, quality of 72
Skin 60, 61, 257
   breakdown 205
   care 273
      and prevention of injury 269
   cleansing supplies 240
   color 12, 251
   probes, application of 27
   substitutes 253
Skinfold thickness 57
Skin-to-skin contact 24
Sleep 12
Slipped capital femur epiphysis 241

Sneezing 16
Soaks 233
Soft palate 14
Sore throat 212
Spine 15, 60, 149
Splints 237
Split Russell's traction 241
Sponge bath 260
Spontaneous breathing 200
Spontaneous respiratory
   activity 208
   distress 195
Square window sign 9, 11*f*
Staple, removal of 255*f*
Steam inhalation 136
   indications 136
   postprocedure care 137
   preparation 136
   procedure 137
   purposes 136
Stent placement 105
Sterile technique 204
   modified 204
Sterile tray containing 182, 228
Steroids 211
Stimulating newborn, techniques for 4*f*
Stimulation 15
Stool specimen collection 95, 96
   aftercare 95
   general instructions 95
   preparation 95
   procedure 95
   purposes 95
Straight single-use catheters 178
Stridor 212
Subcutaneous injection, sites for 162*f*
Subdiaphragmatic abdominal thrusts 196
Subglottic stenosis 212
Succinylcholine 211
Sucking 16
   reflexes 14
Suction apparatus 228
Suction catheter, selection of 2*t*
Suction depths 204
Suction equipment 202
Suction pressure 205
Suctioning procedure 204

Suctioning, correct method for 3f
Sudden infant death syndrome 34
Suprapubic catheter
  home care of 194
  placement of 183f
  set 182f
Suprapubic catheterization 181
  complications 182
  contraindications 182
  equipment needed 182
  home care instructions 184
  indications 181
  nurse's responsibility 184
  patient preparation 182
  postprocedure care 184
  procedure 183
Suprasternal collapse 206
Surgical asepsis 254
Surgical dressing 253
  aftercare 254
  equipment needed 253
  nursing considerations in 254
  preparation 254
  procedure 254
  purposes 253
  types of 253
Swallowing 16
Synchronized intermittent mandatory ventilation 207
  advantages 208
  disadvantages 208
  indications 207
Syringe method 127, 127f

■T

Tachydysrhythmias 105
Tactile stimulation 12
Tap water 185
Teeth 68
Temporal artery 86
Temporal scanning 46, 47f
Tephanie ventilator 268
Testing visual acuity 65
Tetanus 43
Therapeutic hypothermia, eligibility criteria for 271
Therapeutic play 230
Therapeutic purposes 212
Thermometer
  single use 45, 45f
  type of 44
Thermoregulation 266
Thoracentesis 228
  complications 229
  equipment needed 228
  general instructions 228
  indications 228
  postprocedure care 228
  preparation 228
  procedure 228
Thoracic squeezing 148
Throat 68
Thrombocytopenia 224
Thrombotic thrombocytopenic purpura 217
Thumb
  and index finger 204
  over opening 204
Tibial-radialis strength 78
Time-cycled ventilator 207
Time-cycled, pressure-limited ventilation 208
Toddlers and older children 177
Tongue 14
Tonic neck 18
Topical application 171, 172
  forms of 171
Topical steroids 172
Total nutrient admixture 131
Total parenteral nutrition 131, 132f, 134
  administration, methods of 132
  indications 131
  purposes 131
  solution
    components of 131
    type of 131
Toxemia 1
Trach ties 205
Trach tube 204
Tracheal intubation 209
Tracheal wall erosion 206
Tracheocutaneous fistula 206
Tracheoesophageal fistula 205, 206
Tracheostomy 202, 203
  mask 143, 143f
  tube 202, 202f
Tracheostomy care 202
  equipment needed 202
  indications 202
  nurse's responsibility 203
  procedure 203
  techniques, types of 204
Traction 240
  response appearance 14
  types of 241t
Traction care 240
  equipment needed 240
  preparation 242
  procedure 242
  purposes 240
Transcatheter device closure 105
Transcutaneous bilimeter 265
  advantages 265
  disadvantages 265
  guidelines 266
  mode of operation 265
  sites 266
  steps in procedure 266
  unit of measurement 265
Transfusions, types of 220
Transition milk 118
Transport incubator 32
Transpyloric feeding 129
Transureteroureterostomy 191
Traumatic laryngitis 212
Triceps skinfold thickness 57, 57f
Trivandrum developmental screening chart 72
Trouble breathing 203
Tru-cut needle 102
Tube 249
  obstruction 205
  placement, maintaining correct 210
Tube feeding 124, 125
  administering 124
Tuberculosis 43, 146
Tulles 253f
Tumbling E chart 66f
Tuning fork test 68t
Twirl catheter 204
Tympanic membrane 46

■U

Umbilical vein catheterization 226
  complications 227
  contraindications 227

equipment needed 227
indications 227
preparation 227
procedure 227
Umbilical venous catheter 6
Umbilical vessels 1
Umbilicus 15, 258
Upper limb, splints for supporting 237f
Upper respiratory tract infection 64
Ureterostomy 191, 191f, 192
   double-barrel 191
   types of 192
Ureterostomy care 191
   aftercare 191
   complications 192
   equipment needed 191
   indications 191
   nursing considerations 191
   procedure 191
   types 191
Urethra, chronic infection of 181
Urethral obstruction, prevention of 176
Urethral trauma 179
Urinary catheterization 176, 181
   indications 176
Urinary creatinine 281
Urinary obstructions 176
Urinary retention, acute 176
Urinary tract infection 93
Urine 211
   bypasses 191

Urine specimen collection 93, 94
   aftercare 94
   precaution 93
   preparation 93
   procedure 94
   purposes 93
   types 93

■V

Vaccination
   common side effects of 173
   documentation of 81
   general principles in 173
Vaccines
   administration of 152, 173
   dosage of 174t
   reaction 174
   route of 174t
Valvular pulmonic stenosis 105
Vecuronium 211
Vein, puncture of 83, 86
Venipuncture 83, 84f
   site for 84
Venous access devices 132
   type of 133t
Venous catheterization 104
Ventilation
   adequacy of 251
   assisting with 210
   methods 209t
   modes of 207
   timingrate of 4f
Ventilator 141, 207
   pressure-cycled 206

types of 206
volume-cycled 207
Venting tube 128
Ventral suspension 73
Venturi mask 141, 142, 142f, 144
Vertical supine 74
Vessel thrombosis 224
Vest restraint 236
Vibration 148
Vim-Silverman needle 102
Vinel and Ravel's social maturity scale 72
Vision
   acuity of 79
   field of 79
Visual activity 14
Vital signs 44, 60, 220, 251
   assessment of 44
   normal values of 50t
Vocal cord paralysis 202
Vojta technique 72
Vomiting 149

■W

Water play during bath 231
Waterlow classification 54
Weaning and extubation 211
Weighing scale, type of 51
Welcome classification 54
Whole blood 217, 218
Word Side Screening System 72
Wound coverings, type of 253